T0227273

Sudden Cardiac Death

Guest Editors

RANJAN K. THAKUR, MD, MPH, FHRS
ANDREA NATALE, MD, FACC, FHRS

CARDIAC ELECTROPHYSIOLOGY CLINICS

www.cardiacEP.theclinics.com

Consulting Editors

RANJAN K. THAKUR, MD, MPH, FHRS
ANDREA NATALE, MD, FACC, FHRS

December 2009 • Volume 1 • Number 1

SAUNDERS an imprint of ELSEVIER, Inc.

W.B. SAUNDERS COMPANY
A Division of Elsevier Inc.

1600 John F. Kennedy Boulevard • Suite 1800 • Philadelphia, Pennsylvania 19103-2899

http://www.theclinics.com

CARDIAC ELECTROPHYSIOLOGY CLINICS Volume 1, Number 1
December 2009 ISSN 1877-9182, ISBN-13: 978-1-4377-1680-1

Editor: Barbara Cohen-Kligerman
Developmental Editor: Donald Mumford

Cardiac Electrophysiology Clinics (ISSN 1877-9182) is published quarterly by Elsevier Inc., 360 Park Avenue South, New York, NY 10010-1710. Months of issue are March, June, September, and December. Subscription prices are $167.00 per year for US individuals, $250.00 per year for US institutions, $84.00 per year for US students and residents, $187.00 per year for Canadian individuals, $299.00 per year for Canadian institutions, $239.00 per year for international individuals, $299.00 per year for international institutions and $120.00 per year for Canadian and foreign students/residents. To receive student/resident rate, orders must be accompanied by name of affilliated institution, date of term, and the signature of program/residency coordinator on institution letterhead. Orders will be billed at individual rate until proof of status is received. Foreign air speed delivery is included in all Clinics subscription prices. All prices are subject to change without notice. **POSTMASTER:** Send address changes to Cardiac Electrophysiology Clinics, Elsevier Health Sciences Division, Subscription Customer Service, 3251 Riverport Lane, Maryland Heights, MO 63043. **Customer Service: 1-800-654-2452 (US and Canada). From outside of the US and Canada, call 314-477-8871. Fax: 314-447-8029. E-mail: JournalsCustomerService-usa@elsevier.com (for print support); JournalsOnlineSupport-usa@elsevier.com (for online support).**

Reprints. For copies of 100 or more of articles in this publication, please contact the Commercial Reprints Department, Elsevier Inc., 360 Park Avenue South, New York, NY 10010-1710. Tel.: 212-633-3812; Fax: 212-462-1935; E-mail: reprints@elsevier.com.

Printed and bound by CPI Group (UK) Ltd, Croydon, CR0 4YY

Transferred to Digital Print 2011

Contributors

CONSULTING EDITORS

RANJAN K. THAKUR, MD, MPH, FHRS
Professor of Medicine; Director, Arrhythmia
Service, Thoracic and Cardiovascular Institute,
Sparrow Health System, Michigan State
University, Lansing, Michigan

ANDREA NATALE, MD, FACC, FHRS
Executive Medical Director of the Texas
Cardiac Arrhythmia Institute at St David's
Medical Center, Austin, Texas; Consulting
Professor, Division of Cardiology, Stanford
University, Palo Alto, California; Clinical
Associate Professor of Medicine, Case
Western Reserve University, Cleveland, Ohio;
Senior Clinical Director, EP Services, California
Pacific Medical Center, San Francisco;
Department of Biomedical Engineering,
University of Texas, Austin, Texas

GUEST EDITORS

RANJAN K. THAKUR, MD, MPH, FHRS
Professor of Medicine; Director, Arrhythmia
Service, Thoracic and Cardiovascular Institute,
Sparrow Health System, Michigan State
University, Lansing, Michigan

ANDREA NATALE, MD, FACC, FHRS
Executive Medical Director of the Texas
Cardiac Arrhythmia Institute at St David's
Medical Center, Austin, Texas; Consulting
Professor, Division of Cardiology, Stanford
University, Palo Alto, California; Clinical
Associate Professor of Medicine, Case
Western Reserve University, Cleveland, Ohio;
Senior Clinical Director, EP Services, California
Pacific Medical Center, San Francisco;
Department of Biomedical Engineering,
University of Texas, Austin, Texas

AUTHORS

AMIN AL-AHMAD, MD, FACC
Department of Internal Medicine, Division of
Cardiovascular Medicine, Cardiac Arrhythmia
Service, Stanford University School of
Medicine, Stanford, California

TOM P. AUFDERHEIDE, MD, FACEP, FAHA
Professor of Emergency Medicine and
Associate Chair of Research Affairs,
Department of Emergency Medicine, Medical
College of Wisconsin, Milwaukee, Wisconsin

SIVAKUMAR ARDHANARI, MD
Thoracic and Cardiovascular Institute, Sparrow
Health System, Michigan State University,
Lansing, Michigan

CONOR D. BARRETT, MD
Cardiac Arrhythmia Service, Massachusetts
General Hospital and Harvard Medical School
Boston, Massachusetts

MICHAEL L. BERNARD, MD, PhD
Cardiovascular Fellow, Medical University
of South Carolina, Charleston, South Carolina

FRANK BUHTZ, RN
CORIZON GmbH, Kerpen, Germany

J. DAVID BURKHARDT, MD
Texas Cardiac Arrhythmia Institute at
St David's Medical Center, Austin, Texas

OTTO COSTANTINI, MD
Assistant Professor of Medicine; Director,
Arrhythmia Prevention Center, Heart and
Vascular Research Center, MetroHealth
Campus, Case Western Reserve University,
Cleveland, Ohio

IWONA CYGANKIEWICZ, MD
Heart Research Follow-up Program,
University of Rochester Medical Center,
Rochester, New York

LUIGI DI BIASE, MD
Texas Cardiac Arrhythmia Institute at St
David's Medical Center; Department of
Biomedical Engineering, University of Texas,
Austin, Texas; Department of Cardiology,
University of Foggia, Foggia, Italy

KENNETH A. ELLENBOGEN, MD
Kontos Professor of Medicine; Vice Chair,
Department of Internal Medicine, Division
of Cardiology, Cardiac Electrophysiology,
Virginia Commonwealth University,
Richmond, Virginia

AVI FISCHER, MD, FACC
Assistant Professor of Medicine; Director,
Pacemaker and Defibrillator Therapy,
Cardiac Arrhythmia Service, The Zena and
Michael A. Wiener Cardiovascular Institute,
and Marie-Josée and Henry R. Kravis
Center for Cardiovascular Health, Mount
Sinai School of Medicine, New York,
New York

RICHARD I. FOGEL, MD, FACC, FHRS
Clinical Electrophysiology Laboratory, St.
Vincent Hospital, Duke University Medical
Center, Indianapolis, Indiana

VALENTIN FUSTER, MD, PhD
Richard Gorlin MD/Heart Research
Foundation Professor of Cardiology;
Director, The Zena and Michael A. Wiener
Cardiovascular Institute, and Marie-Josée
and Henry R. Kravis Center for Cardiovascular
Health, The Mount Sinai Medical Center,
New York, New York: The Centro Nacional
de Investigaciones Cardiovasculares (CNIC),
Madrid, Spain

NITESH GADEELA, MD
Thoracic and Cardiovascular Institute, Sparrow
Health System, Michigan State University,
Lansing, Michigan

MICHAEL R. GOLD, MD, PhD
Michael E Assey Professor of Medicine,
Chief of Cardiology; and Associate Dean,
Interdisciplinary Clinical Programs, Medical
University of South Carolina, Charleston,
South Carolina

ILAN GOLDENBERG, MD
Associate Professor of Cardiology, Heart
Research Follow-up Program, Cardiology
Division, Department of Medicine, University
of Rochester School of Medicine and Dentistry,
Rochester, New York

DEVI GOPINATH, MD
Electrophysiology Fellow, Heart and Vascular
Center, MetroHealth Campus, Case Western
Reserve University, Cleveland, Ohio

ANURAG GUPTA, MD
Department of Internal Medicine,
Division of Cardiovascular Medicine,
Cardiac Arrhythmia Service, Stanford
University School of Medicine, Stanford,
California

ROBERT G. HAUSER, MD, FACC, FHRS
Senior Consulting Cardiologist, Minneapolis
Heart Institute Foundation, Minneapolis,
Minnesota

SWAPNIL HIREMATH, MD, MPH
Division of Nephrology, University of Ottawa,
Ottawa, Ontario, Canada

CHRISTIAN JONS, MD
Heart Research Follow-up Program, University
of Rochester Medical Center, Rochester,
New York

MARK E. JOSEPHSON, MD
Professor of Medicine; Chief of Cardiology,
Beth Israel Deaconess Medical Center,
Boston, Massachusetts

GAUTHAM KALAHASTY, MD
Assistant Professor of Medicine, Department
of Internal Medicine, Division of Cardiology,
Virginia Commonwealth University,
Richmond, Virginia

HELMUT U. KLEIN, MD
Heart Research Follow-up Program,
University of Rochester Medical Center,
Rochester, New York

KOSTANTINOS KOTSIFAS, MD
Consultant Pulmonary Medicine, Department
of Pulmonary Medicine, Sotiria General
Hospital, Athens, Greece

YOUNGHOON KWON, MD
Staff Physician and Research Fellow,
Healthcare East System, Division of
Cardiology, Department of Medicine,
University of Minnesota, St Joseph Hospital,
St Paul, Minnesota

KEITH G. LURIE, MD
Professor of Medicine and Emergency
Medicine, Department of Emergency
Medicine, Hennepin County Medical Center,
Minneapolis Medical Research Foundation,
University of Minnesota, Minneapolis,
Minnesota

ARTHUR J. MOSS, MD
Professor of Cardiology, Heart Research
Follow-up Program, Cardiology Division,
Department of Medicine, University of
Rochester School of Medicine and Dentistry,
Rochester, New York

ANDREA NATALE, MD, FACC, FHRS
Executive Medical Director of the Texas
Cardiac Arrhythmia Institute at St David's
Medical Center, Austin, Texas; Consulting
Professor, Division of Cardiology, Stanford
University, Palo Alto, California; Clinical
Associate Professor of Medicine, Case
Western Reserve University, Cleveland, Ohio;
Senior Clinical Director, EP Services, California
Pacific Medical Center, San Francisco;
Department of Biomedical Engineering,
University of Texas, Austin, Texas

BENZY J. PADANILAM, MD
Clinical Electrophysiology Laboratory,
St Vincent Hospital, Duke University Medical
Center, Indianapolis, Indiana

RICHARD L. PAGE, MD
Professor of Medicine, Division of Cardiology,
University of Washington School of Medicine;
Robert A. Bruce Endowed Chair in
Cardiovascular Research, Seattle, Washington

**ERIC N. PRYSTOWSKY, MD, FACC,
FAHA, FHRS**
Director, Clinical Electrophysiology
Laboratory: Consulting Professor of Medicine,
St Vincent Hospital, Duke University Medical
Center, Indianapolis, Indiana

ERNEST MATTHEW QUIN, MD
Electrophysiology Fellow, Medical
University of South Carolina, Charleston,
South Carolina

DAVID RARDON, MD, FACC
Clinical Electrophysiology Laboratory,
St Vincent Hospital, Duke University Medical
Center, Indianapolis, Indiana

ROBERT W. RHO, MD
Associate Professor of Medicine, University
of Washington School of Medicine, Seattle,
Washington

JEREMY N. RUSKIN, MD
Cardiac Arrhythmia Service, Massachusetts
General Hospital and Harvard Medical School
Boston, Massachusetts

LUIS CARLOS SAENZ, MD
Fundation Cardio Infantil, Bogota, Colombia

RAHUL SAKHUJA, MD, MPP, MSc
Fellow, Interventional Cardiology,
Massachusetts General Hospital, Boston,
Massachusetts

ASHOK J. SHAH, MD
Fellow, Cardiac Electrophysiology, Thoracic
and Cardiovascular Institute, Sparrow Health
System, Michigan State University, Lansing,
Michigan

STEVEN SZYMKIEWICZ, MD
ZOLL Lifecor Corporation, Pittsburgh,
Pennsylvania

RANJAN K. THAKUR, MD, MPH, FHRS
Professor of Medicine; Director, Arrhythmia
Service, Thoracic and Cardiovascular Institute,
Sparrow Health System, Michigan State
University, Lansing, Michigan

RODERICK TUNG, MD
Assistant Professor of Medicine, Ronald
Reagan UCLA Medical Center, David Geffen
School of Medicine at UCLA; Director,
Specialized Program in VT, UCLA Cardiac
Arrhythmia Center, Los Angeles, California

MIGUEL VACCA, MD, MSc
Fundation Cardio Infantil, Bogota, Colombia

PAUL J. WANG, MD, FACC
Department of Internal Medicine, Division of
Cardiovascular Medicine, Cardiac Arrhythmia
Service, Stanford University School of
Medicine, Stanford, California

DEMETRIS YANNOPOULOS, MD
Assistant Professor of Medicine, Department
of Medicine, Interventional Cardiology,
University of Minnesota, Minneapolis,
Minnesota

Contents

Sudden cardiac death (SCD) is a devastating complication of myocardial infarction. The global incidence of coronary artery disease and heart failure has been increasing greatly in recent years. As a consequence, there is expected to be an increase in the incidence of SCD manifesting as a shared worldwide public health problem. This article summarizes SCD epidemiology, with a focus on the anticipated global rise in incidence.

This article focuses on important advances in the science of cardiopulmonary resuscitation (CPR) in the last decade that have led to a significant improvement in understanding the complex physiology of cardiac arrest and critical interventions for the initial management of cardiac arrest and postresuscitation treatment. Special emphasis is given to the basic simple ways to improve circulation, vital organ perfusion pressures, and the grave prognosis of sudden cardiac death.

In the United States, 250,000 people die from a cardiac arrest every year. Despite a well established emergency medical response system, survival from out-of-hospital cardiac arrest remains poor in United States cities. Paramount to achieving successful resuscitation of a cardiac arrest victim is provision of early defibrillation. Among patients that arrest due to a ventricular fibrillation, the likelihood of survival decreases by 10% for every minute of delay in defibrillation. In 1995, the American Heart Association challenged the medical industry to develop a defibrillator that could be placed in public settings, used safely by lay responders, and provide earlier defibrillation to cardiac arrest victims. Over the last decade, there have been significant technological advancements in automated external defibrillators (AEDs), and clinical studies have demonstrated their benefits and limitations in various public locations. This article discusses the technologic features of the modern AED and the current data available on the use of AEDs in public settings.

The "chain of survival" (early access, early cardiopulmonary resuscitation, early defibrillation, and early advanced care) defines the proven interventions necessary for successful resuscitation and survival of patients with cardiac arrest. Low survival rates from cardiac arrest are not due to lack of understanding of effective interventions, but instead are due to weak links in the chain of survival and the inability of communities to make sure these links function in an efficient, timely, and coordinated fashion. This article reviews how quality is defined for each link, how communities can strengthen each link, and how communities can forge a strong relationship between each link. By optimizing local leadership and stakeholder collaboration, communities have the potential to vastly improve outcomes from this devastating disease.

Sudden cardiac death (SCD) accounts for as many as 450,000 deaths yearly in the United States. Over the last 15 years, many clinical trials have established the effectiveness of an implantable cardioverter-defibrillator (ICD) in reducing sudden and total mortality in patients with structural heart disease. However, controversy remains about exactly how to identify the patients most likely to benefit from an ICD, as well as those who may safely do without an ICD implant. The first primary prevention ICD trials used an abnormal electrophysiological study in addition to a low left ventricular ejection fraction (LVEF) as high-risk markers for SCD. More recent ICD trials selected patients based on the presence of a low LVEF alone. Ideally, noninvasive electrophysiological markers that more directly reflect arrhythmia substrates may better identify patients for prophylactic ICD implant. Several of these markers have been associated with the risk of SCD, but all have yielded contradictory outcome results or have not been tested prospectively. This review focuses on the most promising tests to date, their clinical significance, and their possible use to improve efficacy and efficiency of risk stratification for SCD.

Patients with end-stage renal disease (ESRD) are at a high risk for sudden cardiac death (SCD). SCD is the most common cause of death in this population and, as in the general population, ventricular arrhythmias seem to be the most common cause of SCD. The increased risk of SCD in ESRD is likely due to factors that are unique to the metabolic derangements associated with this state, as well as the increased prevalence of traditional risk factors. Despite this, the evidence base for the assessment and management of SCD in these patients is limited. This article reviews the current data on underlying risk factors for SCD in patients with ESRD, the role of common medical and device-based therapies for the prevention and treatment of SCD, and the applicability of common methods of risk stratification to patients with ESRD.

Patients with ischemic left ventricular dysfunction are at a high risk for ventricular tachyarrhythmias and sudden cardiac death. Randomized clinical trials have demonstrated that pharmacologic management with antiarrhythmic drugs has limited efficacy for the prevention of arrhythmic mortality in this high-risk population, whereas the implantable cardioverter defibrillator (ICD) has significant life-saving benefit in primary and secondary prevention trials. However, secondary analyses of these studies have identified some limitations of the ICD in subsets of patients with coronary artery disease, including limited defibrillator efficacy early after coronary revascularization and acute myocardial infarction. We review current knowledge from primary and secondary prevention clinical trials regarding the benefit and limitations of the ICD in high-risk patients with coronary artery disease.

Sudden cardiac death is the leading cause of death among adults in the United States. Multiple randomized controlled trials have provided clear-cut data on appropriate subgroups of patients whose survival has improved through primary prevention therapy with an implantable cardioverter defibrillator. Current guidelines specify a class I indication in patients with reduced left ventricular ejection fractions with both ischemic and nonischemic cardiomyopathy under various conditions. Cardiac resynchronization therapy has also been demonstrated to reduce mortality in selected patient subgroups and should be combined with an implantable cardioverter defibrillator in appropriate patients. Adherence to these guidelines should result in a reduction in sudden-death mortality.

Although it is estimated that a total of 220,000 patients undergo implantable cardioverter-defibrillator (ICD) implantation per year, only 10% to 20% of these patients experience life-saving therapy; this leaves up to 90% of the targeted population as "nonresponders," who do not derive clinical benefit but incur all of the risks from ICD implantation. This article reviews the landmark primary prevention trials to assess the incidence of sudden death and the absolute magnitude of benefit derived from ICD therapy. The discrepancy between trial patients and real-world implementation of ICD therapy is examined, and the potential for risks incurred from ICD implantation is presented. The natural history of patients who receive appropriate ICD therapy and the durability of ICD benefit with respect to cost-effective analyses are discussed, to support the authors' position that ICD therapy should not be routinely used for the primary prevention of sudden cardiac death.

The implantable cardioverter-defibrillator (ICD) is the standard of care for preventing sudden cardiac death. Contemporary ICDs are capable of providing a variety of therapeutic functions and can automatically gather and store diagnostic data that can guide both device and drug therapy and alert caregivers of impending battery depletion or lead problems. Moreover, much of the diagnostic data can be monitored remotely, so that many patients can be evaluated in their homes. This article, by a former chief executive officer of the first company to commercialize the ICD, traces the history of the device from its beginnings in the early 1980s.

The wearable cardioverter defibrillator (WCD) was introduced into clinical practice about 8 years ago as an alternative approach to protect patients with a temporary high risk of sudden arrhythmic death. The WCD has the characteristics of an implantable defibrillator (ICD) but does not need to be implanted, and it has similarities with an external defibrillator, but does not require a bystander to apply lifesaving shocks when necessary. Based on current clinical experience, the WCD is not an alternative to the ICD, but a device that will contribute to better selection of patients for ICD therapy and may be indicated in case of interrupted protection by an already implanted ICD, temporary inability to implant an ICD, or refusal of an indicated ICD.

The advent of subcutaneous implantable cardioverter-defibrillator (ICD) systems represents a paradigm shift for the detection and therapy of ventricular tachyarrhythmias. Despite advances in transvenous lead technology, problems remain that notably include requirement for technical expertise; periprocedural complications during implantation and explantation; and long-term lead failure. Although subcutaneous ICD systems may mitigate some of these risks, they provide new shortcomings, such as inability to provide pacing therapy for bradyarrhythmias, ventricular tachyarrhythmias, and cardiac resynchronization. Ongoing clinical evaluation and development are required before the role of subcutaneous ICDs as an adjunctive or primary therapy can be defined. This article examines studies investigating the subcutaneous ICD and discusses its possible advantages and disadvantages as compared with current transvenous ICD systems.

Although improvements in implantable cardioverter-defibrillator (ICD) therapy have taken place, many challenges do remain. Inappropriate delivery of therapy is a big problem that impacts the quality of life of ICD recipients. Although there is now a clear understanding that atrial arrhythmias are the main cause of inappropriate ICD therapies, physicians have not been very successful in preventing them. Additionally, although many tachycardia detection discriminators have been shown to be helpful, it is not clear that there is a particular combination that is ideal for all patients. Until such an algorithm is developed (which may not be possible), a detailed knowledge and use of all available programming options, guided by special characteristics of each unique patient, are the only foreseeable solutions. Finally, one must face the prospect that this problem cannot be vanquished, but only ameliorated.

The implantable cardioverter defibrillator (ICD) lead is critical to the function of the ICD system. The mortality reduction associated with ICDs implanted for primary prevention indications has been made possible by the development of effective and reliable transvenous ICD leads. Mortality rates for implantation of transvenous ICD lead systems are currently less than 0.5%. The reliability and functional characteristics of a lead are often not known until it has been in widespread use. An understanding of the mechanism of lead failure is essential for proper patient management. This article describes the design and construction of ICD leads, discusses lead failure, and reviews subsequent management of patients.

Remote monitoring has developed out of the need to accommodate the demand of the growing implantable cardioverter-defibrillator (ICD) and cardiac resynchronization therapy (CRT) population. After several years of clinical use, remote device interrogation systems have demonstrated ease of use for both patient and provider, reliability compared with in-office interrogations, and the ability to detect asymptomatic but clinically significant events. The effect of remote monitoring on morbidity and mortality is currently unknown, but several trials are underway to assess these outcomes. Many devices also have the capacity to remotely track physiologic parameters that may improve the management of heart failure. Remote monitoring of ICD-CRT populations is a promising technological advancement that likely will become the standard of care for ICD follow-up.

This article discusses how ventricular tachycardia ablation should be used, discusses which patients may derive benefit from this treatment, and highlights the best means of implementing it.

Cardiac Electrophysiology Clinics

FORTHCOMING ISSUES

Epicardial Interventions in Electrophysiology
Kalyanam Shivkumar, MD, PhD, and
Noel G. Boyle, MD, PhD, *Guest Editors*

**Advances in Arrhythmia Analyses: A Case-Based
Approach**
Melvin Scheinman, MD, and
Masood Akhtar, MD, *Guest Editors*

Advances in Antiarrhythmic Drug Therapy
Peter R. Kowey, MD, and
Gerald V. Naccarelli, MD,
Guest Editors

THE CLINICS ARE NOW AVAILABLE ONLINE!

Access your subscription at:
www.theclinics.com

Foreword

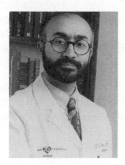
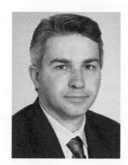

Ranjan K. Thakur, MD, MPH, FHRS   Andrea Natale, MD, FACC, FHRS
Consulting Editors

We are delighted that Elsevier has introduced *Cardiac Electrophysiology Clinics* (*EP Clinics*) for the electrophysiology community. Although we have numerous excellent peer-reviewed journals for new clinical and basic research in electrophysiology, we have lacked a high-quality review journal that all electrophysiologists can use as a reference. Textbooks provide excellent reviews, but because of the long publication process, the newest information is often missing.

The *EP Clinics* will have a much shorter publication time and we hope to bridge the gap between textbooks and peer-reviewed journals. In addition, an editor's job is to filter and focus the literature by selecting article topics, so that busy clinicians can easily review the most pertinent issues of the time, and the *EP Clinics* will certainly do that.

Elsevier has 49 publications in the *Clinics* series for physicians, and the addition of *EP Clinics* brings this total to 50. Publications in the series are indexed by the major indexing services (eg, PubMed, Science Citation Index, Excerpta Medica), and several in the series are published concurrently in other languages. Furthermore, availability of these publications through MD Consult and ScienceDirect increases their reach to millions of readers worldwide.

We are pleased to serve as consulting editors for the *EP Clinics* and hope to bring forth quarterly issues edited by leaders in the field. The goal of this series is to publish issues focused on one topic at a time. The editors will be selected based on their contribution to the particular topic and be responsible for assembling reviews of contemporary issues that are relevant to clinical electrophysiologists and written by thought leaders in the field.

Practicing electrophysiologists and experts in the field will find these reviews useful and authoritative, because even experts in a field have a narrow area of expertise and need colleagues to filter out the most important issues lying outside this field. The wider cardiology community and fellows in training within the various subspecialties of cardiology will find these reviews helpful for keeping abreast of the newest developments. Many of these issues will also be of interest to other physicians and house staff.

We have inaugurated the series with a review on "Sudden Cardiac Death," which is a topic that defined and launched clinical electrophysiology as a specialty more than 3 decades ago. Although it is not possible to cover the entire field, we hope that the readers will find that topics relevant to current practice are well represented.

We thank our contributors for their insightful reviews and our colleagues who are working on editing their own forthcoming issues. We especially want to thank Barbara Cohen-Kligerman at Elsevier who had the vision and provided steadfast support to see this project come to fruition. We have enjoyed working with the staff at Elsevier and look forward to ongoing collaboration in serving the electrophysiology community. We welcome feedback from readers who have ideas for improving the *EP Clinics* or suggestions for topics they would like to see covered in future issues.

Card Electrophysiol Clin 1 (2009) xiii–xv
doi:10.1016/j.ccep.2009.08.017
1877-9182/09/$ – see front matter

Finally, although this has been a labor of love, it has not happened without sacrifices, especially from our families. We acknowledge their love and support and dedicate this issue to them.

Ranjan K. Thakur, MD, MPH, FHRS
Thoracic and Cardiovascular Institute
405 West Greenlawn, Suite 400
Lansing, MI 48910, USA

Andrea Natale, MD, FACC, FHRS
Texas Cardiac Arrhythmia Institute
Center for Atrial Fibrillation at St David's Medical Center
1015 East 32nd Street, Suite 516
Austin, TX 78705, USA

E-mail addresses:
thakur@msu.edu (R.K. Thakur)
andrea.natale@stdavids.com (A. Natale)

DEDICATION

Ranjan Thakur: To my wife Niti, our son Jay, and to my mother.

Andrea Natale: To my wife Marina and our daughters Veronica and Eleonora.

The Changing Epidemiology of Sudden Cardiac Death

Avi Fischer, MD[a], Valentin Fuster, MD, PhD[a,b],*

KEYWORDS

- Sudden cardiac death • Cardiac arrest
- Cardiovascular disease • Global health • SCD risk

Sudden cardiac death (SCD) is a devastating complication of myocardial infarction (MI). Long-term population studies outlining the incidence of SCD after MI in the community are decades old.[1–3] The in-hospital mortality after MI has decreased substantially, and the long-term prognosis after MI has improved greatly, yielding a growing number of MI survivors at risk for sudden cardiac death.[4,5] Patterns of disease progression predict a globally increased incidence of heart disease by 2020.[6–8] Already in the first decade of the new millennium, these predictions are becoming a reality. In the developing world, the greatest increases in prevalence of diabetes, coronary artery disease and heart failure are being seen.[9] As a consequence of the increased prevalence of coronary artery disease and heart failure will be an increasing incidence of SCD. As a result, SCD will manifest as a shared worldwide public health problem. The purpose of this article is to summarize SCD epidemiology, with a focus on the anticipated global rise in incidence.

WHAT IS SCD?

The most widely accepted definition of SCD is the sudden and unexpected death within an hour of symptom onset.[10] Despite a substantial overall decline in morbidity and mortality caused by cardiovascular diseases in the second half of the last century, the survival after an episode of SCD remains in the range of 5%.[11] The sudden nature of this condition, and its occurrence in many instances without warning, are major impediments to improving outcome. Awareness of this important deficiency has led to considerable interest on mechanisms of SCD. Despite a renewed focus, the significant delay in development of effective measures for risk stratification and prevention of SCD can be attributed directly to a poor understanding of mechanisms involved in fatal arrhythmogenesis.[12]

There are several important factors contributing to the challenges faced when assessing true rates of SCD. SCD occurs in the general population in an unpredictable manner, and whenever possible, it is crucial to exclude subjects who are likely to have had a noncardiac cause of sudden death. Additionally, an accurate estimate of SCD incidence requires prospective ascertainment of cases. Studies that have used retrospective analysis of the death certificate to identify cases of SCD likely overestimate SCD incidence by as much as 200% to 300%.[13] Therefore, the US estimates published by the US Centers for Disease Control and Prevention (CDC) (400 to 450 000 per year)[3] are likely significant overestimates.[14]

ARRHYTHMIC MECHANISMS OF SCD

In the last 30 years, there have been important alterations in the prevalence trends of arrhythmias causing SCD (Fig. 1). Early studies reported that ventricular fibrillation (VF) was the initial rhythm in

a The Zena and Michael A. Wiener Cardiovascular Institute, Marie-Josée and Henry R. Kravis Center for Cardiovascular Health, The Mount Sinai Medical Center, One Gustave L Levy Place, Box 1030, New York, NY 10029, USA
b The Centro Nacional de Investigaciones Cardiovasculares (CNIC), Madrid, Spain
* Corresponding author.
E-mail address: valentin.fuster@mssm.edu (V. Fuster).

Card Electrophysiol Clin 1 (2009) 1–11
doi:10.1016/j.ccep.2009.08.004
1877-9182/09/$ – see front matter © 2009 Published by Elsevier Inc.

most SCD cases—75% in a longitudinal study from Seattle[15] and 84% in a series of patients wearing Holter monitors.[16] Despite the spectrum of etiologic conditions, in most cases, SCD results from either ventricular tachycardia (VT)/VF or severe bradycardia/pulseless electrical activity (PEA).[17,18] Of the lethal arrhythmias, VF consistently has been shown to have the highest likelihood of survival. As a result, there has been great emphasis on VF detection and treatment in resuscitation protocols. Since the first descriptions of external defibrillation in the 1960s and the first human implantable cardioverter defibrillator (ICD) in 1980 by Mirowski,[19] the paradigm for the prevention of SCD shifted away from antiarrhythmic drug therapy. Since 1990, however, a declining rate of VF and a rise in prevalence of PEA have been reported (**Fig. 2**). This was reported initially in in-hospital studies and later confirmed in prehospital studies. Data from Seattle from 1990 to 1996 indicated that 41% of SCDs were attributable to VF and 24% to PEA.[20] Another study from Seattle that looked at prevalence trends between 1980 and 2000 reported a 56% decrease in VF as the first identified rhythm from 1980 to 2000 (from 0.85 to 0.38 per 1000 population; relative risk [RR], 0.44; 95% confidence interval [CI], 0.37 to 0.53).[21] Similar reductions were seen in blacks and whites, and the phenomenon was most evident in men (57%; RR, 0.43; 95% CI, 0.35 to 0.53), in whom the baseline incidence was relatively high. An amiodarone versus lidocaine trial reported VF prevalence among prehospital cardiac arrests of only 26%.[22] Similar reports were published from Sweden, documenting a decrease in prevalence of VF by 39% over 17 years despite significant improvements in response time and rates of bystander cardiopulmonary resuscitation.[23] Prevalence of PEA among sudden cardiac arrest cases rose from 6% to 26% from 1980 to 1996.[23] From the mechanistic standpoint, as VF more commonly is related to coronary disease and PEA to noncardiac factors,[24] the significant decrease in age-adjusted mortality from coronary artery disease over the last 50 years[25] may be responsible in part for the decline seen in VF prevalence. As the survival rates from these arrhythmias is markedly different, ongoing investigation focused on improving the understanding of PEA mechanisms and treatment is underway, with the aim of improving current rates of survival from sudden cardiac arrest in the community.

WHO IS AT RISK FOR SCD?

SCD is the consequence of complex interaction between genetic elements, various cardiac conditions, comorbidities, and epidemiologic and environmental factors (**Fig. 3**). Approximately 80% of SCDs are attributed to coronary artery disease.[10,14,26] The two major mechanisms of fatal ventricular arrhythmias include acute coronary ischemia, usually as a result of plaque rupture, and occlusion of an epicardial coronary artery and re-entry associated with areas of slow conduction and previous myocardial scarring. The former is more likely to result in polymorphic VT or VF and may occur in individuals with preserved left ventricular (LV) function. The latter occurs in the setting of an ischemic

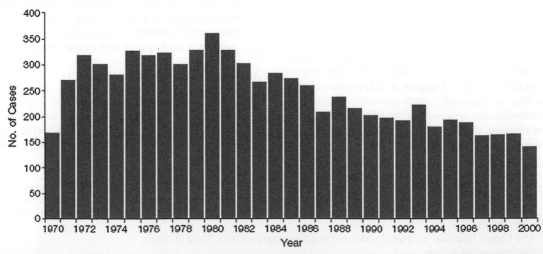

Fig. 1. Annual numbers of all patients treated for out-of-hospital ventricular fibrillation from 1970 to 2000 in Seattle, Washington. (*Modified from* Cobb LA, Fahrenbruch CE, Olsufka M, et al. Changing incidence of out-of-hospital ventricular fibrillation, 1980–2000. JAMA 2002;288:3008; with permission.)

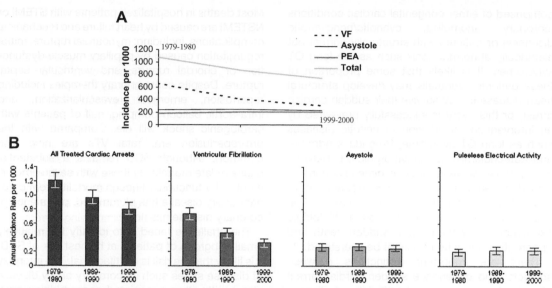

Fig. 2. (*A*) Trends in the mechanism of cardiac arrest from 1980 to 2000 reveals a steady decline in total number of cardiac arrests (*gray hatched line*) largely caused by a decrease in out-of-hospital ventricular fibrillation (*VF, dashed line*). A slight increase in pulseless electrical activity (*PEA, black hatched line*) and asystole (*solid line*) can be seen during this time period. (*B*) Data are mean rates, with 95% confidence intervals (error bars). Rates are adjusted to the Seattle, Washington, in 2000. The first recorded rhythms are represented for a 20-year span. Most of the reduced incidence was because of fewer cases with VF as the first identified cardiac rhythm. The proportion of cases with VF fell from 61% in 1980 to 41% in 2000. (*Modified from* Cobb LA, Fahrenbruch CE, Olsufka M, et al. Changing incidence of out-of-hospital ventricular fibrillation, 1980–2000. JAMA 2002;288:3008; with permission.)

cardiomyopathy after one or more MIs, with re-entrant loops occurring in areas of scarred myocardium. Other etiologies such as hypertrophic cardiomyopathy, dilated cardiomyopathies, arrhythmogenic right ventricular dysplasia, and myocardial infiltrative diseases such as sarcoidosis and amyloidosis account for 10% to 15% of cases. The remaining 5% to 10% of cases are

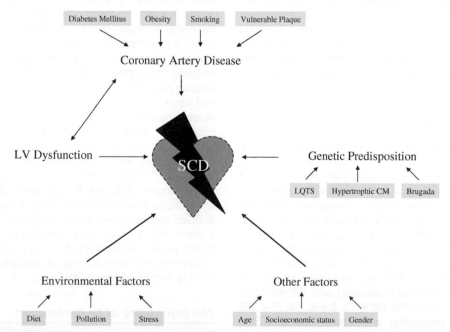

Fig. 3. Sudden cardiac death is multifactorial. There appears to be a genetic component in addition to the interaction between cardiac conditions, comorbidities, and epidemiologic and environmental factors.

comprised of either congenital cardiac conditions (coronary anomalies, cyanotic/noncyanotic diseases) or patients with structurally normal but electrically abnormal heart such as the long QT syndromes. It is likely that some proportion of these patients eventually may develop structural heart disease if they survive their sudden cardiac arrest, or this event is successfully prevented by an intervention. In addition to genetic diseases such as long QT syndrome, Brugada syndrome, and catecholaminergic polymorphic VT, patients with autopsy-negative SCD (no genetic abnormalities identified) may comprise a significant part of this subgroup than previously anticipated.[13] The importance of a careful postmortem histologic examination in patients with sudden death and apparently normal heart cannot be overstated.[26]

There are important distinctions between subjects who experience sudden cardiac arrest after having previously identified heart disease compared with those without previously identified heart disease. Among those without previously documented heart disease, there are many who may have never had symptoms suggestive of heart disease or who were not evaluated for other reasons, such as disparate access to health care. Recent observations such as the recently reported Home Automated External Defibrillation trial[27] have confirmed the remarkably low annual mortality rate (2%) among patients with treated acute anterior MI who did not meet criteria for an implantable defibrillator. This reduction in mortality may have been an important reason that home use of the automated external defibrillator did not benefit this group of patients. These findings underscore the critical need to learn more about patients who have sudden cardiac arrest in the community, particularly when they do not have previously identified heart disease.

Coronary Artery Disease

As mentioned previously, coronary artery disease remains the most common condition associated with SCD, and it has been identified in at least 80% of overall cases. Among all patients with coronary artery disease, however, depending on the age group, only 13% to 20% will have sudden cardiac arrest.[28] Mortality from MI has been decreasing. Data from Global Registry of Acute Coronary Events for 1999 and 2006 reported a 3.9% (95% CI 1.9 to 5.3, $P<.001$) absolute risk reduction in hospital deaths for patients presenting with ST elevation MI (STEMI) and 0.7% (95% CI, 0.3 to 1.7, $P = .02$) for those presenting with non-STEMI (NSTEMI) with a 2.7% (95% CI 0.5 to 4.3, $P = .02$) absolute reduction in cardiogenic shock and heart failure.

Most deaths in hospitalized patients with STEMI or NSTEMI are caused by heart failure and mechanical complications, including: myocardial rupture, mitral regurgitation caused by papillary muscle dysfunction or chordal rupture, and ventricular septal rupture. Despite contemporary therapies including reperfusion, emergent revascularization, and intra-aortic balloon pumping, half of patients with cardiogenic shock will die. Compared with the pre-reperfusion era, fatal VTs are now less common, although SCD remains a substantial cause of late mortality in those with severe impairment of LV function. Although mortality from coronary artery disease has plummeted, prevalence of coronary disease has not.

The challenge faced is to identify the relatively small subgroup of patients at highest risk of SCD. It is likely that the risk is multifactorial. The interplay of disease states such as coronary artery disease along with other associated comorbidities such as diabetes mellitus and congestive heart failure combined with genetic predisposition are likely responsible for the overall risk in the individual patient. There is evidence to suggest that the importance of coronary artery disease in predicting risk of SCD may be related to rupture of the vulnerable plaque. The fact that in the second half of the last century, the significant decrease in mortality from SCD correlated with the overall decrease in mortality from coronary artery disease,[25] supports this possibility. It is likely that treatment and stabilization of the vulnerable plaque were achieved in large measure by treatments such as coronary artery bypass surgery, percutaneous coronary intervention, aspirin use, cholesterol-lowering therapies, and increased awareness of coronary artery disease prevention during this era. There are ongoing attempts to identify risk markers for sudden rupture of the vulnerable plaque but none that have proven definitive. Several epidemiologic studies have evaluated the potential role of total cholesterol levels in predicting sudden cardiac arrest risk, but results have been mixed, with some studies finding a significant role for this condition.[29,30] A cohort study of patients with stable angina followed for 10 years found that low-density lipoprotein (LDL) was a predictor of sudden cardiac arrest in the short term (less than 2 years; RR, 1.8) but not in the long term (greater than 2 years).[31] Further studies may provide further insight into the specific role of predicting plaque rupture and its effect on SCD.

The Importance of LV Dysfunction

Despite various available risk stratifying tests, presently, both in the presence or absence of coronary artery disease, severe LV dysfunction is the most widely used predictor of SCD risk. Based on data from the multicenter primary prevention trials of SCD, the presence of severe LV dysfunction is the main indication for a primary prevention ICD.[32–34] Only 20% to 30% of patients who are implanted with a prophylactic ICD, however, actually receive appropriate therapies over a follow-up period of 4 to 5 years.[32,35] When severe LV dysfunction is used as the criterion for a prophylactic ICD, it takes at least 11 ICD recipients to save one life during a 1-year follow-up period.[35] The high-risk patients in the hospital are likely very different from the outpatients and those who have SCD in the community, often as the very first manifestation of heart disease. Patients who present to health care providers with severely decreased LV dysfunction constitute a high-risk group that is likely to comprise a small proportion of overall SCD cases.[36] This has been observed in community-wide analyses.[37–39] In the Oregon Sudden Unexpected Death Study (Ore-SUDS), severe LV dysfunction predicted SCD but was found to affect less than a third of all SCD cases in the community.[40] Because only a subgroup of symptomatic individuals tend to present for evaluation, this figure is also likely to be an overestimate. Almost half of all SCD cases had normal LV function, and the remaining 20% had either mildly or moderately decreased LV systolic function (LV ejection fraction [LVEF] greater than 0.35 and less than 0.50) (**Fig. 4**). Similar findings were reported from a community-based study in Maastricht, the Netherlands.[37,38] Among 200 cases of SCD with an assessment of LV function available, 101 (51%) had normal LVEF, (greater than or equal to 50%), and 38 (19%) had severely reduced LVEF, (less than or equal to 30%). These findings indicate that although severe LV dysfunction remains a valuable contributor, there is an immediate need to identify clinical and nonclinical predictors that could enhance the process of risk stratification.

Diabetes Mellitus—a High-Risk Marker?

Although diabetes mellitus has been implicated as an important factor in the pathogenesis of SCD, the relationship has yet to be evaluated in prospective, community-wide studies of SCD. The independent role of diabetes mellitus in enhancing risk of SCD has been investigated in a small number of studies. In all studies, diabetes mellitus consistently has been identified as a strong predictor of SCD risk. The Paris Prospective Study enrolled more than 6000 middle-aged, healthy male Parisian civil servants who were followed for more than 23 years.[29] In this cohort, there were a total of 120

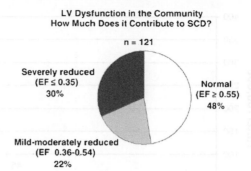

Fig. 4. Severe left ventricular dysfunction, currently the risk predictor most widely used in clinical practice, is likely to affect less than a third of all cases of sudden cardiac death in the general population. (*Data from* Chugh SS, Reinier K, Teodorescu C, et al. Epidemiology of sudden cardiac death: clinical and research implications. Prog Cardiovasc Dis 51:213,2008.)

SCDs, and 192 nonsudden deaths that were related to acute MI. In a multivariate analysis, the presence of diabetes mellitus independently conferred a significant risk for SCD (RR, 2.2) controlling for all other variables (age, body mass index [BMI], tobacco use, medical history, heart rate, systolic blood pressure, cholesterol and triglyceride levels).[29,41] Other large studies, such as the US Nurses Study and the Physicians Health Study[42,43] and a clinical database analysis from Seattle[44] have reported similar findings. Although little is known about the specific mechanism through which diabetes contributes to the pathogenesis of SCD, several postulates exist. First, diabetes mellitus increases the risk of coronary artery disease, but there also may be diabetes-specific accelerated forms of atherosclerosis with enhanced thrombogenicity.[45] Secondly, there is a high prevalence of abnormal prolongation of the corrected QT (QTc) interval on the surface electrocardiogram frequently seen among diabetic individuals.[46] Clinical studies of diabetic individuals also have reported a correlation between prolonged QTc interval and overall cardiac mortality.[47] Several studies have found an association between diabetic autonomic dysfunction and prolongation of the QTc interval.[48–50] The precise mechanisms through which diabetes mellitus increases SCD risk remains unclear; it is likely that a combination of factors exist.

Age and Sex Influences

There are two peaks in the age-related prevalence of SCD, one during infancy representing the sudden infant death syndrome and the second between ages 75 and 85 years (**Fig. 5**). Although the prevalence of SCD in these age groups has persisted over time, the trends seen among males

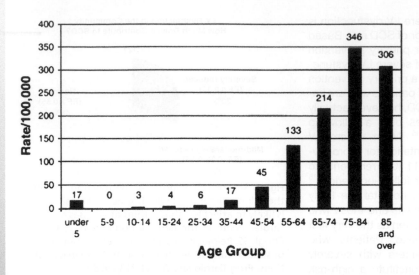

Fig. 5. Age-based annual incidence of sudden cardiac death among residents of Multnomah County, Oregon. (*Data from* Chugh SS, Jui J, Gunson K, et al. Current burden of sudden cardiac death: multiple-source surveillance versus retrospective death certificate-basedreview in a large US community. J Am Coll Cardiol 2004;44: 1268.)

and females has undergone a shift. Females appear to have an increase in the prevalence of SCD, likely as a result of the altered sex distribution in prevalence of and mortality from coronary artery disease (**Fig. 6**).[7] Although earlier studies had reported a 1:3 ratio of females to males, data suggest that females consistently make up approximately 40% of all SCD cases on a yearly basis.[14] The precise reasons for this changing trend warrant further investigation.

Genetic Factors

The association between genetics and sudden death clearly exists in patients with hereditary abnormalities in ion channel function such as the long QT and Brugada syndromes. Other associations are not as clear, but emerging data have provided evidence that genetic factors may contribute to risk of SCD in patients without an

overt channelopathy. The potential association between SCD and history of SCD or coronary artery disease in a first-degree relative was analyzed in a cohort of men and women attended by first responders in King County, Washington.[51] Data from the previously mentioned Paris Prospective Study[29] indicate that the occurrence of SCD in a parent or first-degree relative results in a 1.6- to 1.8-fold increase in SCD susceptibility. In a very small number of cases in this cohort of patients, there was a history of both maternal and paternal SCD events (n = 19). This conferred a ninefold increased risk of SCD. These studies provide evidence of a significant genetic contribution to SCD, and the next step is to identify genetic markers to be used for screening and risk stratification of the high-risk patient. As most patients who have sudden cardiac death have multiple associated comorbidities such as coronary artery disease, diabetes mellitus, obesity, and heart

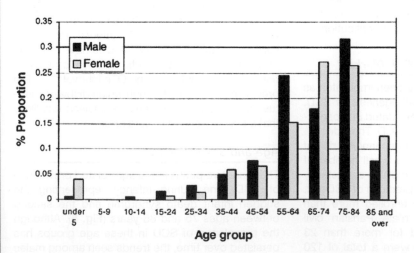

Fig. 6. Sex- and age-based composition of prospectively determined sudden cardiac death population. (*Data from* Chugh SS, Jui J, Gunson K, et al. Current burden of sudden cardiac death: multiple-source surveillance versus retrospective death certificate-based review in a large US community. J Am Coll Cardiol 2004;44:1268.)

failure, each condition may have contributory risk that may be unrelated to the genetic risk of SCD. Therefore, genes that contribute to SCD occurrence have to be separated from genes associated with comorbidities. Additionally, even for the so-called monogenic syndromes such as the long QT syndrome, there may be additional modifier genes and varying degrees of penetrance that are important in determining an individual's risk.[52] For the complex phenotype of overall SCD, it is quite likely that for an individual patient, screening may have to be conducted for a panel of genes instead of a single gene. From a methodological standpoint, approaches that use a very high-resolution map of single nucleotide polymorphisms to search for associations, linkage disequilibrium, or a small shared genomic segment among affected individuals are likely to be necessary.[13,53] Although the search for SCD genes presently do not use community-wide approaches, these studies are likely to be conducted in the very near future.[13,53]

The Socioeconomic Contribution to SCD

With the rising costs of health care and finite availability of resources,[54] the success of current and future strategies for risk stratification and prevention of SCD will depend in large part on how efficiently these strategies are deployed in the community. Assessment of the geographic distribution of SCD incidence in the community is a prerequisite. Although socioeconomic factors are likely to have significant effects on SCD incidence,[55–57] this association has not been evaluated in prospective, population-based studies. Ore-SUDS is a prospective evaluation of sudden cardiac death.[14,40] Originally underwritten by the CDC, this study identifies cases of SCD that occur in metropolitan Portland, Oregon (a population of approximately 1,000,000 residents). A multiple-source method of ascertainment is used to capture all cases of SCD. Cases are reported by first responders (ambulance and emergency medicine personnel, 70%), the state medical examiner or coroner (25%), and from the area hospitals (approximately 5%). The annual incidence of SCD in the first year of this study was 53 per 100,000 residents and accounted for 5.6% of overall deaths.[14] An almost identical incidence was reported in a Canadian survey of out-of hospital cardiac arrests (56 cases per 100,000 population)[58] and in rural Ireland (51.2 cases per 100,000 population).[59] The estimated annual incidence of SCD in the United States based on these figures (total population approximately 300,000,000) would range between 180,000 and 250,000 cases per year.[53] For the world (total population approximately 6,540,000,000), the

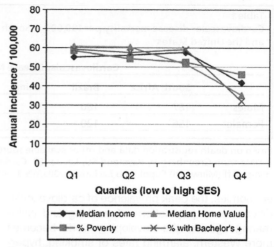

Fig. 7. Annual incidence of sudden cardiac arrest (all ages combined) based on address of residence, grouped by quartiles of socioeconomic status (SES)— low SES to high SES. (*Data from* Chugh SS, Reinier K, Teodorescu C, et al. Epidemiology of sudden cardiac death: clinical and research implications. Prog Cardiovasc Dis 2008;51:213.)

estimated annual burden of SCD would be in the range of 4 to 5 million cases per year.[53]

In Ore-SUDS, the incidence of SCD based on address of residence was 30% to 80% higher in neighborhoods in the lowest socioeconomic quartile compared with those in the highest socioeconomic quartile (**Fig. 7**). The difference was markedly steeper for the age group under age 65 years of age. Identical and significant effects of socioeconomic status were observed for SCD incidence based on geographic location of SCD. Although only 53% of the population lived in the two lowest quartiles, 60% of all SCDs occurred in these quartiles. Among patients younger than 65 years, 66% of all SCDs occurred in these two quartiles. Analysis of age distribution suggests that these disparities potentially could be related to differential access to health care. Socioeconomic disparities may be an important consideration for the implementation of community-wide strategies for prevention of sudden cardiac arrest, especially when considering the problem on a global perspective.[53]

THE GLOBAL OUTLOOK

The increasing prevalence of cardiovascular risk factors has become a threat to economic development in the less-developed world, as trends in global health transform from infectious to chronic diseases.[60] One of the most critical characteristics of the cardiovascular disease epidemic relates to disease prevention. In most less-developed

Table 1
Cardiovascular disease mortality per 100,000 in South Africa, Brazil, China, India, Russia, Portugal, and the United States

	Cardiovascular Disease Mortality Rate, Ages 30–59						
	South Africa	Brazil	China	India	Russia	United States	Portugal
Males	187	180	91	211	576	116	99
Females	156	120	62	139	179	63	62

Based on death registration data and other available sources of information on adult mortality.
Data from Greenberg H, Raymond SU, Leeder SR. Cardiovascular disease and global health: threat and opportunity. Health Aff (Millwood) Suppl Web Exclusives 2005;W5:31–41.

economies, the peak prevalence of cardiovascular disease is in populations of working and child-rearing age. As the developing world becomes more Western, alarming rates of smoking, hypertension, obesity, and diabetes mellitus are seen, with nearly all developing countries demonstrating increased rates of complications as a result of these conditions. Hypertension, elevated lipids, smoking, obesity, sedentary lifestyle, and diabetes account for about 80% of clinical cardiovascular disease in every region of the world.[61,62]

The cardiovascular disease mortality rates in emerging economies, the Russian Federation, and two Western economies can be seen in (**Table 1**).[60] Mortality rates for South Africa, Brazil, and India all exceed those of the United States and Portugal. In the Russian Federation, the cardiovascular mortality rate is five times that seen in the United States. China has not caught up yet; however, cardiovascular death has risen from 12.1% in 1957 to 35.8% in 2001. In China, high blood pressure was present in 7.7% of people age 15 and older from 1979 to 1980, 50% higher than from 1958 to 1959. Sixty-one percent of men and 7% of women in China smoke, and one third of all adults are overweight.[60] The prevalence of type 2 diabetes mellitus increased nearly threefold from 1980 to 1994, and the ongoing increase in obesity will only exacerbate this.[63] In Brazil, 10% of the population is obese (BMI greater than 30 kg/m^2), and another 25% to 30% overweight (BMI greater than 25 kg/m^2).[64] More than one third of the population is hypertensive, and 40% of men and 25% of women smoke.[65] In India, the prevalence of hypertension increased from 1% to 3% in 1950 to 10% to 30% in 2000.[66] The prevalence of type 2 diabetes mellitus has more than doubled in India's urban areas in the past 20 years.[67] In South Africa, the evidence points to a sizable rise in the incidence of type 2 diabetes.[68] With current understandings of the pathophysiology of cardiovascular disease, risk factor modulation and appropriate medication use can alter the trajectory of disease progression favorably.

With the decreased mortality from coronary artery disease in the United States during the second half of the 20th century, there is evidence suggesting a significant decrease in rates of SCD.[53] This likely is the result of prevention of mortality from coronary disease through the use of medications such as aspirin, beta-blockers, angiotensin-converting enzyme (ACE) inhibitors, and statins. Additionally, more widespread availability and use of coronary interventions, and dietary and lifestyle changes such as weight loss and smoking cessation have added to the reduction.[53] There is an alarming rise in the prevalence of obesity and diabetes in the first decade of the new millennium in the United States and worldwide, however. A resurgence of coronary artery disease and heart failure can be expected, and a worldwide public health problem is likely. An estimate for global annual incidence of SCD is in the range of 4 to 5 million cases per year.[53] In near future, as incidence of VF among cases of sudden cardiac arrest continues to fall and PEA continues to rise, advances in resuscitation efforts are likely to focus on mechanisms and treatment of PEA. The important goal of preventing SCD, however, will depend heavily on enhancement of risk stratification techniques. Therefore, discovery of novel risk stratification markers and methods has become the top priority in the field of sudden cardiac arrest investigation. Physicians are also learning that although severe LV dysfunction is a useful predictor for a subgroup of patients who will have future SCD, the specificity of this predictor is significantly lower than anticipated, and the search must be extended beyond the ejection fraction.

Among the strategies previously used to identify predictors of SCD, there has been a significant lack of community-wide analyses. Studies that use hospital- and clinic-based ascertainment of SCD patients will still have a role, but meaningful predictors of SCD are most likely to be discovered by prospective, community-wide investigations. There are several clinical and nonclinical predictors that already have shown promise in longitudinal cohort or community-wide studies. Specific examples from relatively recent studies are a diagnosis of diabetes mellitus, prolonged QTc interval on the surface electrocardiogram, and low socioeconomic status. Sudden cardiac arrest in patients with coronary artery disease that was previously silent still constitutes the largest and proportion of patients, however. Factors that determine rupture of the vulnerable plaque have been the target of intensive ongoing investigation and are likely to still have the highest yield for determinants of sudden cardiac arrest. It is clear that genetic factors play a role in the occurrence of SCD, and rapid advancements in the field of gene technology indicate that identification of putative genetic predictors is imminent. For risk stratification of SCD to be comprehensive, factors as diverse as genomics and socioeconomic status may have to be taken into consideration. All of these predictors require validation in diverse groups of individuals to ensure their relevance across populations. The ultimate goal of preventing SCD is likely to be attained only through a continued, focused refinement of interactions between substrates critical in the pathogenesis of SCD, particularly in the context of the global population.

REFERENCES

1. Cooper R, Cutler J, Desvigne-Nickens P, et al. Trends and disparities in coronary heart disease, stroke, and other cardiovascular diseases in the United States: findings of the National Conference on Cardiovascular Disease Prevention. Circulation 2000;102(25):3137–47.
2. Kuisma M, Repo J, Alaspaa A. The incidence of out-of-hospital ventricular fibrillation in Helsinki, Finland, from 1994 to 1999. Lancet 2001;358:473–4.
3. Zheng ZJ, Croft JB, Giles WH, et al. Sudden cardiac death in the United States, 1989 to 1998. Circulation 2001;104(18):2158–63.
4. Gillum RF. Trends in acute myocardial infarction and coronary heart disease death in the United States. J Am Coll Cardiol 1994;23(6):1273–7.
5. Weaver WD, Hill DL, Fahrenbruch C, et al. Automatic external defibrillators: importance of field testing to evaluate performance. J Am Coll Cardiol 1997;10:1259–64.
6. Murray CJ, Lopez AD. Alternative projections of mortality and disability by cause 1990–2020: Global Burden of Disease Study. Lancet 1997;349:1498–504.
7. Murray CJ, Lopez AD. Global mortality, disability, and the contribution of risk factors: Global Burden of Disease Study. Lancet 1997;349:1436–42.
8. Murray CJ, Lopez AD. Mortality by cause for eight regions of the world: Global Burden of Disease Study. Lancet 1997;349:1269–76.
9. Okrainec K, Banerjee DK, Eisenberg MJ. Coronary artery disease in the developing world. Am Heart J 2004;148:7–15.
10. Myerburg RJ, Castellanos A. Cardiac arrest and sudden cardiac death. In: Zipes DP, Libby P, Bonow RO, et al, editors. Braunwald's heart disease. A textbook of cardiovascular medicine. Philadelphia: Elsevier Saunders; 2005. p. 865.
11. Myerburg RJ. Sudden cardiac death: exploring the limits of our knowledge. J Cardiovasc Electrophysiol 2001;12:369–81.
12. Myerburg RJ. Scientific gaps in the prediction and prevention of sudden cardiac death. J Cardiovasc Electrophysiol 2002;13:709–23.
13. Arking DE, Chugh SS, Chakravarti A, et al. Genomics in sudden cardiac death. Circ Res 2004;94:712–23.
14. Chugh SS, Jui J, Gunson K, et al. Current burden of sudden cardiac death: multiple-source surveillance versus retrospective death certificate-based review in a large US community. J Am Coll Cardiol 2004;44:1268–75.
15. Greene HL. Sudden arrhythmic cardiac death—mechanisms, resuscitation, and classification: the Seattle perspective. Am J Cardiol 1990;65:4–12.
16. Bayes de Luna A, Coumel P, Leclercq JF. Ambulatory sudden cardiac death: mechanisms of production of fatal arrhythmia on the basis of data from 157 cases. Am Heart J 1989;117:151–9.
17. Myerburg RJ, Castellanos A. Cardiac arrest and sudden cardiac death. In: Braunwald E, editor. Heart disease: a textbook of cardiovascular medicine. 5th edition. Philadelphia: W.B. Saunders; 1997. p. 742.
18. Zipes DP, Wellens HJ. Sudden cardiac death. Circulation 1998;98:2334–51.
19. Mirowski M, Reid PR, Mower MM, et al. Termination of malignant ventricular arrhythmias with an implanted automatic defibrillator in human beings. N Engl J Med 1980;303:322–4.
20. Cobb LA, Fahrenbruch CE, Walsh TR, et al. Influence of cardiopulmonary resuscitation prior to defibrillation in patients with out-of-hospital ventricular fibrillation. JAMA 1999;281:1182–8.
21. Cobb LA, Fahrenbruch CE, Olsufka M, et al. Changing incidence of out-of-hospital ventricular fibrillation, 1980–2000. JAMA 2002;288:3008–38.
22. Dorian P, Cass D, Schwartz B, et al. Amiodarone as compared with lidocaine for shock-resistant ventricular fibrillation. N Engl J Med 2002;346:884–90.
23. Herlitz J, Andersson E, Bang A, et al. Experiences from treatment of out-of-hospital cardiac arrest during 17 years in Goteborg. Eur Heart J 2000;21:1251–8.
24. Parish DC, Dinesh Chandra KM, Dane FC. Success changes the problem: why ventricular fibrillation is declining, why pulseless electrical activity is

emerging, and what to do about it. Resuscitation 2003;58:31–5.

25. Fox CS, Evans JC, Larson MG, et al. Temporal trends in coronary heart disease mortality and sudden cardiac death from 1950 to 1999: the Framingham Heart Study. Circulation 2004;110:522–7.

26. Chugh SS, Kelly KL, Titus JL. Sudden cardiac death with apparently normal heart. Circulation 2000;102:649–54.

27. Bardy GH, Lee KL, Mark DB, et al. Home use of automated external defibrillators for sudden cardiac arrest. N Engl J Med 2008;358:1793–804.

28. Kannel WB, Cupples LA, D'Agostino RB. Sudden death risk in overt coronary heart disease: the Framingham Study. Am Heart J 1987;113:799–804.

29. Jouven X, Desnos M, Guerot C, et al. Predicting sudden death in the population: the Paris Prospective Study I. Circulation 1999;99:1978–83.

30. Thorgeirsson G, Sigvaldason H, Witteman J. Risk factors for out-of-hospital cardiac arrest: the Reykjavik Study. Eur Heart J 2005;26:1499–505.

31. Benchimol D, Dubroca B, Bernard V, et al. Short- and long-term risk factors for sudden death in patients with stable angina. Int J Cardiol 2000;76:147–56.

32. Bardy GH, Lee KL, Mark DB, et al. Amiodarone or an implantable cardioverter–defibrillator for congestive heart failure. N Engl J Med 2005;352:225–37.

33. Buxton AE, Lee KL, Fisher JD, et al. A randomized study of the prevention of sudden death in patients with coronary artery disease. Multicenter Unsustained Tachycardia Trial Investigators. N Engl J Med 1999;341:1882–90.

34. Moss AJ, Hall WJ, Cannom DS, et al. Improved survival with an implanted defibrillator in patients with coronary disease at high risk for ventricular arrhythmia. Multicenter Automatic Defibrillator Implantation Trial Investigators. N Engl J Med 1996;335:1933–40.

35. Moss AJ, Zareba W, Hall WJ, et al. Prophylactic implantation of a defibrillator in patients with myocardial infarction and reduced ejection fraction. N Engl J Med 2002;346:877–83.

36. Myerburg RJ, Mitrani R, Interian A Jr, et al. Interpretation of outcomes of antiarrhythmic clinical trials: design features and population impact. Circulation 1998;97:1514–21.

37. de Vreede-Swagemakers JJ, Gorgels AP, Dubois-Arbouw WI, et al. Out-of-hospital cardiac arrest in the 1990s: a population-based study in the Maastricht area on incidence, characteristics, and survival. J Am Coll Cardiol 1997;30:1500–5.

38. Gorgels AP, Gijsbers C, de Vreede-Swagemakers J, et al. Out-of-hospital cardiac arrest—the relevance of heart failure. The Maastricht Circulatory Arrest Registry. Eur Heart J 2003;24:1204–9.

39. Reinier K, Stecker EC, Vickers C, et al. Incidence of sudden cardiac arrest is higher in areas of low

socioeconomic status: a prospective two-year study in a large United States community. Resuscitation 2006;70:186–92.

40. Stecker EC, Vickers C, Waltz J, et al. Population-based analysis of sudden cardiac death with and without left ventricular systolic dysfunction: two-year findings from the Oregon Sudden Unexpected Death Study. J Am Coll Cardiol 2006;47:1161–6.

41. Balkau B, Jouven X, Ducimetiere P, et al. Diabetes as a risk factor for sudden death. Lancet 1999;354:1968–9.

42. Albert CM, Chae CU, Grodstein F, et al. Prospective study of sudden cardiac death among women in the United States. Circulation 2003;107:2096–101.

43. Albert CM, Mittleman MA, Chae CU, et al. Triggering of sudden death from cardiac causes by vigorous exertion. N Engl J Med 2000;343:1355–61.

44. Jouven X, Lemaitre RN, Rea TD, et al. Diabetes, glucose level, and risk of sudden cardiac death. Eur Heart J 2005;26:2142–7.

45. Beckman JA, Creager MA, Libby P. Diabetes and atherosclerosis: epidemiology, pathophysiology, and management. JAMA 2002;287:2570–81.

46. Veglio M, Borra M, Stevens LK, et al. The relation between QTc interval prolongation and diabetic complications. The EURODIAB IDDM Complication Study Group. Diabetologia 1999;42:68–75.

47. Rana BS, Lim PO, Naas AA, et al. QT interval abnormalities are often present at diagnosis in diabetes and are better predictors of cardiac death than ankle brachial pressure index and autonomic function tests. Heart 2005;91:44–50.

48. Lloyd-Mostyn RH, Watkins PJ. Defective innervation of heart in diabetic autonomic neuropathy. Br Med J 1975;3:15–7.

49. Pourmoghaddas A, Hekmatnia A. The relationship between QTc interval and cardiac autonomic neuropathy in diabetes mellitus. Mol Cell Biochem 2003;249:125–8.

50. Veglio M, Chinaglia A, Borra M, et al. Does abnormal QT interval prolongation reflect autonomic dysfunction in diabetic patients? QTc interval measure versus standardized tests in diabetic autonomic neuropathy. Diabet Med 1995;12:302–6.

51. Friedlander Y, Siscovick DS, Weinmann S, et al. Family history as a risk factor for primary cardiac arrest. Circulation 1998;97:155–60.

52. Benhorin J, Moss AJ, Bak M, et al. Variable expression of long QT syndrome among gene carriers from families with five different HERG mutations. Ann Noninvasive Electrocardiol 2002;7:40–6.

53. Chugh SS, Reinier K, Teodorescu C, et al. Epidemiology of sudden cardiac death: clinical and research implications. Prog Cardiovasc Dis 2008;51:213–28.

54. Bodenheimer T. High and rising health care costs. Part 1: seeking an explanation. Ann Intern Med 2005;142:847–54.

55. Escobedo LG, Zack MM. Comparison of sudden and nonsudden coronary deaths in the United States. Circulation 1996;93:2033–6.

56. Hemingway H, Malik M, Marmot M. Social and psychosocial influences on sudden cardiac death, ventricular arrhythmia, and cardiac autonomic function. Eur Heart J 2001;22:1082–101.

57. Mensah GA, Mokdad AH, Ford ES, et al. State of disparities in cardiovascular health in the United States. Circulation 2005;111:1233–41.

58. Vaillancourt C, Stiell IG. Cardiac arrest care and emergency medical services in Canada. Can J Cardiol 2004;20:1081–90.

59. Byrne R, Constant O, Smyth Y, et al. Multiple-source surveillance incidence and aetiology of out-of-hospital sudden cardiac death in a rural population in the west of Ireland. Eur Heart J 2008;29:1418–23.

60. Greenberg H, Raymond SU, Leeder SR. Cardiovascular disease and global health: threat and opportunity. Health Aff (Millwood) Suppl Web Exclusives 2005;W5:31–41.

61. Ezzati M, Hoorn SV, Rodgers A, et al. Estimates of global and regional potential health gains from reducing multiple major risk factors. Lancet 2003; 362:271–80.

62. Yusuf S, Hawken S, Ounpuu S, et al. Effect of potentially modifiable risk factors associated with myocardial infarction in 52 countries (the INTERHEART study): case–control study. Lancet 2004;364: 937–52.

63. Bennett PH, Li G, Xiaoren P. China. In: Ekoe J, Zimmet P, Williams R, editors. The epidemiology of diabetes mellitus: an international perspective. Chichester, England and New York: J. Wiley; 2001. p. 247.

64. Monteiro CA, Conde WL, Popkin BM. Independent effects of income and education on the risk of obesity in the Brazilian adult population. J Nutr 2001;131:881S–6S.

65. Fuchs SC, Petter JG, Accordi MC, et al. Establishing the prevalence of hypertension. Influence of sampling criteria. Arq Bras Cardiol 2001;76:445–52.

66. Padmavati S. Prevention of heart disease in India in the 21st century: need for a concerted effort. Indian Heart J 2002;54:99–102.

67. Ramachandran A, Snehalatha C, Latha E, et al. Rising prevalence of NIDDM in an urban population in India. Diabetologia 1997;40:232–7.

68. Motala AA. Diabetes trends in Africa. Diabetes Metab Res Rev 2002;18(Suppl 3):S14–20.

Advances in Cardiopulmonary Resuscitation

Demetris Yannopoulos, MD[a],*, Kostantinos Kotsifas, MD[b],
Keith G. Lurie, MD[c]

KEYWORDS

- CPR • Circulation • Cardiac arrest • Hypothermia
- Ventilation • Compression • Devices • Blood flow

Sudden cardiac death is one of the most common causes of death, accounting for approximately 1,000,000 deaths yearly in North America and Europe.[1,2] This clinical toll is enormous; more than 1000 adults die each day in the United States from an out-of-hospital cardiac arrest and a similar number die from in-hospital cardiac arrest. Survival from out-of-hospital and in-hospital cardiac arrest remains poor despite a significant improvement in many aspects of treatment of emergency clinical situations. Even in the most advanced emergency medical systems in Western societies[1] neurologically intact survival rates remain less than 20%. This article focuses on important advances in the science of cardiopulmonary resuscitation (CPR) in the last decade that have led to a significant improvement in understanding the complex physiology of cardiac arrest and critical interventions for the initial management of cardiac arrest and postresuscitation treatment. Special emphasis is given to the basic simple ways to improve circulation, vital organ perfusion pressures, and the grave prognosis of sudden cardiac death.

The complexity of cardiac arrest has led to a study theory that divides it into 3 phases. Although the existence of the 3 phases is not scientifically proven, they provide a useful construct for a more comprehensive understanding of the complexities of cardiac arrest.

Specific treatments targeting the pathophysiology of each phase increase the chances of a meaningful recovery.[3] The first phase after cardiac arrest is termed "the electrical phase." This lasts about 4 minutes after cardiac arrest; most patients present with ventricular fibrillation (VF) initially and often respond to immediate defibrillation. The second phase, called "the circulatory phase" begins at minute 4 and lasts to minute 10, depending on the surrounding temperature and conditions. High-quality CPR, with emphasis on improvement of the delivery of oxygenated blood to the brain and heart before defibrillation, is paramount, and techniques that increase circulation have been shown to improve outcomes. The third phase, or "metabolic phase," usually begins after 10 minutes. Current treatment strategies for patients in the metabolic phase are poor. These late efforts generally target the metabolic derangements associated with prolonged ischemia. Survival is inversely related to the time of untreated cardiac arrest. Most of the patients in cardiac arrest receive professional assistance during the second phase because of delays in arrival of paramedics or lack of bystander CPR. This is one of the reasons that extra emphasis has been placed on improving circulation and simplifying the delivery of compressions and ventilations in recent American Heart Association (AHA) Guidelines.

[a] Department of Medicine, Interventional Cardiology, University of Minnesota, 420 Delaware Street, MMC 508, Minneapolis, MN 55455, USA
[b] Department of Pulmonary Medicine, Sotiria General Hospital, Goudi 10928, Athens, Greece
[c] Department of Emergency Medicine, Hennepin County Medical Center, Minneapolis Medical Research Foundation, University of Minnesota, 914 South 8th Street, 3rd Floor, Minneapolis, MN 55404, USA
* Corresponding author.
E-mail address: yanno001@umn.edu (D. Yannopoulos).

Card Electrophysiol Clin 1 (2009) 13–31
doi:10.1016/j.ccep.2009.08.009
1877-9182/09/$ – see front matter © 2009 Published by Elsevier Inc.

IMMEDIATE CPR

The earlier the intervention and targeted therapies are delivered after cardiac collapse, the higher the chances of survival. Because most patients in cardiac arrest are initially found by laypersons, a renewed emphasis has been placed on increasing bystander CPR. Studies have shown that when operators who receive 911 calls provide instruction by phone on how to provide CPR to lay rescuers who have not been previously trained in CPR, teaching only chest-compression CPR results in no worse outcomes compared with teaching mouth-to-mouth technique and chest compression.[4] This simplified approach to teaching CPR has only been shown to result in no harm in long-term outcomes. However, prolonged periods of chest-compression-only CPR have been shown to be dangerous in some animal studies, and high-quality studies are lacking in humans. Despite a lack of substantial improvement in outcomes with chest-compression-only CPR, fear of disease transmission from mouth-to-mouth ventilation and the challenges of trying to teach mouth-to-mouth by telephone have shifted the emphasis of phone instructions before arrival of the emergency medical services (EMS) to focus rescuers on chest compressions only. These efforts increase the chances of successful defibrillation because the "no-flow" state is reduced. Without bystander CPR the likelihood of neurologically intact survival is significantly reduced.

Early defibrillation is an essential therapy for the electrical phase of cardiac arrest. Direct current defibrillation can restore a perfusing rhythm in 80% of patients within 1 to 2 minutes. However, after 10 minutes the success rate falls to less than 5%. That is one of the reasons that broad deployment of public-access defibrillators in places where large numbers of people are likely to congregate has been encouraged. In one study that tested early defibrillation in casinos in the United States the survival of patients suffering VF was 50% overall. Patients who received defibrillation within 3 minutes of collapse had a 75% hospital discharge rate.[5] Based on a solid body of evidence, early defibrillation in a witnessed arrest is a class I recommendation based on the 2005 AHA CPR Guidelines.[6] Other studies have not shown so much promise for use of automated external defibrillators (AEDs).[7] The public-access defibrillation study funded by the US National Institutes of Health found a small but statistically significant difference in outcomes when thousands of AEDs were deployed and compared with defibrillation by first responders. In an equally important study from Seattle, Cobb and colleagues[8] showed that survival rates decreased by 30% when AEDs were placed on all first-responder vehicles in Seattle. These investigators demonstrated that 90 seconds of CPR before delivery of a shock resulted in a significant increase in survival. These data stressed, for the first time, the importance of priming the pump to clear lactate and circulate blood through the heart before defibrillation.

Other issues related to defibrillation remain complicated. For example, Bardy and colleagues[9] showed that in survivors of anterior-wall myocardial infarction who were not candidates for implantation of a cardioverter-defibrillator, access to a home AED did not significantly improve overall survival, compared with reliance on conventional resuscitation methods, despite the higher theoretic probability for sudden cardiac death than controls. Similarly, although there are no clinical data demonstrating improved long-term survival rates between the monophasic and biphasic waveforms for treatment of VF during the electrical phase of cardiac arrest, a single high-energy (150–200 J) biphasic defibrillation shock is believed to be the treatment of choice of in- and out-of-hospital VF.

One of the biggest changes in cardiac arrest science in the past 15 years is that the frequency of VF as the initial cardiac arrest rhythm has decreased from about 50% to less than 30%.[10] The reasons for this change remain unknown but use of implantable defibrillators in high-risk patients and more aggressive preventative care with cholesterol-lowering agents, β-blockers and interventional cardiology procedures may contribute to this epidemiologic change. There are animal data to suggest that some drugs, including β-blockers and angiotensin-converting enzyme (ACE) inhibitors may decrease the duration of VF. Regardless of the cause, the change in the frequency of VF as the initial presenting rhythm to asystole (nearly 50%) and pulseless electrical activity focuses even more attention on finding better ways to improve circulation, as described in the next section.

IMPROVING CIRCULATION

Most prehospital cardiac arrests cannot be treated within 4 minutes from the time of arrest. Initiation of therapy for cardiac arrest after 4 to 5 minutes of a nonperfusing rhythm calls for immediate compressions to generate blood flow and partially replete the membrane energy required for generation of an organized rhythm. When the time between the 911 call and paramedic arrival is longer than 4 to 5 minutes, CPR before shock significantly improves survival and hospital discharge rates up to 5-fold (from 4% to 22%). If the time to defibrillation is less than 5 minutes, there are no differences in survival.[11]

The focus of modern CPR is on improved circulation during CPR; this means more effective compressions, fewer interruptions, and less frequent ventilations. For basic life support (BLS) the compression/ventilation ratio is 30:2, to provide fewer interruptions of compressions for ventilation. During CPR, even in the best of circumstances, the generated cardiac output is less than 20% of normal. Respiratory exchange is adequate with less-than-normal minute ventilation, in part because gas exchange is limited by the severely reduced pulmonary flow. For advanced life support (ALS), continuous chest compressions without interruption for ventilations are strongly recommended to improve circulation and enhance vital-organ perfusion and oxygenation. Equally important is starting chest compressions immediately, as soon as they are indicated.

This recommendation is based on a consensus of experts in CPR. However, it has been shown in pigs that with the shift from a 15:2 to a 30:2 compression/ventilation ratio the common carotid blood flow doubles and there is a 25% increase in cardiac output without any compromise in oxygenation and acid-base balance (**Fig. 1**).[12] Further efforts to reduce the ventilation frequency are harmful in animals, as described later.[13,14]

During ALS uninterrupted compressions with a rate of 100/min are recommended. The rescuers that are responsible for the ventilation should deliver 8 to 10 breaths/min with special care not to hyperventilate. Continuous delivery of high-quality chest compressions with attention to full chest-wall recoil is tiring and rescuers should rotate frequently (every 2–3 minutes) to avoid excessive fatigue, which diminishes the quality of CPR.[15]

VENTILATIONS

Periodic positive-pressure ventilation during CPR is fundamental to providing oxygen to the blood and tissues.[16] Recent studies have shown that each positive-pressure ventilation is associated with an increase in intrathoracic pressure, which

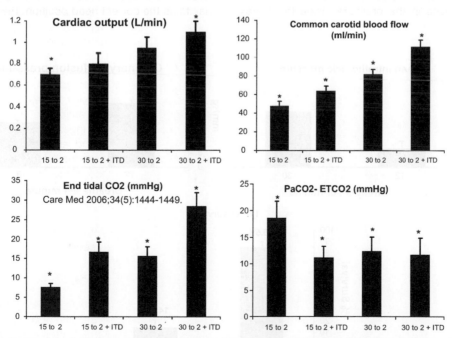

Fig. 1. After 6 minutes of untreated VF 6 minutes of either 15:2 or 30:2 compression/ventilation ratio CPR was performed. At the end the inspiratory ITD was added for another 4 minutes. There was a significant increase of cardiac output, common carotid artery flow, end tidal CO_2 in the animals that received 30:2 C/V ratio. There was a further increase with the addition of an ITD although it was applied late. $Paco_2$-$Etco_2$ is a marker of pulmonary ventilation/perfusion matching. * means statistically significant difference when compared with the ratio of 15:2 with a $P<.05$. (*From* Yannopoulos D, Aufderheide TP, Gabrielli A, et al. Clinical and hemodynamic comparison of 15:2 and 30:2 compression-to-ventilation ratios for cardiopulmonary resuscitation. Crit Care Med 2006;34:1444; with permission.)

increases intracranial pressure and decreases cardiac filling; the hemodynamic consequences reduce cerebral and coronary perfusion. Too frequent or too few ventilations can be harmful, if not deadly.[17,18] The frequency of ventilation during CPR should be reduced to 8 to 10 breaths/min once the airway has been secured, and each 500-mL tidal-volume breath should be delivered rapidly (in <1 second) to minimize the duration of positive airway pressures. These subtle but fundamental changes in ventilation technique ensure optimal circulation during conventional, manual, closed-chest CPR.[19] The benefits of positive-pressure ventilation must be weighed against the harm associated with too much ventilation. In addition, the unwillingness of the layperson to provide CPR because of the fear of communicating diseases and the inherent aversion to mouth-to-mouth ventilation should be taken into consideration.

Excessive ventilation rates and volumes increase intrathoracic pressure and intracranial pressures and concomitantly decrease coronary perfusion pressure, mean arterial pressure, and survival rates in animals (**Fig. 2**).[18] Intracranial pressures are regulated, in part, by intrathoracic pressures: each time ventilation is delivered there is an increase in the pressure inside the thorax and the brain, which reduces cardiac and cerebral perfusion pressures.[19]

Maintaining an open and secure airway is paramount during CPR. However, stopping chest compressions and taking time to intubate stops all circulation. Techniques and devices that allow rescuer personnel to provide ventilation without having to interrupt chest compressions, including use of a 2-handed face-mask technique and some of the supraglottic airway devices, are simple but significant advances. Thus, although endotracheal intubation is still recommended, many advanced EMS systems perform CPR with a face-mask technique or supraglottic airway initially and then intubate 10 minutes later or after a return of spontaneous circulations. Thus, use of a Combitube or other supraglottic airway device (eg, KING LTS-D, King Systems, Noblesville, IN, USA), which are placed in the oropharyngeal cavity and allow for nonselective airway isolation for the purpose of ventilation, and the laryngeal mask airway, is recommended. These devices have not been shown to alter outcomes after cardiac arrest but they do maintain airway patency.

When using a face-mask for ventilation, a 2-person technique is recommended. One person maintains the correct head position, the complete

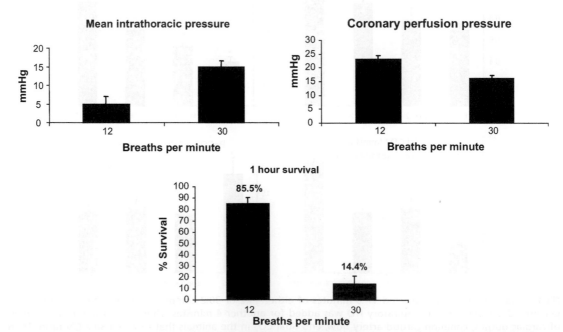

Fig. 2. Hyperventilation and survival. When after 6 minutes of untreated VF pigs received CPR with either 12 or 30 breaths/min (as observed frequently in a clinical trial), the mean intrathoracic pressure was inversely related to coronary perfusion pressure and 1-hour survival rates; $P<.05$. (*From* Aufderheide TP, Sigurdsson G, Pirrallo RG, et al. Hyperventilation-induced hypotension during cardiopulmonary resuscitation. Circulation 2004;109:1960; with permission.)

seal, and a jaw thrust to maintain airway patency, and the second person squeezes the resuscitator bag. This approach can be used for a more prolonged period when adequate personnel are available as it enables rescuers to perform high-quality CPR without stopping compressions and interrupting circulation to place an advanced airway device. This approach works well when using an impedance threshold device (ITD), as described later in this article, and is inexpensive. Delaying intubation by providing good face-mask ventilation technique is an important way to maximize chest compression time.

COMPRESSIONS

Chest compressions or "external cardiac massage" was first introduced into the modern medical literature by Kouwenhoven and colleagues in 1960.[20] Generation of blood flow during compressions results from an increase in intrathoracic pressure (thoracic pump theory), the mechanical effect of compressing the heart between the sternum and spine (cardiac pump theory), and the cardiac valvular system, which allows mainly unidirectional flow. The recommendation for pushing "hard and fast" results from the understanding of the importance of compressions during CPR. However, pushing too hard and too fast can be harmful; like the ventilation frequency, understanding the subtleties of the chest-compression technique is essential for good outcomes. A depth of 3 to 5 cm is considered adequate compression depth (**Fig. 3**).[21] The rate should be 100 compressions/min because lower rates decrease forward blood flow.[22] Interruptions should be minimized, because every time compressions are stopped, it takes a significant amount of time to reestablish adequate aortic pressure and coronary perfusion pressure.[23] For example, pulse checks should not last more than 10 seconds. CPR should be

delivered continuously for 2 minutes before pulse or rhythm checks. In observational studies the average time without compressions during resuscitation varies from 25% to 50% (**Fig. 4**).[24] This variation can be extremely detrimental as no compressions means no perfusion.

One of the recommendations by the AHA is that uninterrupted chest compressions should be delivered before the delivery of a shock, and chest compressions should be resumed immediately thereafter for 2 minutes. Although performing chest compression immediately after direct current shock was based on consensus opinion, the overall thrust of the recommendation is the importance of circulation before defibrillation (**Fig. 5**). Chest compressions for 90 seconds to 3 minutes before defibrillation help to "prime" the pump, making successful return of spontaneous circulation most likely after defibrillation. Chest compressions for 60 seconds to 2 minutes immediately after defibrillation are believed to help prevent the hypotension and asystole that is often observed when a defibrillation shock is delivered. As a result, rather than check for a pulse after a defibrillation shock in a patient who has been in VF for more than 4 minutes, the rescuers should immediately resume CPR to maintain circulation, even if the heart is spontaneously beating. Although a theoretic risk of reinducing fibrillation with chest compression exists, there are no human data to support a significant risk or benefit in performing 2 minutes of CPR immediately after defibrillation and before checking for rhythm and pulses.

COMPRESSION-ONLY (HANDS-ONLY) CPR

Because uninterrupted chest compressions are easier to perform and possibly a more attractive and simpler method to teach bystander CPR (as

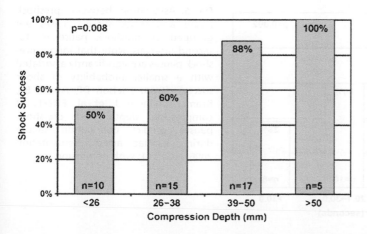

Fig. 3. Association between chest compression depth and shock success. Cases are grouped by 30-second average compression depth in approximately 11-mm (0.5-in) intervals. Chest compression depth of 38 to 50 mm (1.5–2 in) represents current CPR guidelines recommendations. Deeper chest compressions are significantly associated with increased probability of shock success. (*From* Edelson DP, Abella BS, Kramer-Johansen J, et al. Effects of compression depth and pre-shock pauses predict debrillation failure during cardiac arrest. Resuscitation 2006;71(2):141; with permission.)

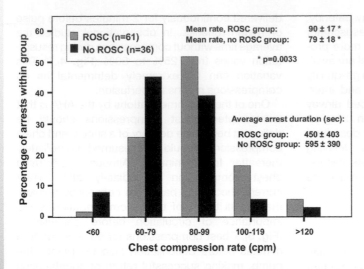

Fig. 4. Chest compression rates correlation with initial resuscitation outcome. Subgroup of patients attaining ROSC is shown in gray; subgroup that did not, in black. Note 2 overlapping but distinct distributions, with mean rates for each group shown. Note mean durations of resuscitation for 2 groups, demonstrating that the group that expired received longer resuscitation efforts on average, arguing against a "slow-code" bias. Asterisk denotes statistical significance from a 2-tailed *t*-test as shown. (*From* Abella BS, Sandbo N, Vassilatos P, et al. Chest compression rates during cardiopulmonary resuscitation are suboptimal: a prospective study during in-hospital cardiac arrest. Circulation 2005;111:428; with permission.)

shown by the Survey of Survivors of Out-of-Hospital Cardiac Arrest in the Kanto Region of Japan [SOS-KANTO] study[25] the Emergency Cardiovascular Care Committee of the AHA has released a science advisory recommending an alternative strategy of compression-only or "hands-only" CPR for layperson bystanders witnessing an adult cardiac arrest.[4]

The recommendations summarized include the following 3 possibilities: (1) If an adult suddenly collapses, trained or untrained bystanders should (at a minimum) activate their community emergency medical response system (call 911) and provide high-quality chest compressions by pushing hard and fast in the center of the chest, minimizing interruptions according to the published guidelines (class I). (2) If a bystander has not received training in CPR, then hands-only CPR is strongly encouraged (class IIa). The

rescuer should continue hands-only CPR until an AED arrives and is ready for use or EMS providers take over care of the victim. (3) When the bystander has received training in CPR, he or she can provide conventional CPR using a 30:2 compression/ventilation ratio (class IIa) or hands-only CPR (class IIa). CPR with either of the 2 techniques should be continued until defibrillation is possible or EMS providers take over. When the bystander, regardless of training status, is not confident in his or her ability to provide conventional CPR, including high-quality chest compressions with rescue breaths (compressions of adequate rate and depth with minimal interruptions), then hands-only CPR is recommended (class IIa).

There is no evidence to support the adoption of this approach by trained EMS paramedics. There is, on the contrary, a significant body of evidence

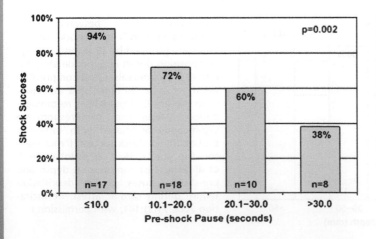

Fig. 5. Association between preshock pause and shock success. Cases are grouped by preshock pause in 10-second intervals. Note that longer preshock pauses are significantly associated with a smaller probability of shock success. (*From* Edelson DP, Abella BS, Kramer-Johansen J, et al. Effects of compression depth and pre-shock pauses predict debrillation failure during cardiac arrest. Resuscitation 2006;71(2):141; with permission.)

that disputes the notion that prolonged CPR can be performed without the presence of ventilation. It has recently been shown that when delivered ventilations decrease from 10 beats/min to 2 beats/min, a significant decrease in brain tissue oxygen tension and carotid blood flow occurs.[13] In addition, in a 24-hour neurologic and survival evaluation study, animals with no assisted ventilation had significantly worse neurologic outcomes with evidence of significant respiratory and metabolic acidosis and profound hypoxemia within the first of 4 minutes of chest-compression-only CPR despite open airways compared with standard CPR (**Fig. 6**).[14] This new investigation is in concordance with 2 previously published studies that showed worsening rates of return of spontaneous circulation (ROSC) and evidence of severe respiratory acidosis and hypoxemia when prolonged CPR is performed without ventilations.[16,26] There are data in support of a chest-compression-only strategy for lay rescuers, but there are no prospective randomized trials that demonstrate a benefit to this approach by professional first responders. By contrast, EMS systems in Europe

and the United States that follow the AHA Guidelines on compressions show the highest survival rates in the history of CPR (Rae, King County, WA, USA; White, Rochester, MN, USA; Sunde, Oslo, Norway).

CHEST-WALL DECOMPRESSION

With each chest-wall decompression, the negative intrathoracic pressure naturally generated by the elastic recoil properties of the chest wall promotes venous return to the heart, thereby increasing preload for the next compression cycle. The decompression-induced vacuum within the chest is transmitted to the brain and as a result intracranial pressure is transiently reduced, thereby reducing resistance to forward brain flow. Incomplete decompression, like hyperventilation, is a common mistake and is harmful. Incomplete chest-wall recoil decreases blood flow to the heart and brain during CPR. Fatigue and ineffective technique, inappropriate hand positioning, or poorly designed mechanical CPR adjuncts can result in incomplete chest-wall recoil. Data from recent trials

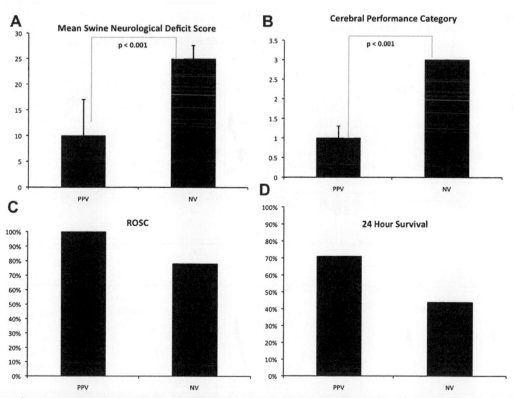

Fig. 6. After 8 minutes of untreated VF, animals were treated for another 8 minutes with either 10 positive-pressure ventilation (PPV)/min or with no assisted ventilation (NAV) before defibrillation. Survivors were followed for 24 hours. *A*, Mean neurologic score; *B*, CPC score; *C*, rate of return to spontaneous circulation; *D*, 24-hour survival rate in percentage. The number of animals that survived of the total number of animals in the group is shown in parentheses.

demonstrated that many rescuers fail to decompress completely,[27,28] which results in a sustained end diastolic increase of intrathoracic pressure. This phenomenon, when examined in a porcine model of cardiac arrest, revealed 2 fundamental effects. First, incomplete chest-wall recoil caused a significant decrease of mean arterial pressure, an increase in right atrial pressure, and thus decreased coronary perfusion pressures. Second, incomplete chest-wall recoil led to a significant increase in intracranial pressure and a decrease in cerebral and systemic perfusion pressures (**Fig. 7**).[19] When incomplete decompression and positive-pressure ventilation occurred simultaneously, cerebral perfusion ceased; the cerebral perfusion gradient was essentially zero for at least 3 to 4 compression-decompression cycles (**Fig. 8**).

Devices

Mechanical devices have been developed with the intent to improve circulation and promote air exchange and ventilation. Those devices are discussed in detail in this section.

Harnessing negative intrathoracic pressure to increase venous return and increase vital organ perfusion during CPR

Inspiratory ITD The dynamic energy of the expanding chest wall during the decompression phase can be harnessed to increase venous return, increase aortic pressure, lower intracranial pressure, and increase circulation to the heart and brain. The inspiratory ITD regulates the entry of air through the airways into the chest during the decompression phase of CPR. It causes a decrease in intrathoracic pressure of −2 to 10 mmHg, depending on the method used to perform chest compressions. The intrathoracic vacuum that develops with the ITD helps to draw blood back to the heart and lower intracranial pressure during the recoil phase of CPR.[29] Although this device is attached to an airway, it is used during CPR to enhance circulation (**Fig. 9**).

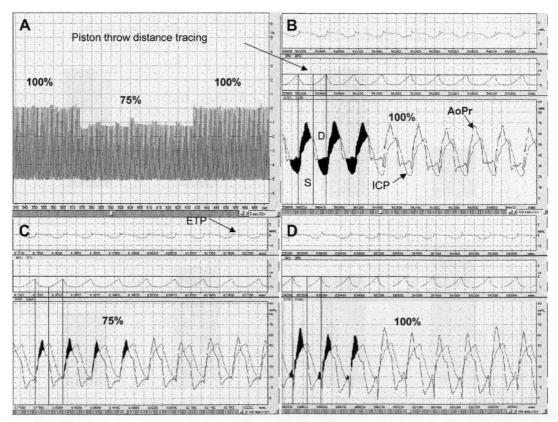

Fig. 7. The effect of incomplete chest-wall recoil on cerebral perfusion pressure (A–D). (*From* Yannopoulos D, McKnite S, Aufderheide TP, et al. Effects of incomplete chest wall decompression during cardiopulmonary resuscitation on coronary and cerebral perfusion pressures in a porcine model of cardiac arrest. Resuscitation 2005;64:363; with permission.)

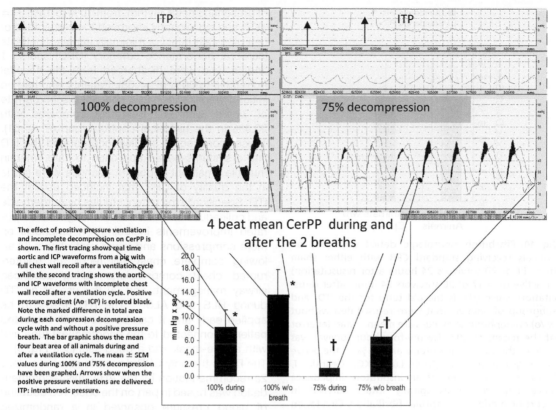

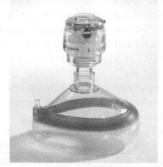

The effect of positive pressure ventilation and incomplete decompression on CerPP is shown. The first tracing shows real time aortic and ICP waveforms from a pig with full chest wall recoil after a ventilation cycle while the second tracing shows the aortic and ICP waveforms with incomplete chest wall recoil after a ventilation cycle. Positive pressure gradient (Ao ICP) is colored black. Note the marked difference in total area during each compression decompression cycle with and without a positive pressure breath. The bar graphic shows the mean four beat area of all animals during and after a ventilation cycle. The mean ± SEM values during 100% and 75% decompression have been graphed. Arrows show when the positive pressure ventilations are delivered. ITP: intrathoracic pressure.

Fig. 8. Effect on cerebral perfusion pressure when positive-pressure ventilations are added to incomplete chest decompressions. (*From* Yannopoulos D, McKnite S, Aufderheide TP, et al. Effects of incomplete chest wall decompression during cardiopulmonary resuscitation on coronary and cerebral perfusion pressures in a porcine model of cardiac arrest. Resuscitation 2005;64:363; with permission.)

Demonstration of ITD benefit in animal and clinical studies form the basis for the level IIa recommendation for the ITD in the 2005 AHA Guidelines. One of the first animal studies performed with the ITD demonstrated that use of the active ITD increased 24-h survival and preserved neurologic function after induced cardiac arrest in pigs.[30]

There was a statistically significant increase in these key outcome parameters, as shown in **Fig. 10**. There was improved neurologic function in the overall study group, and in the subset of pigs that were resuscitated with defibrillation shock therapy and epinephrine. Blood gas data demonstrated that relative tissue oxygenation was

- Concept: Lower intrathoracic pressure in the chest during the decompression phase of CPR enhances venous return to the thorax.

- Design: Each time the chest wall recoils following a compression, the ITD transiently blocks air/oxygen from entering the lungs, creating a small vacuum in the chest, resulting in improved preload.

Fig. 9. The concept and design of the inspiratory ITD. The ITD can be placed on an endotracheal tube or on a specially designed face-mask for bag- mask ventilation provided that a good air seal is applied. Timing lights flash at a rate of 10/min to guide ventilations and compressions (10 compressions between 2 flashes).

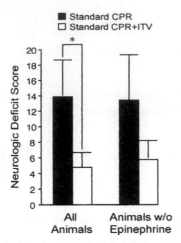

Fig. 10. Pittsburgh neurologic deficit score for all animals receiving standard CPR with either sham (n = 11 of 20 survivors 24 hours after resuscitation) or active (n = 17 of 20 survivors 24 hours after resuscitation) valve (ITV is the old term for the ITD) and subgroup of animals that were resuscitated without (w/o) epinephrine. All values are mean ± stander error of the mean; *P<.03. Twenty-four-hour survival was 55% in the sham valve group and 85% in the active valve group (P<.05). (*From* Lurie KG, Zielinski T, McKnite S, et al. Use of an inspiratory impedance valve improves neurologically intact survival in a porcine model of ventricular fibrillation. Circulation 2002;105:124; with permission.)

considered adequate in both groups and no differences were observed between groups on autopsy. The intrathoracic pressures were significantly lower in the ITD group. Subsequent studies have demonstrated that use of the ITD lowers intracranial pressures more rapidly than in pigs treated with standard CPR alone. It is hypothesized that this observation helps to explain the markedly improved neurologic outcomes in this porcine survival study.

After the animal studies, Pirrallo and colleagues[31] demonstrated with a double-blind, randomized, control trial that systolic blood pressures were twice as high with an active ITD when compared with a sham device. A concurrent study demonstrated that 24-hour survival rates were twice as high in patients presenting with pulseless electrical activity with the active device.[32] More recently, Aufderheide and colleagues[33] reported beneficial outcomes from the use of the ITD in 5 US EMS systems and Davis and colleagues[34] showed a nearly 2-fold survival improvement when the ITD was used on patients with an in-hospital cardiac arrest. Aufderheide and colleagues[33] showed that the changes in CPR practice resulted in a significant increase of hospital discharge rates for all patients, regardless

of presenting heart rhythm, from 10% to 13% (P = .007) and significantly improved the percentage of neurologically intact or minimally impaired patients (cerebral performance category [CPC] scores 1 and 2) who were discharged from the hospital from 33% to 60% (P = .03). Patients who had an initial rhythm of VF had a hospital discharge rate of 31.1% with ITD treatment compared with 20.4% in the historical control group (P = .01). These more recent studies incorporated the ITD into a systems-based approach to care wherein multiple small but important changes were made in the quality of CPR that included use of the ITD. Specifically the recent studies by Aufderheide and colleagues and Davis and colleagues incorporated improvements including: (1) emphasis on more compressions and fewer ventilations; (2) allowing complete chest-wall recoil; (3) uninterrupted chest compressions during advanced airway management; and (4) the use of an ITD during BLS and ALS.[33] The ITD needs to be applied early and it can be used with intubated patients connected to the endotracheal tube and with a face-mask and a good seal (see **Fig. 9**).[35] The ITD is the only CPR device to receive a class 2a recommendation by the AHA; this recommendation was based in part on the observed doubling of blood pressure observed in a randomized double-blind, out-of-hospital, cardiac arrest trial with the ITD.[15,31] It is important to emphasize that no device, including the ITD, is a panacea; this and other new technologies need to be used in a systems-based approach to improve survival rates significantly.

Intrathoracic pressure regulator The second generation of intrathoracic pressure regulation devices to improve cardiorespiratory interactions during CPR is the intrathoracic pressure regulator (ITPR). This device is not dependent on the elastic properties of the expanding chest wall to generate negative intrathoracic pressure. The device provides continues negative airway pressure in intubated animals and allows for positive-pressure ventilation delivery. This device improves all basic hemodynamic parameters during CPR and the rates of return to spontaneous circulation. In addition. it has shown significant improvement in hemodynamic parameters during hypovolemic cardiac arrest (hemorrhage).[36] This device is cleared for sale by the US Food and Drug Administration and clinical trials are under way to determine its potential benefit.

Compression devices

The load-distributing band (LDB) device (Autopulse, Zoll Circulation, Sunnyvale, CA, USA), an automated band-compression device, has been shown to increase perfusion pressures in animals and humans.[37,38] It is based on the physiologic principal that circumferential thoracic compression increases intrathoracic pressure without significant cardiac compression and can effectively produce forward flow. Increasing intrathoracic pressure results in forward blood flow. There is some controversy, however, as use of this device has been reported to be associated with positive and adverse outcomes. For example, a recent large randomized trial (ASPIRE) was prematurely stopped because of safety concerns. Rates of survival to discharge from hospital were found to be lower in the LDB-CPR group (5.8% vs 9.9% [$P = .04$]; adjusted for covariates and clustering, $P = .06$). In addition, survival with a CPC score of 1 or 2 was recorded in 7.5% (28 of 371) of patients in the manual CPR group compared with 3.1% (12 of 391) in the LDB-CPR group ($P = .006$).[39] In contrast, a second nonrandomized historical control based study on the LDB-CPR, published in the same issue of *JAMA*, showed that when the LBD-CPR device was used in a systems-based approach to care that included CPR before shock and therapeutic hypothermia, survival rates increased. The second study compared resuscitation outcomes before and after an urban EMS system switched from manual CPR to LDB-CPR. A total of 499 patients were included in the manual CPR phase (2001–2003) and 284 patients in the LDB-CPR phase (2003–2005); of these latter patients, the LDB device was applied in 210 patients. Patients in the manual CPR and LDB-CPR phases were comparable except for more EMS-witnessed arrests (18.7% vs 12.6%) with LDB. Rates of survival to discharge from hospital were poor in the historical phase (2.9%) and increased to 9.7% ($P<.01$) with the new system. In a secondary analysis of the 210 patients in whom the LDB device was applied, 38 patients (18.1%) survived to hospital admission, and only 12 patients (5.7%) survived to hospital discharge. Among patients in the manual CPR and LDB-CPR groups who survived to discharge from hospital, there was no significant difference between groups in CPC or overall performance category. Thus, in a nonrandomized study a new resuscitation strategy that included using LDB-CPR on EMS ambulances was associated with improved survival to discharge from hospital in adults with out-of-hospital nontraumatic cardiac arrest, but the study design was controversial.[40] Based on the fundamental physiologic relationships described earlier in this article related to the importance of incomplete chest-wall recoil and potential

harm associated with increasing the intrathoracic pressure too much, the authors speculate that better regulation of changes in intrathoracic pressure with LBD-CPR types of devices would result in more consistent results (**Fig. 11**).

Active compression decompression device

The active compression decompression (ACD) CPR device turns the thorax into an active bellows, drawing respiratory gases into the lungs with each decompression, along with a small amount of blood back to the heart. With each compression air and blood are propelled out of the thorax.[41] Multiple out-of-hospital and in-hospital hemodynamic and survival studies have been performed with ACD CPR. Some have shown significant improvements in up to 1-year survival, whereas others have shown no significant benefit with the device.[42] The combination of an ACD device with the inspiratory ITD offers significant hemodynamic improvement during CPR.[43] The ITD activates ACD CPR by harnessing the bellowslike action of the thorax. The device combination results in a significant augmentation in coronary and cerebral circulation. The device combination was shown to improve short-term survival outcomes: 24-hour survival rates were increased by 50% in 2 separate randomized controlled trials.[42,44] At present the manual ACD CPR device is not approved by the US Food and Drug Administration (FDA) for sale in the United States.

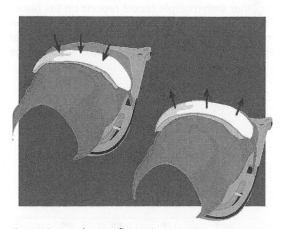

Fig. 11. Autopulse configuration. During compression (*left*) the band is tightened by the motor, and compression force is directed inward. During relaxation (*right*), the band is released, and the chest expands. (*From* Halperin HR, Paradis N, Ornato JP, et al. Cardiopulmonary resuscitation with a novel chest compression device in a porcine model of cardiac arrest: improved hemodynamics and mechanisms. J Am Coll Cardiol 2004;44:2214; with permission.)

Another ACD device, which is automated rather than manual, is the Lund University Compression Assist Device or LUCAS device. There are no randomized controlled trials with this device. However, this device provides an alternative to manual CPR and allows for complete chest-wall recoil with some degree of active decompression. FDA regulations currently limit the decompression phase forces to 3 pounds (1.3 kg).

THERAPEUTIC HYPOTHERMIA

Although the benefits of therapeutic hypothermia were first described 50 years ago for patients after cardiac arrest, only recently have clinicians adopted this postresuscitation technique to help preserve brain function.[45] Animal and humans studies have shown that the rapid lowering of core temperature to 33°C for 24 hours improves neurologically intact survival rates for patients with an initial rhythm of VF. Two randomized human trials published in the New England Journal of Medicine in 2002 demonstrated that mild to moderate hypothermia (32–34°C), post resuscitation, resulted in an improvement (16%–23% absolute risk reduction) for poor neurologic outcomes in patients who had a witnessed VF arrest. There was a significant improvement in 6-month survival rates in the hypothermic groups (**Fig. 12** and **Table 1**).[46,47] Current AHA Guidelines support this approach, with a level 2a recommendation for patients who present with a witnessed arrest and VF as the presenting rhythm. These data, together with multiple recent reports on the benefits of therapeutic hypothermia, have resulted in more widespread use of therapeutic hypothermia for any patient after a cardiac arrest who remains comatose. The authors strongly support this more liberalized approach to this significant clinical advance.

Recent studies have shown that it is possible to cool during CPR before reperfusion is achieved to further minimize tissue damage before it occurs. Cooling during CPR in animals with venovenous access systems or with cold intravenous saline and use of ACD CPR plus the ITD may eventually offer a means to rapidly decrease cerebral temperatures during CPR and improve neurologic outcomes.[48,49] Based on data in support of therapeutic hypothermia, the guidelines recommend cooling of comatose patients after successful resuscitation when possible, as long as there is a protocol in place to assure careful monitoring of core temperatures and hemodynamics, prevention of shivering, and maintenance of adequate perfusion pressures during the recommended 24-hour period of cooling. Further study is needed to evaluate the therapeutic potential of early cooling and to investigate the best way of achieving cerebral hypothermia in a timely and practical manner.

PHARMACOLOGIC MANAGEMENT

There have been few advances in the pharmacologic management of patients in cardiac arrest.

Vasoactive Medications

Evidence for the broad use of vasoactive medication during CPR comes primarily from animal studies. There are no placebo-controlled trials to demonstrate long-term benefit of epinephrine or vasopressin. The 2005 AHA Guidelines recommend the use of either of these agents with a class IIb level of recommendation.

Epinephrine is the most commonly used vasopressor during CPR. The beneficial hemodynamic effects of epinephrine during CPR are caused by its potent α-adrenergic effects. The significant increase in central aortic pressures results in significant increase in coronary and cerebral perfusion pressures and possibly rates of successful resuscitation.[50]

However, based on multiple clinical trials, use of high-dose epinephrine is contraindicated and harmful in patients in cardiac arrest (class III recommendation). The guidelines continue to recommend 1 mg of epinephrine every 3 to 5 minutes (recommendation class IIb) for adults in cardiac arrest. If no venous access has been obtained, endotracheal or intraosseous administration can be effective.

Vasopressin is recommended as an alternative vasopressor during CPR. It too has potent

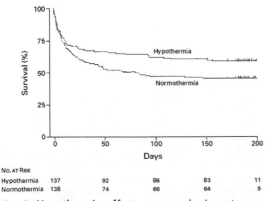

NO. AT RISK

Hypothermia	137	92	86	83	11
Normothermia	138	74	66	64	9

Fig. 12. Hypothermia effect on neurologic outcomes and survival. Censored data are indicated by tick marks. (*From* Hypothermia after Cardiac Arrest Study Group. Mild therapeutic hypothermia to improve the neurologic outcome after cardiac arrest. N Engl J Med 2002;346:549; with permission.)

Table 1
Neurologic outcome and mortality at 6 months

Outcome	Normothermia	Hypothermia	Risk Ratio (95% CI)[a]	P Value[b]
	Number/Total Number (%)			
Favorable neurologic outcome[c]	54/137 (39)	75/136 (55)	1.40 (1.08–1.81)	0.009
Death	76/138 (55)	56/137 (41)	0.74 (0.58–0.95)	0.02

[a] The risk ratio was calculated as the rate of a favorable neurologic outcome or the rate of death in the hypothermia group divided by the rate in the normothermia group. CI denotes confidence interval.
[b] Two-sided P values are based on Pearson's χ^2 tests.
[c] A favorable neurologic outcome was defined as a cerebral-performance category of 1 (good recovery) or 2 (moderate disability). One patient in the normothermia group and 1 in the hypothermia group were lost to neurologic follow-up.
From Hypothermia after Cardiac Arrest Study Group. Mild therapeutic hypothermia to improve the neurologic outcome after cardiac arrest. N Engl J Med 2002;346:549; with permission.

vasoconstricting properties. No study has shown that vasopressin use increases hospital discharge rates when used in patients in cardiac arrest. A recent study showed the combination of epinephrine plus vasopressin resulted in higher rates of ROSC, and no increase in long-term survival rates, but a strong trend toward worsening of neurologic outcomes, except in those with an initial rhythm of asystole arrest.[51] However, the quality of CPR was an important uncontrolled variable in that study. Another more recent randomized clinical trial showed no significant benefit with the combination of epinephrine plus vasopressin compared with epinephrine alone.[52] The authors of this article recommend that 1 to 2 doses of epinephrine are used before using vasopressin, given the lack of definitive data and levels of recommendation in

the new guidelines to epinephrine and vasopressin.

There is no good treatment of asystole. Atropine, a vagolytic medication, has no known negative effects in patients with asystole, and can be given for severe bradycardiac and asystole with doses of 1 mg intravenously every minute to a total dose of 3 mg. There is no randomized animal or human study to support the administration of atropine for improvement of outcomes.

Antiarrhythmic Agents

As with the other intravenous medications, there are insufficient levels of data or consensus among the experts regarding the use of antiarrhythmic agents during CPR. Amiodarone is

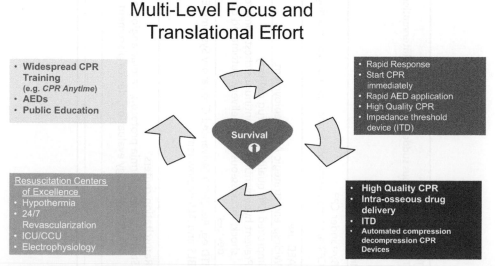

Fig. 13. A systems-based approach to resuscitation.

Table 2
The effect of various sudden cardiac arrest interventions: a combination of all of the interventions could theoretically result in a 24% to 37% increase in survival

Intervention	Effect	Expected Absolute Survival Rate ↑ Compared with Baseline (%)
Bystander CPR CPR anytime in schools, homes, and public meeting places	□ Rapid EMS notification □ Start circulation	2–5[58-61]
AED use Widespread strategic AED deployment	□ Reduce time to first shock in VF patients	4–6[6,62-66]
Improved CPR quality and drug delivery Prevent hyperventilation, continuous chest compressions, CPR pre/post shock, intraosseous drug delivery, automated compression-decompression devices	□ Increase circulation to heart and brain □ Increase oxygen and drug delivery	6–10[17,27,67,68]
ITD eg, ResQPOD (Advanced Circulatory Systems, Eden Prairie, MN, USA) BLS and ALS deployment	□ Increase circulation to heart and brain □ Increase oxygen and drug delivery	5[31,32,44,69]
Resuscitation centers Standard hypothermia protocols, cardiac angiography, intensive care/ electrophysiology evaluation, device placement	□ Revascularization □ Organ preservation □ Prevent sudden cardiac death	5–10[46,47,70-73]
		Total: 22–36

considered the drug of choice and as an intravenous bolus of 150 to 300 mg for VF or pulseless ventricular tachycardiac that are unresponsive to the initial sequences of CPR-shock-CPR-vasoconstrictors. The recommendation is based on limited clinical trials,[53,54] showing improvement in hospital admission but no definitive increase in hospital discharge rates, when compared with placebo or lidocaine. Given the lack of definitive data, lidocaine (initial dose of 1–1.5 mg/kg intravenously) can also be used in patients in cardiac arrest.

REPERFUSION THERAPY

Because of the high incidence of obstructive coronary artery disease (70% of autopsy patients document active thrombus in the coronary tree and from patients undergoing cardiac catheterization another 70% show evidence of severe coronary artery stenosis) in the cardiac arrest population and the inability to make the diagnosis of ST elevation myocardial infarction based on the postresuscitation ECG, elective angiogram and

primary angioplasty should be considered in all survivors without any other clear cause for the cardiac arrest.[55] Long-term prognosis after primary percutaneous coronary intervention (PCI) in survivors of cardiac arrest is good, with 2-year survival rates reported up to 70%.[56] A body of evidence that primary PCI should be considered in survivors of cardiac arrest is currently being evaluated and will be addressed in the next AHA/ECC Guidelines in 2010. In a recent study, reperfusion therapy (PCI or coronary artery bypass graft) had the most profound effect on outcome (adjusted odds ratio = 4.47) when compared with no reperfusion therapy. Patients were transported directly from the emergency department to the PCI suite when clinically stable.[57]

SYSTEMS-BASED APPROACH TO RESUSCITATION

Perhaps one of the biggest advances in CPR is the systems-based approach. The notion that one single intervention can significantly improve outcomes in cardiac arrest has been fading because of the complexity and severity of

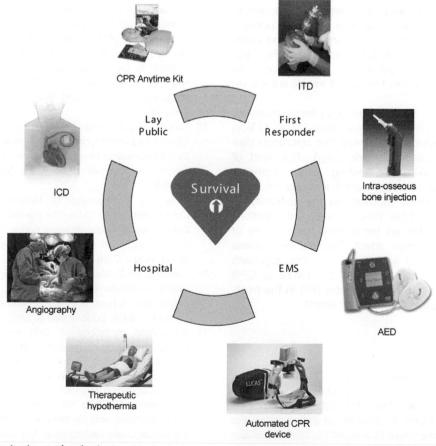

Fig. 14. Resuscitation technologies.

multiorgan dysfunction that develops from the systemic hypoperfusion and hypoxemia. Data from Seattle demonstrating that the introduction of AEDs in all of the first-responder vehicles resulted in a decrease in survival rates for nearly a decade was a warning of the importance of circulation during resuscitation. When CPR was performed for 90 seconds before defibrillation, survival rates were shown to improve with AED implementation. Different efforts to address the issue have shown promise, with significant improvement in mortality and hospital discharge. Application of good-quality CPR, limitation of compression interruptions and ventilations, addition of an inspiratory ITD, and early postresuscitation hypothermia and reperfusion therapies have shown promise when implemented as a system rather than unique interventions.[57]

One program that focuses on this systems-based approach is called Take Heart America. The approach is shown in **Fig. 13**. This technology-based approach implements all of the most highly recommended changes in the 2005 AHA Guidelines. **Table 2** describes the key interventions and their anticipated benefits. This approach includes using new techniques and devices to train lay and professional rescuers in a faster and more reliable way on how to perform CPR, increase circulation during CPR, and focus on skilled postresuscitation care (see **Fig. 14**). Some of these technologies, which have been available only within the past 5 years, are shown in **Fig. 14**.

When these technologies have been deployed, survival rates have increased from 9% to 17% in sites that have implemented this approach (see http://www.takeheartamerica.org/). This kind of approach, akin to treating other complex diseases like cancer or human immunodeficiency virus syndromes, focuses on the criticality of integrating multiple time-sensitive interventions with state-of-the art technology for the care of patients in cardiac arrest. The authors believe that the synergy associated with this approach underlies the foundation for the future of CPR and will result in a fundamental shift in the treatment of all patients in cardiac arrest.

REFERENCES

1. Cobb LA, Fahrenbruch CE, Olsufka M, et al. Changing incidence of out-of-hospital ventricular fibrillation, 1980–2000. JAMA 2002;288:3008–13.
2. Zheng ZJ, Croft JB, Giles WH, et al. Sudden cardiac death in the United States, 1989 to 1998. Circulation 2001;104:2158–63.
3. Weisfeldt ML, Becker LB. Resuscitation after cardiac arrest: a 3-phase time-sensitive model. JAMA 2002; 288:3035–8.
4. Sayre MR, Berg RA, Cave DM, et al. Hands-only (compression-only) cardiopulmonary resuscitation: a call to action for bystander response to adults who experience out-of-hospital sudden cardiac arrest: a science advisory for the public from the American Heart Association Emergency Cardiovascular Care Committee. Circulation 2008;117:2162–7.
5. Valenzuela TD, Roe DJ, Nichol G, et al. Outcomes of rapid defibrillation by security officers after cardiac arrest in casinos. N Engl J Med 2000;343:1206–9.
6. Caffrey SL, Willoughby PJ, Pepe PE, et al. Public use of automated external defibrillators. N Engl J Med 2002;347:1242–7.
7. Marijon E, Combes N, Boveda S. Home automated defibrillators after myocardial infarction. N Engl J Med 2008;359:533–4.
8. Cobb LA, Fahrenbruch CE, Walsh TR, et al. Influence of cardiopulmonary resuscitation prior to defibrillation in patients with out-of-hospital ventricular fibrillation. JAMA 1999;281:1182–8.
9. Bardy GH, Lee KL, Mark DB, et al. Home use of automated external defibrillators for sudden cardiac arrest. N Engl J Med 2008;358:1793–804.
10. Nichol G, Thomas E, Callaway CW, et al. Regional variation in out-of-hospital cardiac arrest incidence and outcome. JAMA 2008;300:1423–31.
11. Wik L, Hansen TB, Fylling F, et al. Delaying defibrillation to give basic cardiopulmonary resuscitation to patients with out-of-hospital ventricular fibrillation: a randomized trial. JAMA 2003;289: 1389–95.
12. Yannopoulos D, Aufderheide TP, Gabrielli A, et al. Clinical and hemodynamic comparison of 15:2 and 30:2 compression-to-ventilation ratios for cardiopulmonary resuscitation. Crit Care Med 2006;34: 1444–9.
13. Lurie KG, Yannopoulos D, McKnite SH, et al. Comparison of a 10-breaths-per-minute versus a 2-breaths-per-minute strategy during cardiopulmonary resuscitation in a porcine model of cardiac arrest. Respir Care 2008;53:862–70.
14. Yannopoulos D, Matsuura T, McKnite S, et al. No assisted ventilation CPR and 24-hour neurological outcomes in a porcine model of cardiac arrest. Crit Care Med 2009. Epub ahead of print.
15. 2005 AHA guidelines of CPR and emergency cardiovascular care. Circulation 2005;112.
16. Idris AH, Becker LB, Fuerst RS, et al. Effect of ventilation on resuscitation in an animal model of cardiac arrest. Circulation 1994;90:3063–9.
17. Aufderheide TP, Lurie KG. Death by hyperventilation: a common and life-threatening problem during cardiopulmonary resuscitation. Crit Care Med 2004; 32:S345–51.

18. Aufderheide TP, Sigurdsson G, Pirrallo RG, et al. Hyperventilation-induced hypotension during cardiopulmonary resuscitation. Circulation 2004; 109:1960–5.

19. Yannopoulos D, McKnite S, Aufderheide TP, et al. Effects of incomplete chest wall decompression during cardiopulmonary resuscitation on coronary and cerebral perfusion pressures in a porcine model of cardiac arrest. Resuscitation 2005;64:363–72.

20. Kouwenhoven WB, Jude JR, Knickerbocker GG. Closed-chest cardiac massage. JAMA 1960;173: 1064–7.

21. Halperin HR, Tsitlik JE, Guerci AD, et al. Determinants of blood flow to vital organs during cardiopulmonary resuscitation in dogs. Circulation 1986;73: 539–50.

22. Kern KB, Sanders AB, Raife J, et al. A study of chest compression rates during cardiopulmonary resuscitation in humans. The importance of rate-directed chest compressions. Arch Intern Med 1992;152: 145 9.

23. Berg RA, Sanders AB, Kern KB, et al. Adverse hemodynamic effects of interrupting chest compressions for rescue breathing during cardiopulmonary resuscitation for ventricular fibrillation cardiac arrest. Circulation 2001;104:2465–70.

24. Abella BS, Sandbo N, Vassilatos P, et al. Chest compression rates during cardiopulmonary resuscitation are suboptimal: a prospective study during in-hospital cardiac arrest. Circulation 2005;111: 428–34.

25. SOS-KANTO study group. Cardiopulmonary resuscitation by bystanders with chest compression only (SOS-KANTO): an observational study. Lancet 2007;369:920–6.

26. Idris AH, Banner MJ, Wenzel V, et al. Ventilation caused by external chest compression is unable to sustain effective gas exchange during CPR: a comparison with mechanical ventilation. Resuscitation 1994;28:143–50.

27. Aufderheide TP, Pirrallo RG, Yannopoulos D, et al. Incomplete chest wall decompression: a clinical evaluation of CPR performance by EMS personnel and assessment of alternative manual chest compression-decompression techniques. Resuscitation 2005;64:353–62.

28. Aufderheide TP, Pirrallo RG, Yannopoulos D, et al. Incomplete chest wall decompression: a clinical evaluation of CPR performance by trained laypersons and an assessment of alternative manual chest compression-decompression techniques. Resuscitation 2006;71:341–51.

29. Aufderheide TP, Alexander C, Lick C, et al. From laboratory science to six emergency medical services systems: New understanding of the physiology of cardiopulmonary resuscitation increases survival rates after cardiac arrest. Crit Care Med 2008;36:S397.

30. Lurie KG, Zielinski T, McKnite S, et al. Use of an inspiratory impedance valve improves neurologically intact survival in a porcine model of ventricular fibrillation. Circulation 2002;105:124–9.

31. Pirrallo RG, Aufderheide TP, Provo TA, et al. Effect of an inspiratory impedance threshold device on hemodynamics during conventional manual cardiopulmonary resuscitation. Resuscitation 2005;66: 13–20.

32. Aufderheide TP, Pirrallo RG, Provo TA, et al. Clinical evaluation of an inspiratory impedance threshold device during standard cardiopulmonary resuscitation in patients with out-of-hospital cardiac arrest. Crit Care Med 2005;33:734–40.

33. Aufderheide TP, Birnbaum M, Lick C, et al. A tale of seven EMS systems: an impedance threshold device and improved CPR techniques double survival rates after out-of-hospital cardiac arrest. Circulation 2007;116(Suppl II):II936–7.

34. Davis S, Thigpen K, Basol R, et al. Implementation of the 2005 American Heart Association Guidelines together with the Impedance Threshold Device improves hospital discharge rates after in-hospital cardiac arrest. Circulation 2008;118:S765.

35. Plaisance P, Soleil C, Lurie KG, et al. Use of an inspiratory impedance threshold device on a facemask and endotracheal tube to reduce intrathoracic pressures during the decompression phase of active compression-decompression cardiopulmonary resuscitation. Crit Care Med 2005;33:990–4.

36. Yannopoulos D, Nadkarni VM, McKnite SH, et al. Intrathoracic pressure regulator during continuous-chest-compression advanced cardiac resuscitation improves vital organ perfusion pressures in a porcine model of cardiac arrest. Circulation 2005;112:803–11.

37. Halperin HR, Paradis N, Ornato JP, et al. Cardiopulmonary resuscitation with a novel chest compression device in a porcine model of cardiac arrest: improved hemodynamics and mechanisms. J Am Coll Cardiol 2004;44:2214–20.

38. Halperin HR, Tsitlik JE, Gelfand M, et al. A preliminary study of cardiopulmonary resuscitation by circumferential compression of the chest with use of a pneumatic vest. N Engl J Med 1993;329:762–8.

39. Hallstrom A, Rea TD, Sayre MR, et al. Manual chest compression vs use of an automated chest compression device during resuscitation following out-of-hospital cardiac arrest: a randomized trial. JAMA 2006;295:2620–8.

40. Ong ME, Ornato JP, Edwards DP, et al. Use of an automated, load-distributing band chest compression device for out-of-hospital cardiac arrest resuscitation. JAMA 2006;295:2629–37.

41. Shultz JJ, Coffeen P, Sweeney M, et al. Evaluation of standard and active compression-decompression CPR in an acute human model of ventricular fibrillation. Circulation 1994;89:684–93.

42. Plaisance P, Lurie KG, Vicaut E, et al. A comparison of standard cardiopulmonary resuscitation and active compression-decompression resuscitation for out-of-hospital cardiac arrest. French Active Compression-Decompression Cardiopulmonary Resuscitation Study Group. N Engl J Med 1999; 341:569–75.

43. Lurie KG, Coffeen P, Shultz J, et al. Improving active compression-decompression cardiopulmonary resuscitation with an inspiratory impedance valve. Circulation 1995;91:1629–32.

44. Wolcke BB, Mauer DK, Schoefmann MF, et al. Comparison of standard cardiopulmonary resuscitation versus the combination of active compression-decompression cardiopulmonary resuscitation and an inspiratory impedance threshold device for out-of-hospital cardiac arrest. Circulation 2003;108: 2201–5.

45. Benson DW, Williams GR Jr, Spencer FC, et al. The use of hypothermia after cardiac arrest. Anesth Analg 1959;38:423–8.

46. Hypothermia after Cardiac Arrest Study Group. Mild therapeutic hypothermia to improve the neurologic outcome after cardiac arrest. N Engl J Med 2002; 346:549–56.

47. Bernard SA, Gray TW, Buist MD, et al. Treatment of comatose survivors of out-of-hospital cardiac arrest with induced hypothermia. N Engl J Med 2002; 346:557–63.

48. Nozari A, Safar P, Stezoski SW, et al. Critical time window for intra-arrest cooling with cold saline flush in a dog model of cardiopulmonary resuscitation. Circulation 2006;113:2690–6.

49. Srinivasan V, Nadkarni VM, Yannopoulos D, et al. Rapid induction of cerebral hypothermia is enhanced with active compression-decompression plus inspiratory impedance threshold device cardiopulmonary resusitation in a porcine model of cardiac arrest. J Am Coll Cardiol 2006;47: 835–41.

50. Michael JR, Guerci AD, Koehler RC, et al. Mechanisms by which epinephrine augments cerebral and myocardial perfusion during cardiopulmonary resuscitation in dogs. Circulation 1984;69:822–35.

51. Wenzel V, Krismer AC, Arntz HR, et al. A comparison of vasopressin and epinephrine for out-of-hospital cardiopulmonary resuscitation. N Engl J Med 2004; 350:105–13.

52. Gueugniaud PY, David JS, Chanzy E, et al. Vasopressin and epinephrine vs. epinephrine alone in cardiopulmonary resuscitation. N Engl J Med 2008; 359:21–30.

53. Dorian P, Cass D, Schwartz B, et al. Amiodarone as compared with lidocaine for shock-resistant ventricular fibrillation. N Engl J Med 2002;346:884–90.

54. Kudenchuk PJ, Cobb LA, Copass MK, et al. Amiodarone for resuscitation after out-of-hospital cardiac arrest due to ventricular fibrillation. N Engl J Med 1999;341:871–8.

55. Spaulding CM, Joly LM, Rosenberg A, et al. Immediate coronary angiography in survivors of out-of-hospital cardiac arrest. N Engl J Med 1997;336: 1629–33.

56. Bendz B, Eritsland J, Nakstad AR, et al. Long-term prognosis after out-of-hospital cardiac arrest and primary percutaneous coronary intervention. Resuscitation 2004;63:49–53.

57. Sunde K, Pytte M, Jacobsen D, et al. Implementation of a standardised treatment protocol for post resuscitation care after out-of-hospital cardiac arrest. Resuscitation 2007;73:29–39.

58. Holmberg M, Holmberg S, Herlitz J. Factors modifying the effect of bystander cardiopulmonary resuscitation on survival in out-of-hospital cardiac arrest patients in Sweden. Eur Heart J 2001;22: 511–9.

59. Holmberg M, Holmberg S, Herlitz J, et al. Survival after cardiac arrest outside hospital in Sweden. Swedish Cardiac Arrest Registry. Resuscitation 1998;36:29–36.

60. Larsen MP, Eisenberg MS, Cummins RO, et al. Predicting survival from out-of-hospital cardiac arrest: a graphic model. Ann Emerg Med 1993; 22:1652–8.

61. Valenzuela TD, Roe DJ, Cretin S, et al. Estimating effectiveness of cardiac arrest interventions: a logistic regression survival model. Circulation 1997;96:3308–13.

62. Auble TE, Menegazzi JJ, Paris PM. Effect of out-of-hospital defibrillation by basic life support providers on cardiac arrest mortality: a metaanalysis. Ann Emerg Med 1995;25:642–8.

63. Stiell IG, Wells GA, DeMaio VJ, et al. Modifiable factors associated with improved cardiac arrest survival in a multicenter basic life support/defibrillation system: OPALS Study Phase I results. Ontario Prehospital Advanced Life Support. Ann Emerg Med 1999;33:44–50.

64. Stiell IG, Wells GA, Field BJ, et al. Improved out-of-hospital cardiac arrest survival through the inexpensive optimization of an existing defibrillation program: OPALS study phase II. Ontario Prehospital Advanced Life Support. JAMA 1999;281:1175–81.

65. Weaver WD, Hill D, Fahrenbruch CE, et al. Use of the automatic external defibrillator in the management of out-of-hospital cardiac arrest. N Engl J Med 1988; 319:661–6.

66. White RD, Bunch TJ, Hankins DG. Evolution of a community-wide early defibrillation programme

experience more than 13 years using police/fire personnel and paramedics as responders. Resuscitation 2005;65:279–83.

67. Abella BS, Alvarado JP, Myklebust H, et al. Quality of cardiopulmonary resuscitation during in-hospital cardiac arrest. JAMA 2005;293:305–10.

68. Wik L, Kramer-Johansen J, Myklebust H, et al. Quality of cardiopulmonary resuscitation during out-of-hospital cardiac arrest. JAMA 2005;293:299–304.

69. Plaisance P, Lurie KG, Vicaut E, et al. Evaluation of an impedance threshold device in patients receiving active compression-decompression cardiopulmonary resuscitation for out of hospital cardiac arrest. Resuscitation 2004;61:265–71.

70. Bernard S, Buist M, Monteiro O, et al. Induced hypothermia using large volume, ice-cold intravenous fluid in comatose survivors of out-of-hospital cardiac arrest: a preliminary report. Resuscitation 2003;56:9–13.

71. Lurie KG, Idris A, Holcomb JB. Level 1 cardiac arrest centers: learning from the trauma surgeons. Acad Emerg Med 2005;12:79–80.

72. Merchant RM, Abella BS, Khan M, et al. Cardiac catheterization is underutilized after in-hospital cardiac arrest. Resuscitation 2008;79:398–403.

73. Yannopoulos D, Aufderheide T. Acute management of sudden cardiac death in adults based upon the new CPR guidelines. Europace 2007;9:2–9.

Public Access Defibrillation

Robert W. Rho, MD[a,b,*], Richard L. Page, MD[a,c]

KEYWORDS
- Ventricular fibrillation • Defibrillation • Cardiac arrest
- Resuscitation • Automated external defibrillator

In the United States, 50 to 60 people suffer a cardiac arrest each hour, amounting to approximately 250,000 deaths every year. In the first 5 minutes of a cardiac arrest, ventricular tachycardia and ventricular fibrillation (VF) are the most frequent cardiac arrhythmias encountered. Despite emergency medical response systems, the long-term survival from out-of-hospital cardiac arrest remains poor in most United States cities. Paramount to achieving successful resuscitation of a cardiac arrest victim is providing early defibrillation. The likelihood of survival decreases by 7% to 10% for every 1-minute delay in defibrillation. If defibrillation is delayed more than 10 minutes, the likelihood of survival is very poor. Modern living with vertical high-rise buildings, heavy traffic, and sprawling suburbs pose significant obstacles to emergency medical services (EMS) within cities. In 1995, in response to the abysmal survival of out-of-hospital cardiac arrest, the American Heart Association challenged the medical industry to develop a defibrillator that could be placed in public settings, used safely by lay responders, and provide earlier defibrillation to cardiac-arrest victims. Over the last decade, there have been significant technological advancements in automated external defibrillators (AEDs) and clinical studies have demonstrated their benefits and limitations in public locations. This article discusses the modern AED and the data to support public access defibrillation (PAD).

THE MODERN AUTOMATED EXTERNAL DEFIBRILLATOR

The AED is designed to accurately analyze electrocardiograms obtained via defibrillation pads placed by lay responders on an arrest victim's chest. The device was first clinically introduced in 1979 by Diack and colleagues.[1] This "automatic cardiac resuscitator" was field tested in 21 cardiac-arrest victims in VF and resulted in 35 successful defibrillations to sinus rhythm.

Since this original "proof of concept" report, significant important advancements in AEDs have occurred. Today, the AED is a lightweight, small, portable device designed to be safe, reliable, and easy to use. The device is equipped with a highly accurate algorithm that accurately detects ventricular tachycardia and VF and is able to distinguish it from supraventricular arrhythmias and artifact with nearly 100% sensitivity and specificity. The device provides visual instructions and voice prompts to the lay responder as to whether a shock is advised. When a shock is advised, the responder pushes a button on the unit to deliver the shock. Many modern devices are programmed to comply with the most recent International Liaison Committee on Resuscitation–American College of Cardiology–American Heart Association (ILCOR/ACC/AHA) guidelines for cardiac resuscitation and can coach the responder through cardiopulmonary resuscitation (CPR), sensing and adapting to the responder's actions.[2] Modern devices also have

a Department of Medicine, University of Washington, Seattle, WA, 98195-6422, USA
b Division of Cardiology, University of Washington Medical Center, 1959 NE Pacific Street, HSB, Room AA121C, Box 356422, Seattle, WA 98195-6422, USA
c Division of Cardiology, University of Washington Medical Center, 1959 NE Pacific Street, HSB, Room AA510A, Box 356422, Seattle, WA 98195-6422, USA
* Corresponding author. Division of Cardiology, University of Washington Med Center, 1959 NE Pacific Street, Room AA121C, Box 356422, Seattle, WA 98195-6422.
E-mail address: rrho@u.washington.edu (R.W. Rho).

Card Electrophysiol Clin 1 (2009) 33–40
doi:10.1016/j.ccep.2009.08.005
1877-9182/09/$ – see front matter © 2009 Published by Elsevier Inc.

automatic self-tests ensuring that the battery and all other components of the AED are operational when it is needed.

THE USE OF AUTOMATED EXTERNAL DEFIBRILLATORS BY LAY RESPONDERS

To achieve shorter call-to-defibrillation times, many communities have equipped nontraditional first responders (eg, police officers, firefighters) with AEDs. These nontraditional first responders are able to arrive at the scene of a cardiac-arrest victim before paramedics and, therefore, provide earlier defibrillation. Additionally, these nontraditional first responders may be the first to arrive at other situations where a cardiac arrest may have occurred, such as at the scene of an accident, and can administer early defibrillation. Investigators have reported significant improvements in survival when earlier defibrillation was achieved by nontraditional emergency-response personnel equipped with an AED. Weaver and colleagues[3] demonstrated that among 276 cardiac-arrest victims treated initially by firefighters, 84 (30%) survived to hospital discharge. This is compared to the survival of 44 of 228 (19%) victims when firefighters performed CPR only and defibrillation was performed only after arrival of paramedics (odds ratio, 1.8; 95% CI, 1.1–2.9). The average call-to-defibrillation time was 3.6 minutes with firefighters compared to 5.1 minutes with paramedics. This study and others[4,5] demonstrated that non–emergency medical team rescuers were able to safely and effectively provide earlier defibrillation with an AED and improve survival significantly.

Further insights on the use of AEDs by lay responders have been gained from experience of AED use in aircrafts and casinos, locations where traffic is heavy and stressful situations are common. The recognition and resuscitation of patients aboard an aircraft pose significant challenges. Until recently, victims of cardiac arrest aboard aircraft suffered from significant delays in defibrillation and therefore rarely survived. Quantas Airlines had a limited program that provided AEDs on some international flights. Results were promising.[6] American Airlines was the first carrier to equip all aircraft with AEDs and train all flight attendants in their use. Over a 2-year period, the AED was used in 200 instances, 191 events in aircraft and 9 events in the airport terminal. Electrocardiographic data was available in 185 patients. The AED advised a shock in 14 of 14 patients who had VF diagnosed as their initial arrhythmia. No shock was advised in the remaining patients. The sensitivity and specificity of identifying VF was 100%. The first shock successfully

defibrillated 13 of 14 patients and defibrillation was withheld in 1 patient at the request of the family. The rate of survival to hospital discharge after defibrillation was 40%.[7]

These studies demonstrate the feasibility, efficacy, and safety of the AED and its use by lay persons on aircraft and in airport terminals (**Fig. 1**). Subsequently, in April 2001, the US Federal Aviation Administration made AEDs

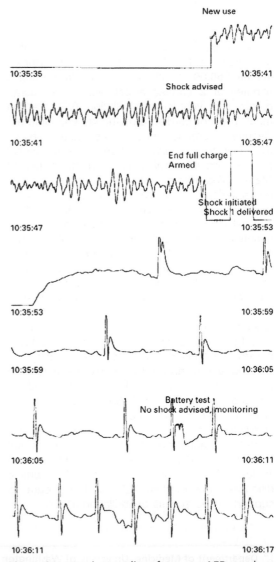

Fig. 1. An actual recording from an AED used on a passenger found to be in VF. A shock is advised, delivered, and followed by a pause, then sinus rhythm with 2:1 conduction, and eventual sinus rhythm with 1:1 conduction. The patient survived to hospital discharge. (*From* Page RL, Joglar JA, Kowal RC, et al. Use of automated external defibrillators by a U.S. airline. N Engl J Med 2000;343:1212; with permission.)

mandatory on all United States domestic and international flights.

Another important study assessed the feasibility, safety, and efficacy of AEDs used by trained security officers in casinos. AEDs were placed in locations where a rescuer could retrieve the AED and apply it to a victim within 3 minutes of an arrest. Because all casinos are equipped with surveillance cameras, investigators were able to report accurate times from collapse to defibrillation. One hundred and forty-eight patients had a cardiac arrest. VF was the initial rhythm in 105 patients and shock was advised in all cases. Four patients (4%) were pronounced dead at the scene, 35 patients (33%) died in the emergency department, and 56 patients (53%) survived to hospital discharge. The mean time from collapse to attachment of the AED was 3.5 ± 2.9 minutes; the mean time from collapse to first defibrillation shock was 4.4 ± 2.9 minutes; and the mean time from collapse to arrival of paramedics was 9.8 ± 4.3 minutes. Among patients with witnessed cardiac arrest and defibrillation no later than 3 minutes after collapse, the survival rate to hospital discharge was 74%.[8]

These studies illustrate the feasibility, safety, and efficacy of the use of the AED in specific environments characterized by heavy traffic of people under stressful situations and the presence of trained lay-rescuers.

The effectiveness of AEDs placed in more general public locations as part of an integrated PAD system has also been studied. Capucci and colleagues[9] reported the experience of the Piacenza Progetto Vita (PPV), a PAD system in which 12 AEDs were placed in high-risk locations, 12 were placed in lay-staffed ambulances, and 15 were placed in police cars serving the Piacenza region of Italy. In this study, 1287 lay volunteers were trained in the use of AEDs and responded to all cases of suspected cardiac arrest. The time from emergency call to arrival on the scene was 4.8 ± 1.2 minutes for the PPV responders versus 6.2 ± 2.3 minutes for EMS ($P = .05$). Survival to hospital discharge was 10.5% for the PPV group versus 3.3% for the EMS-treated group ($P = .006$). A "shockable" rhythm (ventricular tachycardia or VF) was present in 23.8% of the PPV group versus 15.6% for the EMS group ($P = .05$), probably because the PPV responder was able to arrive sooner than the EMS. This study demonstrated that a PAD system manned by lay-responders could triple overall survival above and beyond a well-developed EMS system by providing defibrillation approximately 1.5 minutes earlier than the EMS system.

In Austria, a national PAD program was initiated in 2002. During the study period, 1865 devices were deployed and, over a 2-year period, the use of an AED was documented in 73 cases. Eleven cases were excluded from the analysis because the devices were activated by EMS dispatchers and considered part of the local EMS system. Survival to hospital discharge was 17 of 62 (27%) among patients who required use of the AED. Evaluation of a historical control prior to the PAD system demonstrated a survival to hospital discharge rate of 4.3%.[10] In the United Kingdom, the government decided in 1999 that PAD should become a part of a core service provision under the National Health Service. Results of the initial phase of the implementation, which placed AEDs in fixed sites at airports and railway stations, have been reported. Out of 172 patients in whom the AED was used, a shockable rhythm was detected in 135 (78%). Thirty-eight of 172 (28%) persons who suffered a cardiac arrest in these locations survived to hospital discharge.[11]

The first randomized study of AEDs was the PAD (Public Access Defibrillation) trial, a National Institutes of Health–sponsored, prospective, multicenter trial of AEDs placed in prespecified public places. Community units were assigned to a structured emergency-response system involving lay volunteers trained in CPR, with half the community units being provided with AEDs. The primary outcome was survival to hospital discharge. This study included 19,000 volunteer responders in 993 community units in 24 North American regions. A total of 30 of 128 arrests (23%) survived to hospital discharge in the CPR + AED arm of the study compared to 15 of 107 (14%) in the CPR-only arm ($P = .03$; relative risk, 2.0; 95% CI, 1.07–3.77). Although large, multiunit, residential complexes represented 16% of the study locations, 28% of all cardiac arrests occurred at these locations. This finding is important because survival from cardiac arrest in residential locations was very poor in this study (0.6%).[12]

An important observation relevant to the overall impact of AEDs in public places is that over 75% of out-of-hospital cardiac arrests occur in the home.[13,14] Given the high frequency of arrest in the home, and the poor survival in residential units in the PAD trial, the Home AED Trial (HAT) was undertaken. HAT enrolled 7001 patients who had suffered an anterior myocardial infarction but were not candidates for an implantable cardiac defibrillator. In each case, someone in the home was instructed in CPR and activation of EMS, but half were randomized to receive a home AED. During a median follow-up of 37.3 months, 450 patients died (6.5% in the control group and 6.4% in the AED group; $P = .77$). The average mortality in this study was 2.1% in the control group and 2.0% in the AED group, which were lower than the historical data employed to calculate the power of the study. This reduced overall mortality is attributed to better medical management and high rate of revascularization following the index myocardial infarction. Among patients with death from tachyarrhythmias, less than one half of arrests that occurred at home were witnessed (58 of 160). Among all patients who died, only 41% died at home in this study. The AED was used in 32 patients in the study. A shock was advised for 13 patients and delivered in 12 patients. Five patients survived to hospital discharge but 1 died several days later. Overall, 4 of 14 (28.6%) patients who had VF and were shocked by the AED survived long term. Interestingly, the AED was used in 7 neighbors who had suffered a cardiac arrest but were not enrolled in the study. A shock was advised in 4 of 7 patients and 2 of 4 survived to hospital discharge. There were no documented inappropriate shocks in this study. Although the HAT study demonstrated no significant difference in mortality with home AEDs, it is important to re-emphasize that the study population had an event rate that was considerably lower than expected. Whether the home AED would be more effective in a higher-risk population remains unknown. The HAT study also demonstrated (1) that cardiac arrests occur less often in the home (41%) than what has been reported previously, (2) that the usefulness of home AEDs is limited because many arrests in the home are not witnessed despite the best-case scenario of a spouse educated in sudden death and the use of an AED, and (3) that, when the AED was used, it was accurate and effective and resulted in a long-term survival of 33%. Furthermore, neighbors of homes with AEDs also benefited with 2 of 4 patients in whom a shock was advised surviving to hospital discharge.[15]

Based on the HAT data, patients who wish to have an AED at home should not be discouraged, but general policy decisions or third-party coverage about home AEDs cannot be supported by the available data on home AEDs. On the other hand, in households that include a higher-risk patient (eg, patients with myocardial infarction with severely depressed ejection fraction refusing a defibrillator, patients with long-QT syndrome, patients with arrhythmogenic right ventricular cardiomyopathy, and patients with hypertrophic cardiomyopathy) along with a motivated and educated companion, a home AED may be reasonable. In addition, homeowners who frequently entertain large numbers of older guests may consider providing the added security of an AED.

PUBLIC ACCESS DEFIBRILLATION PROGRAMS: WHERE DO WE BEGIN?

Several variables influence the potential impact that an AED will have in a given location. These include (1) the likelihood that a cardiac arrest would be witnessed and a potential rescuer would be present in that location, (2) the EMS response time to that location, and (3) the demographics and number of patients in that location. Simply having an AED present does not save lives if a cardiac arrest is not likely to be witnessed, even if that locale has very heavy traffic (such as public restrooms or residential complexes). At a population level, to make any significant impact on the total number of cardiac arrests due to ventricular arrhythmias, it would seem reasonable to conclude that an AED should be disseminated widely throughout the community. However, the issues discussed above, along with cost constraints, suggest that initial efforts in any community should focus first on locations where AEDs are most likely to be used. The American Heart Association suggests that such a place should be defined as a location where at least one cardiac arrest is likely to occur every 2 years. In a study by Becker and colleagues[12] conducted in King County, Washington, from 1990 to 1994, public sites where cardiac arrests may occur were divided into 23 location categories. Ten sites were found to have a "high" incidence of cardiac arrests, although only the international airport, county jail, and a large shopping mall reached the American Heart Association threshold. The placement of 276 AEDs in the 172 high-incidence sites was estimated to provide treatment for 134 cardiac-arrest patients in a 5-year period. Because 80 of 134 (60%) of patients were found to be in VF, assuming a survival rate of between 10% and 40%, the investigators estimated that between 8 and 32 lives might have been saved over a period of 5 years. However, to cover the remaining 347 arrests that occurred in public, AEDs would have to have been placed in more than 70,000 sites. In the PAD study, AEDs were placed only in locations thought to be generally suitable for AEDs. Among these prespecified sites, cardiac arrest occurred most frequently in fitness centers (5.1 per 1000 persons) and golf courses (4.8 per 1000 persons) and least frequently in office complexes (0.7 per 1000 persons) and hotels (0.7 per 1000 persons). Survival in PAD sites from treatable cardiac arrest was highest in recreational complexes, public transportation sites, and fitness centers. Survival was poor in residential facilities, reflecting the low likelihood that a bystander rescuer will be available at these sites.[12]

Based on the data available, communities establishing a PAD program should focus initial efforts on placing AEDs at locations where cardiac arrests are most likely to occur, especially where emergency medical team response times of less than 5 minutes cannot be reliably achieved. This may include large transportation terminals, exercise facilities, sports complexes, golf courses, and shopping centers. Ideally, the work of planning and maintaining the PAD program and the job of training individuals in the program should be supervised and coordinated by the local EMS and supervised by a physician. The PAD program should be integrated and coordinated through the local EMS system and each AED should be registered and "on-line" so that the local EMS system is aware of any instance that the AED is in use as well as its precise location. The precise location within each venue for each AED should be carefully selected to allow for the most efficient use of the AED for that location (ie, reached within 3 minutes) and the location of the AED should be clearly marked.

The cost for such a system does not need to be assumed entirely by local government but can be shared by local businesses who may benefit from the worthy charitable donation and "good will" advertisement that the AED may provide. As an example of some innovations in widespread dissemination of AEDs, Japan has placed AEDs in vending machines situated in locations where people congregate. The AED is installed behind an unlocked, transparent door and clearly marked. The cost of the AED is shared by the manufacturer of the drinks, the provider of the vending machine, the distributor of the AED, and the proprietor of the vending machine. Another innovative way to help pay for AEDs is through paid advertising above boxes in which AEDs are stored.[16]

An area of significant attention has been the placement of AEDs at elementary and high schools. Despite parental expectation that teachers and staff be trained in CPR, most surveys of elementary and high schools demonstrate that up to one third of teachers have no training in CPR.[17] In a cross-sectional survey of high schools in Washington state, the principal at each high school in the Washington Interscholastic Activities Association (n = 407) was asked to complete a Web-based questionnaire. One hundred and eighteen (29%) completed the survey. Sixty-four (54%) schools reported having at least one AED on school grounds (mean 1.6, range 1–4 AEDs). As for funding for the AEDs, 60% came from donations, 27% came from the school district, and 11% came from individual schools or athletic departments. AED training was completed by 78% of coaches, 72% of administrators, 70% of school nurses, and 48% of teachers. Only 25% of schools coordinated the implementation of AEDs with an outside medical agency and only 6% of schools coordinated the AED with the local EMS system. One school used the AED on a basketball official, who survived after a single shock. This study illustrates that significant improvements need to made to the structuring and coordination of emergency response plans in public high schools.[18] The placement of AEDs at National Collegiate Athletic Association Division I universities may also benefit spectators, coaches, and referees in that up to 77% of sudden cardiac arrests in college sporting venues occur in older non-students.[19]

Data on the efficacy of AEDs on young athletes are limited but raise some concern regarding the low survival rate. In a study by Drezner and Rogers,[20] the timing and detail of nine athletes who had a sudden cardiac arrest was analyzed. All nine athletes had a witnessed cardiac arrest and seven athletes received immediate defibrillation with an average time to defibrillation of 3.1 minutes. Despite early defibrillation, only one of the nine athletes survived. The lower-than-expected survival rates may be due to structural heart disease (hypertrophic cardiomyopathy and arrhythmogenic right ventricular cardiomyopathy), which is common among young athletes who present with a sudden cardiac arrest. These findings should not discourage the implementation of PAD programs in school athletic venues but should stimulate increased work in improving on existing emergency action plans at athletic events.

Teachers, physical education instructors, and administrators should all be trained and certified in basic life support. Emergency response systems for cardiac-arrest scenarios on campus should be carefully planned, and those plans should be carefully reviewed and integrated with the local EMS system. Goals of these response plans should strive for a collapse-to-EMS-call time of less than 1 minute and a collapse-to-first-shock time of less than 3 minutes. Because the sudden death of a child is an especially tragic event for a family and community, the carefully planned distribution of AEDs on school campuses and athletic venues may be justified even though cardiac arrests are rare. Many states have legislation supporting the placement of AEDs in schools and at school sporting events.[21]

PUBLIC AWARENESS AND EDUCATION

A critical factor in the success of a PAD program is public awareness and widespread training in basic life support and in the basic operation of an AED. Strong evidence shows that lay responders are capable of safely and effectively administering treatment with an AED. Even naïve sixth graders have been demonstrated to perform well in mock simulations of the use of the AED and, in some cases, performed better than trained professionals.[22] The importance of broad public awareness and training cannot be overemphasized because of the high likelihood that a non–medically trained bystander will be responsible for the initial treatment of cardiac-arrest victims.

AUTOMATED EXTERNAL DEFIBRILLATORS AND CIVIL LIABILITY

A potential barrier to the effectiveness of a PAD program is the fear of lawsuits that may arise because of complications during the resuscitation attempt. To protect layperson responders involved in the resuscitation attempts of a cardiac-arrest victim, state and federal legislators have been actively involved in providing "good Samaritan" liability protection to organizations and individuals. The Aviation Medical Assistance Act (Public Law 105–170) was signed by President Clinton on April 24, 1998, and provided liability protection to airlines and individuals attempting to obtain or provide medical assistance on airplanes. On November 13, 2000, President Clinton signed the Cardiac Arrest Survival Act, now Public Law 106–505, which requires the placement of AEDs in federal buildings and provides civil immunity to users of the AED. The Cardiac Arrest Survival Act has played a pivotal role in setting the standards for immunity protection for rescuers using AEDs and for those who acquire an AED. As of 2001, all 50 states passed laws providing limited immunity protection for lay rescuers using AEDs to resuscitate a cardiac-arrest victim. A complete list of state legislation and regulations regarding AED and PAD programs can be obtained on the Internet.[21,23]

ADVANCED DIRECTIVES

With the implementation of an aggressive resuscitation system within communities, it is important for patients with chronic or terminal illnesses and for our extremely elderly patients to carefully consider advanced directives. Physicians should remind such patients to carefully consider whether they wish to be resuscitated in the event of a cardiac arrest. Aggressive resuscitation of a patient who has little chance at long-term survival may lead to unnecessary morbidity, unnecessary physical and psychological distress to the patient and family, and unnecessary health-care expenditures. Patients who do not wish to be resuscitated should have this clearly marked on a necklace or bracelet.

COST-EFFECTIVENESS

PAD programs will be more cost-effective in regions where the likelihood is high that an AED will be used and where survival from the standard EMS system is very poor (<5%). Cram and colleagues[24] estimated that in locations where an AED would be used at a rate of once every 5 years as recommended by the American Heart Association, each AED in a public place would cost $30,000 per each quality-adjusted life-year (QALY) gained compared to EMS response alone. The AED would be much more cost-effective in some locations, such as international airports, public sports venues, golf courses, jails, health clubs, and large shopping malls. The AED would be less cost-effective in community centers, primary care centers, and hotels, where the cost is estimated to be more than $200,000 per QALY gained. However, the analysis of the cost-effectiveness of AEDs in PAD programs has significant limitations. The cost of these programs will vary from community to community. Every location has unique characteristics influencing the cost-effectiveness of an AED at that location, such as frequency of events (number of times the AED is likely to be used related to the demographics and number of people frequenting this location), likelihood of an available rescuer at the location, local EMS response times to that location, and the impact the AED would have on survival at that location. Even the likelihood of vandalism requiring replacement of the AED at the location should be taken into consideration. Determining which entities (private or public) may contribute to the cost of implementing such a program further complicates assessment of the cost of a PAD program.

KEEPING PACE WITH THE SCIENCE OF RESUSCITATION

In November 2005, the International Liaison Committee on Cardiac Resuscitation and the American Heart Association (ILCOR/AHA) published new guidelines for CPR and emergency cardiac care. These updated guidelines were based on the evaluation of 22,000 peer-reviewed publications conducted by 281 physicians and scientists from the international resuscitation community.[2]

After an updated review of the literature and science of resuscitation, the guidelines committee recommended the following:

An emphasis on good quality CPR and minimizing interruptions

In the case of a witnessed cardiac arrest, a one-shock protocol followed by five cycles of CPR (one cycle equals 30 compressions to two breaths) before checking for a pulse

In the case of an unwitnessed cardiac arrest, five cycles of CPR preceding defibrillation

Since publication of these guidelines in 2005, all AEDs manufactured currently are in compliance. Changes to the programming of AEDs have included a one-shock protocol and the addition of voice prompts to continue CPR immediately after the first shock.

SUMMARY

The AED is a safe and effective tool that can significantly improve survival of cardiac-arrest victims. However, the effectiveness of this device depends on it being available at the site of arrest. Based on solid clinical evidence of the safety, accuracy, and effectiveness of AED use by lay responders, many communities are adopting PAD programs. These efforts have been supported in the United States with legislation at the state and federal level mandating the placement of AEDs in selected locations, providing funding for the development of local PAD programs, and providing liability protection to organizations and individuals who become involved in the execution of PAD. Further research into the relative effectiveness of AEDs in specific locations, financial support from private sources, improvements in public awareness and education on the use of AEDs will guide the development of community PAD programs and save lives that may otherwise be lost prematurely.

REFERENCES

1. Diack AW, Welborn WS, Rullman RG, et al. An automatic cardiac resuscitator for emergency treatment of cardiac arrest. Med Instrum 1979;13:78–83.
2. 2005 American Heart Association guidelines for cardiopulmonary resuscitation and emergency cardiovascular care. Circulation 2005;112(24 Suppl):IV1–IV203.
3. Weaver WD, Hill D, Fahrenbuch CE, et al. Use of automated external defibrillators in the management of out-of-hospital cardiac arrest. N Engl J Med 1988;319:661–6.
4. White RD, Vukov LF, Bugliosi TF. Early defibrillation by police: initial experience with measurement of critical time intervals and patient outcome. Ann Emerg Med 1994;23:1009–13.
5. Mossesso VN Jr, Davis EA, Auble TE, et al. Use of automated external defibrillators by police officers for treatment of out-of-hospital cardiac arrest. Ann Emerg Med 1998;32:200–7.
6. O'Rourke MF, Donaldson E, Geddes JS. An airline cardiac arrest program. Circulation 1997;96:2849–53.
7. Page RL, Joglar JA, Kowal RC, et al. Use of automated external defibrillators by a U.S. airline. N Engl J Med 2000;343:1210–6.
8. Valenzuela TD, Roe DJ, Nichol G, et al. Outcomes of rapid defibrillation by security officers after cardiac arrest in casinos. N Engl J Med 2000;343:1206–9.
9. Capucci A, Aschieri D, Piepoli MF, et al. Tripling survival from sudden cardiac arrest via early defibrillation without traditional education in cardiopulmonary resuscitation. Circulation 2002;106:1065–70.
10. Fleischhackl R, Roessler B, Domanovits H, et al. Results from Austria's nationwide public access defibrillation (ANPAD) programme collected over 2 years. Resuscitation 2008;77:195–200.
11. Davies CS, Colquhoun MC, Boyle R, et al. A national programme for on-site defibrillation by lay persons in selected high risk areas: initial results. Heart 2005;91:1299–302.
12. Hallstrom A, Ornato JP, Weisfeldt M, et al. Public-access defibrillation and survival after out-of-hospital cardiac arrest. N Engl J Med 2004;351:637–46.
13. Becker LB, Eisenberg M, Fahrenbruch C, et al. Public locations of cardiac arrest: implications for public access defibrillation. Circulation 1998;97:2106–9.
14. Pell JP, Sirel JM, Marsden AK, et al. Potential impact of public access defibrillators on survival after out of hospital cardiopulmonary arrest: retrospective cohort study. Br Med J 2002;325:515.
15. Bardy GH, Lee KL, Mark DB, et al. Home use of automated external defibrillators for sudden cardiac arrest. N Engl J Med 2008;358:1793–804.
16. Mitamura H. Public access defibrillation: advances from Japan. Nat Clin Pract Cardiovasc Med 2008;5(11):690–2.
17. Gagliardi M, Neighbors M, Spears C, et al. Emergencies in the school setting: Are public school teachers adequately trained to respond? Prehosp Disaster Med 1994;9:222–5.
18. Rothmier JD, Drezner JA, Harmon KG. Automated external defibrillators in Washington State high schools. Br J Sports Med 2007;41:301–5.
19. Drezner JA, Rogers KJ, Zimmer RR, et al. Use of automated external defibrillators at NCAA Division I universities. Med Sci Sports Exerc 2005;37:1487–92 State Legislation.
20. Drezner JA, Rogers KJ. Sudden cardiac arrest in intercollegiate atheletes: detailed analysis and outcomes of resuscitation in nine cases. Heart Rhythm 2006;3:755–9.

21. National Conferences of State Legislatures Web site. Health care program state laws on heart attacks: cardiac arrest and defibrillators. Available at: http://www.ncsl.org/programs/health/aed.htm. Accessed March 31, 2009.

22. Gundry JW, Comess KA, DeRook FA, et al. Comparison of naïve sixth grade children with trained professionals in the use of an automated external defibrillator. Circulation 1999;100:1703–7.

23. Department of Health and Human Services Program Support Center Web site. Guidelines for public access defibrillation programs in federal facilities. Available at: http://www.foh.dhhs.gov/public/whatwedo/AED/HHSAED.asp. Accessed May 31, 2009.

24. Cram P, Vijan S, Fendrick AM. Cost effectiveness of automated external defibrillator deployment in selected public locations. J Gen Intern Med 2003; 18:745–54.

Optimizing Community Resources to Address Sudden Cardiac Death

Younghoon Kwon, MD[a], Tom P. Aufderheide, MD, FACEP, FAHA[b],*

KEYWORDS

- Sudden cardiac death • Cardiac arrest
- Community resources
- Cardiopulmonary resuscitation (CPR)
- Bystander CPR • Public access defibrillation

Sudden cardiac arrest occurring outside the hospital is one of the leading causes of death in the developed world and claims 350,000 to 450,000 lives per year in the United States.[1] Despite recent advancements in resuscitative care and continuing efforts to improve public awareness of sudden cardiac arrest in the community, overall survival still remains low.[2]

The well-established "chain of survival" (early access, early cardiopulmonary resuscitation [CPR], early defibrillation, and early advanced care) incorporates scientifically proven interventions necessary for successful resuscitation and survival for patients with cardiac arrest (**Fig. 1**).[3,4] It is becoming increasingly evident, however, that low survival rates from cardiac arrest are not due to lack of understanding of effective interventions, but instead are due to weak links in the chain of survival and the inability of communities to ensure these links function in an efficient, timely, and coordinated fashion.

This article identifies for each link in the chain of survival aspects that define the link's quality, explains how communities can strengthen each link, and describes how communities can optimize local leadership and community stakeholder collaboration to forge a strong relationship between each link so that the sequence of interventions provided to patients with cardiac arrest are consistently efficient, timely, and well coordinated.

EARLY ACCESS—BYSTANDER CARDIOPULMONARY RESUSCITATION

Studies have demonstrated convincingly that the odds of surviving out-of-hospital cardiac arrest (OHCA) increase two to four times when bystander CPR occurs before the arrival of emergency medical services (EMS).[5–7] Both the quality of bystander CPR and the interval from collapse to initiation of CPR have been associated with survival and good quality of life in survivors.[8,9] Therefore, the frequency of early initiation of bystander CPR significantly influences a community's overall performance in achieving successful outcome from cardiac arrest.

Despite these proven and marked benefits, rates of bystander CPR in communities are low.[10] The bystander CPR rate in most communities is less than 20%—in some it is only a few percent—and the variation between communities is large. Proposed theories to explain the low rate of bystander CPR include unpreparedness and lack of knowledge of the bystander to implement appropriate actions,[11,12] fear during the emergency, fear of causing harm, unfounded fear of legal consequences,[13] and unfounded fear of contracting a communicable disease by providing mouth-to-mouth breathing.[14–16] Although actual barriers may be a combination of these factors, all of them derive from the lack of public awareness of sudden cardiac arrest and lack of training

[a] Healthcare East System, Division of Cardiology, Department of Medicine, University of Minnesota, 45 West 10th Street, St Joseph Hospital, St Paul, MN 55102, USA
[b] Department of Emergency Medicine, Medical College of Wisconsin, 9200 W. Wisconsin Avenue, FH/Pavilion 1P, Milwaukee, WI 53226, USA
* Corresponding author.
E-mail address: taufderh@mcw.edu (T.P. Aufderheide).

Card Electrophysiol Clin 1 (2009) 41–50
doi:10.1016/j.ccep.2009.08.014
1877-9182/09/$ – see front matter © 2009 Published by Elsevier Inc.

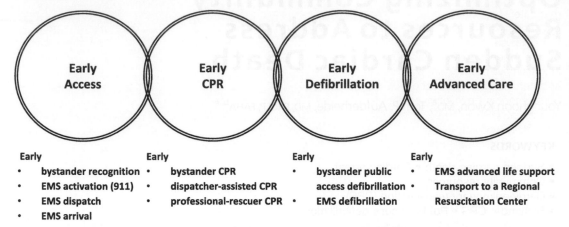

Early
- bystander recognition
- EMS activation (911)
- EMS dispatch
- EMS arrival

Early
- bystander CPR
- dispatcher-assisted CPR
- professional-rescuer CPR

Early
- bystander public access defibrillation
- EMS defibrillation

Early
- EMS advanced life support
- Transport to a Regional Resuscitation Center

Fig. 1. The chain of survival. The chain of survival defines the proven interventions necessary for successful resuscitation and survival for patients with cardiac arrest. (*Adapted from* Cummins RO, Ornato JP, Thies WH, et al. Improving survival from sudden cardiac arrest: the "chain of survival" concept. A statement for health professionals from the Advanced Cardiac Life Support Subcommittee and the Emergency Cardiac Care Committee, American Heart Association. Circulation 1991;83:1833; with permission.)

in CPR. Although American Heart Association CPR courses train more than 8 million Americans each year in CPR, this represents only between 2% to 3% of the American public. Clearly, more efficient and effective methods to train the public are required to comprehensively train a community and national population in bystander CPR.

Bystander Cardiopulmonary Resuscitation Training

It is now recognized that it is impossible to train large populations using classroom-based CPR training methods.[17] The time demands of most American lifestyles preclude taking a 4-hour CPR course for all but those with an employment obligation for formal CPR training and certification. Recognizing these barriers, alternative training formats and materials have been developed and proposed to make training shorter, more accessible, and cost-effective.

Video self-instruction (VSI) is a successful alternative to traditional CPR courses for laypersons. This approach includes compact training materials combined in an inexpensive "CPR kit" (including an inflatable CPR manikin and training CD or video) that allows the participant to train in the privacy of his or her home at any time and that teaches high-quality CPR skills in approximately 20 minutes. Studies comparing CPR training with VSI versus a traditional 4-hour CPR course demonstrated VSI training resulted in similar, if not superior, CPR performance and skills retention initially and at 2 and 6 months.[18,19] The educational materials also provide permanent access to intermittent refresher training, when desired.

Furthermore, VSI participants provide the training materials to two to three additional family members or friends, significantly multiplying the educational impact of this approach.[18,19]

Thus, for the first time, VSI provides a proven, effective CPR training approach that enables communities to train a significantly larger portion of the layperson population in these basic life-saving skills and increases the community's incidence of bystander CPR.

Cardiopulmonary Resuscitation in the Schools

Mandating CPR training in the schools holds the potential to train a generation of Americans in CPR. With time, the entire United States population could be trained in CPR (and in the use of automated external defibrillators [AEDs]).[20] Video-mediated instruction, no longer than a total of 30 minutes, now makes training possible in a single classroom period. This short time of training has removed a previous barrier (a 4-hour course) to widespread implementation of CPR in the schools.

Communities with receptive school boards that have adopted this approach (such as the Take Heart America [THA] project) have significantly increased the portion of the community trained in CPR.[21] Use of video-mediated instruction "CPR kits" further expands the impact of this approach as junior and senior high school students can take the materials home and train additional family and friends.

Although low, the cost of training materials (CPR kits) continues to be a potential barrier to budget-challenged school boards. The lack of a federal mandate for CPR in the schools currently precludes universal national implementation. Nonetheless, this concept, rigorously supported by the American Heart Association, is becoming increasingly popular in schools that are early adopters and that have recognized its importance. Such schools have enjoyed the success of this approach. CPR in the schools, then, is another potentially effective tool for communities to increase citizen CPR training.

Simplified Cardiopulmonary Resuscitation Technique

Simplifying the CPR technique used by laypersons has the potential to increase the frequency of citizen action in an emergency and pave the way for innovative and new methods for mass CPR training. Animal studies have demonstrated that continuous chest compressions without rescue breathing are effective for a witnessed arrest during the first several minutes of CPR.[22,23] Clinical studies subsequently have confirmed that outcomes are acceptable after 'hands-only" bystander CPR (compared with bystander CPR with rescue breathing in untrained and trained laypersons).[24,25] This new concept removes the potential barriers to layperson action during an emergency, including fear of contracting a communicable disease by providing mouth-to-mouth breathing and concern by laypersons for the complexity of administering CPR. The American Heart Association recently published a recommendation that bystanders who witness a sudden collapse in an adult should perform chest-compression-only CPR if the rescuer is a bystander without CPR training or is previously trained but not confident in his or her ability to provide conventional CPR, including high-quality chest compressions with rescue breathing.[26]

Mass Cardiopulmonary Resuscitation Training

The demonstrated success of VSI[18,19] and simplification of layperson CPR technique[26] has opened a window of opportunity for effective and simple mass training in CPR. Training the public to recognize cardiac arrest, call 911, and perform chest-compression-only CPR is now possible in 30-second public service announcements on television or shown at innovative locations, such as doctors' offices and emergency department waiting rooms. These short video clips, which also can be downloaded to cell phones and other electronic devices used by most Americans, have the potential to vastly increase public awareness as well as the rate of bystander CPR in the community. Such approaches are being studied in selected communities and hold promise to train entire populations in this life-saving technique. Communities should consider this as a potential option to improve the rate of bystander CPR locally.

EARLY DEFIBRILLATION—PUBLIC ACCESS DEFIBRILLATION

Early defibrillation is a critical link in the chain of survival that can significantly improve outcome from OHCA.[27] For ventricular fibrillation cardiac arrest, the likelihood of survival substantially decreases for every minute of delay to defibrillation from the onset of cardiac arrest.[3,28] The concept of public access defibrillation (PAD) has emerged with advances in technology that have made AEDs reliable and simple to operate, enabling trained lay rescuers to perform early defibrillation (if they have access to an AED at the site of the cardiac arrest).[29]

PAD programs, which place AEDs in public locations throughout the community and train lay rescuers in CPR and use of the AEDs, incorporate an effective internal emergency response plan linked with the local EMS system. PAD programs are a crucial adjunct to a community's EMS-based efforts to achieve earlier defibrillation. They have been demonstrated to be safe, to consistently provide effective defibrillation minutes earlier than the EMS system, and to double survival rate from ventricular fibrillation OHCA.[30–33]

The American Heart Association recommends the following critical elements to achieve high-quality PAD programs[34]:

- The community should focus on strengthening each link in the chain of survival.
- Ideally, the PAD program should be under the supervision of a qualified health care provider with expertise in emergency cardiac care. The PAD director can optimize and coordinate training, site evaluation, AED placement, communication with the EMS system, lay-rescuer retraining, and quality-improvement monitoring.
- All lay rescuers should be trained in both CPR and AED use. Members of the PAD program should practice their internal emergency response several times each year, with unannounced drills.
- A written response plan should be implemented at each site, targeting a collapse-to-first-shock time of 4 to 5 minutes or less.
- The AED should be placed in a central, highly visible, and accessible location near a telephone. Residents or employees at

the site should be aware of the location. AEDs should ideally be placed no farther than a 1- to 1.5-minute walk from any location in the PAD site. AEDs should not be placed in locked offices or cabinets.

- The PAD program should be integrated with the local EMS system.
- The program should include a method to ensure data retrieval and quality assurance review of any AED use.
- The AED should be maintained according to manufacturer's recommendations.

Priority of PAD implementation should be given to public locations in the community expected to have the highest frequency of cardiac arrest. Locations where large crowds gather, such as public transportation terminals (eg, airports and train stations), sports arenas, shopping malls, recreational complexes, large industrial complexes, and federal buildings, should be considered strongly for PAD programs. Other public locations expected to have a relatively higher frequency of cardiac arrest due to physical activity or higher-risk populations include golf courses, health clubs, medical offices, and non–patient care areas of hospitals.[35,36]

Automated External Defibrillators in the School

Most pediatric cardiac arrests occur among adolescents with previously undiagnosed congenital heart abnormalities in the setting of rigorous sports activity.[37–39] Although the incidence of pediatric cardiac arrest is low, the consequences are devastating.[40] When prompt and effective resuscitation is given, pediatric cardiac arrest survivors have the highest number of life-years salvaged. Furthermore, many at-risk adults are located at schools, including faculty, parents, and members of the community attending extramural activities.[20] As with CPR, the school is an ideal place to implement training programs in AED use, since students are more willing to learn and have the potential to spread the knowledge they have acquired.[41]

One example of successful PAD program implementation in the schools is Project ADAM (Automated Defibrillators in Adam's Memory), which began after a series of sudden deaths among high school athletes in Wisconsin.[42] This project has facilitated PAD program implementation in schools nationally by providing comprehensive resources that schools need to plan, fund, and implement a PAD program.

Automated External Defibrillators in the Home

The most common location of OHCA is the home.[43] While the PAD Trial doubled ventricular fibrillation survival rate by placing AEDs in public locations, it also demonstrated a markedly low survival rate in residential facilities.[33] The subsequent Home AED Trial (HAT) failed to demonstrate a survival benefit by placing AEDs in the home compared with reliance on conventional resuscitation methods.[44] Given these results, placement of AEDs in the home is considered an ineffective strategy and should not be pursued by communities at this time.

Communities and Public Access Defibrillation Programs

Despite these proven and marked benefits, PAD programs in communities remain underutilized. PAD programs are typically implemented by early-adopting companies and organizations. The programs (although highly effective) are independent, sporadically implemented, and variably maintained. Communities lack local leadership to champion strategic development of PAD programs, optimize locations of highest incidence of cardiac arrest in the community, and provide comprehensive coverage to the community. Moreover, communities lack public awareness of the importance of these programs, initiatives to generate funding to support these programs, and the administrative and political will to support a comprehensive community initiative. Thus, this proven and effective intervention, which doubles survival rate from cardiac arrest, remains grossly underutilized and prohibited from realizing its survival potential.

EARLY ADVANCED CARE—EMERGENCY MEDICAL SERVICES
The Coordinating Role of Emergency Medical Services in the Community

The EMS system represents a pivotal and coordinating component in the care of cardiac arrest for the community. As such, it is critically important to the community's cardiac arrest survival performance. EMS implements and coordinates crucial, time-sensitive interventions, including facilitating early access through 911, deploying rapid EMS, providing dispatcher-assisted bystander CPR, integrating with local PAD programs, delivering high-quality professional resuscitation, and selecting optimal hospital transport destinations for resuscitated cardiac arrest patients. Accordingly, the local EMS cardiac arrest survival rate is an accurate reflection of community performance and should be evaluated continuously as a community's quality assurance measure.[45]

Dispatcher-assisted Telephone Cardiopulmonary Resuscitation

Communities should implement every strategy to encourage laypersons to perform CPR until EMS arrives. One of the most effective ways to immediately increase the incidence of bystander CPR in the community is to provide verbal instruction by the EMS dispatcher over the telephone. Dispatcher-assisted CPR dramatically increases the rate and quality of bystander-delivered CPR.[46] More importantly, dispatcher-assisted bystander CPR has been shown to improve survival in OHCA compared with no bystander CPR.[7] Since most bystanders are untrained in CPR and must provide this intervention during the initial few minutes before EMS arrival, simple instructions are necessary. Under these circumstances, chest-compression-only CPR has been shown to be just as effective (if not more so) for untrained laypersons.[26]

Communities should implement aggressive dispatcher-assisted bystander CPR programs. Success of the program requires training, retraining, and continuous quality improvement.

Professional Cardiopulmonary Resuscitation

The quality of CPR delivered by trained medical professionals directly correlates with successful resuscitation.[47] However, the quality of CPR delivered varies. When electronically recorded and then evaluated, well-established, excellent EMS systems have been shown to provide chest compressions that are too shallow, long interruptions in chest compressions, incomplete chest-wall recoil, and excessive ventilation rates.[48–50] Because the quality of CPR provided correlates with successful resuscitation, it is a critical component of the community's cardiac arrest survival performance.

Accordingly, every EMS director should comprehensively educate and train first- and second- responding EMS personnel to provide high-quality CPR. Equally important, the quality of CPR needs to be electronically measured to provide real-time feedback to rescuers (while resuscitative efforts are being performed) and to provide continuous quality improvement for the EMS system. EMS directors can use readily available equipment now capable of electronically monitoring CPR performance during resuscitation.[51]

A suggested list of the important components of high-quality CPR (many of which have been demonstrated to be correlated with improved hemodynamics during CPR) include[52]:

- Chest compression depth: 1.5 to 2 in
- Chest compression rate: 100/min
- Ventilation rate: 6 to 10 breaths/min; ventilation duration: no more than 1 s/breath; tidal volume: 500 to 600 mL/breath
- Complete chest recoil following each compression
- Maximize hands-on time; minimize interruptions to CPR; no pauses in chest compressions more than 10 seconds
- CPR immediately before and immediately after defibrillation
- Use of Impedance Threshold Device (ITD; Advanced Circulatory Systems, Inc, Eden Prairie, Minnesota)
- Minimization of rescuer fatigue

OPTIMIZING POSTARREST CARE— REGIONALIZATION OF RESUSCITATION CENTERS
Postarrest Cardiac Care

Optimizing hospital-based care for patients resuscitated from cardiac arrest has been shown to increase survival rate greater than any single intervention the community can make. One-year neurologically intact survival was more than doubled (from 26% to 56%) after implementing optimal postresuscitation care.[53]

There is wide variation in hospital-based survival rates following treatment of patients resuscitated from OHCA.[54–59] In-hospital factors found to be associated with improved survival include increased size of the hospital, availability of a cardiac catheterization laboratory, increased volume of patients treated for cardiac arrest, and available staffing (ratio of beds to nurses).[57–59] Furthermore, optimal postarrest cardiac care is complex and requires sophisticated hospital-based capabilities as well as protocol-driven, comprehensive care delivered by a coordinated, multidisciplinary team. The demands of such optimal care are often beyond the capabilities of most paramedic-receiving hospitals.

Optimized postarrest hospital-based care should include (1) therapeutic hypothermia, (2) hemodynamic support, (3) services of a cardiac catheterization laboratory, (4) optimal intensive care unit care, (5) option of using implantable cardioverter-defibrillators, and (6) social services.

Therapeutic hypothermia
The most significant advance in postarrest cardiac care is implementation of therapeutic hypothermia

(rapidly reducing core body temperature to 32°C to 34°C for 12 to 48 hours followed by controlled re-warming). This novel therapy significantly reduces mortality and improves neurologic outcome in comatose survivors of OHCA.[60,61] Therapeutic hypothermia should be an integral part of a standardized treatment strategy. Numerous techniques are available to induce and maintain hypothermia. These techniques include topical application of ice, use of cutaneous cooling devices, and intravascular cooling. Implementation of therapeutic hypothermia requires planning, education, and integration of emergency medicine, cardiology, and intensive care unit services within an institution.

Hemodynamic support
Post–cardiac arrest myocardial dysfunction, which is common and usually transient in patients resuscitated from cardiac arrest, requires appropriate (and sometimes aggressive) hemodynamic support. Treatment often requires use of inotropes and vasopressors to maintain hemodynamic stability. Mechanical hemodynamic support, including an intra-aortic balloon pump, should be available and implemented if pharmacologic measures fail. Other measures include percutaneous cardiopulmonary bypass, extracorporeal membrane oxygenation, and the use of transthoracic ventricular assist devices.[62,63]

Services of cardiac catheterization laboratory
Because the majority of OHCA patients have coronary artery disease that often precipitates cardiac arrest, prompt coronary arteriography followed by percutaneous intervention is life-saving in appropriate patients. Immediate access to interventional cardiology and availability of a cardiac catheterization laboratory at the treating hospital are essential.[64,65]

Optimal intensive care unit care
Post–cardiac arrest patients are at risk of developing multiorgan dysfunction. Accordingly, they require optimal intensive care, including advanced hemodynamic monitoring, neurologic assessment, hemodynamic optimization, and the highest standards of critical care.

Expert neurologic prognostication
Early determination of outcome after OHCA is a complicated issue requiring expert neurologic care. Accurate neurologic outcome prediction requires neurologists experienced in treating patients resuscitated from cardiac arrest and additionally may require electrophysiological examinations and neuroimaging tests. Comatose survivors of cardiac arrest often take longer than other patient populations to regain consciousness and achieve return to neurologic baseline (especially with therapeutic hypothermia treatment). Decisions to withdraw life support are critically important and need to be based on extensive experience with these newer treatments in the cardiac arrest patient population.[66,67]

Implantable cardioverter-defibrillators
Insertion of implantable cardioverter-defibrillators is indicated in many patients who survive cardiac arrest. Such therapy is lifesaving, potentially increases quality of life, and should be implemented in all appropriate cardiac arrest survivors.[68]

Social services
The complex nature of postarrest cardiac care demands appropriate psychosocial support for patients and their families throughout their hospitalization. Social service care should be integrated into optimal hospital-based care of cardiac arrest patients.

Regionalization of Postarrest Hospital-based Care

Given the profound variability in hospital-based survival rates and the need for sophisticated hospital-based capabilities to optimize outcome for patients resuscitated from OHCA, communities should establish selected resuscitation centers regionally and transport resuscitated OHCA patients directly and exclusively to those resuscitation centers. Using the successful concept of the trauma center, local regionalization of resuscitation centers will provide resuscitated victims of OHCA with the highest quality hospital-based care and the community with a doubling of survival rates.[53,69,70] Establishing regional resuscitation centers requires a community-wide plan and collaboration among EMS directors, hospital administrators, emergency departments, cardiologists, and intensive care specialists throughout the community.

A COMMUNITY-WIDE APPROACH TO CARDIAC ARREST

A very successful model of a community-wide approach to cardiac arrest is the THA Project.[21] THA is a demonstration project designed to show how cardiac arrest survival rates in America's cities can be significantly increased through a comprehensive, community-wide approach. THA has deployed state-of-the art resuscitation science strategies and outreach programs in four demonstration communities: St Cloud, Minnesota;

Anoka County, Minnesota; Columbus, Ohio; and Austin, Texas.

Key aspects of the THA approach are centered on strengthening and coordinating each link in the chain of survival throughout an entire community by increasing community awareness of cardiac arrest; implementing innovative CPR training programs in schools and media to increase the rate of bystander CPR; comprehensively implementing PAD programs in high-risk public locations; improving the quality of resuscitation skills of professional rescuers; and establishing resuscitation centers to optimize care of patients resuscitated from OHCA.

Combining the efforts of doctors, nurses, paramedics, health educators, and community leaders, THA already has demonstrated the validity of this general concept by increasing community-wide survival rates from OHCA more than two-fold.

COORDINATION AND ADMINISTRATION OF COMMUNITY RESOURCES
What a Community Needs to Succeed

Cardiac arrest registry
Without an established cardiac arrest registry (capturing outcome of all cardiac arrests in the community), it is impossible to identify the current performance of the community and barriers to potential improvement. The CARES (Cardiac Arrest Registry to Enhance Survival) project is an excellent example of an immediately available cardiac arrest database that can be adopted by any community interested in improving outcome from cardiac arrest. It captures all essential data elements for OHCA events using an Internet-based network. The program is rapidly being adopted in many communities.[71]

Cardiac arrest champion
To implement and coordinate a sustained and effective program to significantly improve the local survival rate from cardiac arrest, a community needs a cardiac arrest champion. This individual should have knowledge and expertise in the field of cardiac arrest as well as passion for improving cardiac arrest outcome. An effective community program needs this leadership to succeed.

Medical leadership and collaboration
A community also needs an EMS medical director who has the will and capacity to provide medical leadership, oversight, and coordination to ensure the highest quality care for cardiac arrest patients. This person should take responsibility for training EMS rescuers in high-quality CPR, acquiring EMS equipment to electronically monitor the

performance of CPR, and implementing a CPR continuous quality-assurance program. The EMS medical director is pivotal in optimizing rapid access through 911, implementing dispatcher-assisted CPR, minimizing EMS response time, integrating EMS response with PAD programs, and establishing EMS transport policy to resuscitation centers. The EMS medical director also plays a collaborative role in working with community hospitals that receive EMS patients (heightening awareness of the medical community to optimal standards of practice).

Collaboration among hospitals and medical specialties can be challenging. Lack of collaboration and competing interests frequently represent barriers to a coordinated community plan. Common ground should be established in a genuine interest in improving outcome from cardiac arrest and a community-wide multidisciplinary committee instituted to meet on a regular basis. The formation of such a committee is a necessity for community progress. Continued communication and established common interests eventually achieve consensus on an action plan for improved cardiac arrest care in the community.

Political leadership
Efforts to improve care of OHCA cannot be maximized unless there is support from local government, including the mayor's office and city council. In general, governmental departments recognize the public health impact of cardiac arrest and the potential benefit to local citizens of improved care. Communities should contact the appropriate local governmental agencies once a community plan has been defined.[72]

Community support
Promoting CPR training in the schools, video-mediated CPR instruction, and innovative media techniques heightens awareness of cardiac arrest in the community. Every member of the community should be encouraged to actively participate in the chain of survival.

The community should establish a cardiac arrest survivors' network. Cardiac arrest survivors can promote a community initiative better than any other spokespeople. Fund-raising campaigns can be responsibly linked to public cardiac arrest survivor events to generate income for PAD programs and other critical initiatives.

Administrative assistance
A dedicated administrative assistant is a necessity for scheduling, for organizational planning, and for maintaining continuous progress on multiple

initiatives. Communities must find creative ways to initially fund and maintain this critically important support.

Communication and collaboration

For communities to forge a strong relationship between each link so that efficient, timely, and coordinated sequences of interventions can be provided to patients with cardiac arrest, community stakeholders must establish an infrastructure for scheduled meetings on an ongoing basis. Stakeholders at these regularly scheduled meetings should include (but not necessarily be limited to) EMS directors, hospital administrators, EMS personnel, emergency physicians, and community leaders. Collectively, this consortium of stakeholders should identify weaknesses in the community's links in the chain of survival and implement appropriate short-term and long-range action plans. Coordination among the sequences of cardiac arrest interventions should be continually addressed. A community-wide continuous quality-assurance program should be implemented to continuously evaluate the community's performance. Although other interests will compete, commitment and collaboration among stakeholders will result in transformation of the community's survival rate from cardiac arrest.

Additional resources

Such organizations as the Citizen CPR Foundation (http://www.citizencpr.org), whose mission is to save lives from sudden death by stimulating citizen and community action, represent a valuable and comprehensive resource to communities and community leaders interested in improving outcome from cardiac arrest.

SUMMARY

The chain of survival (early access, early CPR, early defibrillation, and early advanced care [see **Fig. 1**]) defines the proven interventions necessary for successful resuscitation and survival of patients with cardiac arrest. Low survival rates from cardiac arrest are not due to lack of understanding of effective interventions but are instead due to weak links in the chain of survival and the inability of communities to make certain these links function in an efficient, timely, and coordinated fashion. This article has reviewed how quality is defined for each link, how communities can strengthen each link, and how communities can forge a strong relationship between each link. By optimizing local leadership and stakeholder collaboration, communities have the potential to vastly improve outcomes from this devastating disease.

ACKNOWLEDGMENTS

We gratefully acknowledge Ms Dawn Kawa for her valuable and gracious assistance in preparation of this manuscript.

REFERENCES

1. Callans DJ. Out-of-hospital cardiac arrest—the solution is shocking. N Engl J Med 2004;351:632–4.
2. Rea TD, Eisenberg MS, Becker LJ, et al. Temporal trends in sudden cardiac arrest: a 25-year emergency medical services perspective. Circulation 2003;107:2780–5.
3. Cummins RO, Ornato JP, Thies WH, et al. Improving survival from sudden cardiac arrest: the "chain of survival" concept. Circulation 1991;83:1832–47.
4. ECC Committee, Subcommittees and Task Forces of the American Heart Association. 2005 American Heart Association guidelines for cardiopulmonary resuscitation and emergency cardiovascular care. Circulation 2005;112(24 Suppl):IV1–203.
5. Gallagher EJ, Lombardi G, Gennis P. Effectiveness of bystander cardiopulmonary resuscitation and survival following out-of-hospital cardiac arrest. JAMA 1995;274:1922–5.
6. Cummins RO, Eisenberg MS, Hallstrom AP, et al. Survival of OHCA with early initiation of cardiopulmonary resuscitation. Am J Emerg Med 1985;3:114–9.
7. Rea TD, Eisenberg MS, Culley LL, et al. Dispatcher-assisted cardiopulmonary resuscitation and survival in cardiac arrest. Circulation 2001;104(21):2513–6.
8. Stiell IG, Wells GA, De Maio VJ, et al. Modifiable factors associated with improved cardiac arrest survival in a multicenter basic life support/defibrillation system: OPALS study phase I results. Ann Emerg Med 1999;33:44–50.
9. Stiell IG, Nichol G, Wells G, et al. Health-related quality of life is better for cardiac arrest survivors who received citizen cardiopulmonary resuscitation. Circulation 2003;08:1939–44.
10. De Maio VJ, Stiell IG, Spaite DW, et al. OPALS study group. CPR-only survivors of OHCA: implications for out-of-hospital care and cardiac arrest research methodology. Ann Emerg Med 2001;37:602–8.
11. Swor R, Khan I, Domeier R, et al. CPR training and CPR performance: do CPR-trained bystanders perform CPR? Acad Emerg Med 2006;13:596–601.
12. Coon SJ, Guy MC. Performing bystander CPR for sudden cardiac arrest: behavioral intentions among the general adult population in Arizona. Resuscitation 2009;80(3):334–40.
13. Nolan RP, Wilson E, Shuster M, et al. Readiness to perform cardiopulmonary resuscitation: an emerging strategy against sudden cardiac death. Psychosom Med 1999;61:546–51.

14. Locke CJ, Berg RA, Sanders AB, et al. Bystander cardiopulmonary resuscitation—concerns about mouth-to-mouth contact. Arch Intern Med 1995; 155:938–43.
15. Shibata K, Taniguchi T, Yoshida M, et al. Obstacles to bystander cardiopulmonary resuscitation in Japan. Resuscitation 2000;44:187–93.
16. Johnston TC, Clark MJ, Dingle FA, et al. Factors influencing Queenslanders' willingness to perform bystander cardiopulmonary resuscitation. Resuscitation 2003;56:67–75.
17. Flint LS, Billi JE, Kelly K, et al. Education in adult basic life support training programs. Ann Emerg Med 1993;22:468–74.
18. Lynch B, Einspruch EL, Nichol G, et al. Effectiveness of a 30-minute CPR self-instruction program for lay responders: a controlled randomized study. Resuscitation 2005;67(1):31–43.
19. Einspruch EL, Lynch B, Aufderheide TP, et al. Retention of CPR skills learned in a traditional Heartsaver course versus 30-minute video self-training: a controlled randomized study. Resuscitation 2007; 74(3):476–86.
20. Lotfi K, White L, Rea T, et al. Cardiac arrest in schools. Circulation 2007;116:1374–9.
21. Take Heart America. Available at: http://takeheart america.org. Accessed September 15, 2009.
22. Berg RA, Kern KB, Hilwig RW, et al. Assisted ventilation does not improve outcome in a porcine model of single-rescuer bystander cardiopulmonary resuscitation. Circulation 1997;95(6):1635–41.
23. Chandra NC, Gruben KG, Tsitlik JE, et al. Observations of ventilation during resuscitation in a canine model. Circulation 1994;90(6):3070–5.
24. SOS-KANTO Study Group. Cardiopulmonary resuscitation by bystanders with chest compression only (SOS-KANTO): an observational study. Lancet 2007;369(9565):920–6.
25. Hallstrom A, Cobb L, Johnson E, et al. Cardiopulmonary resuscitation by chest compression alone or with mouth-to-mouth ventilation. N Engl J Med 2000;342(21):1546–53.
26. Sayre MR, Berg RA, Cave DM, et al. Hands-only (compression-only) cardiopulmonary resuscitation: a call to action for bystander response to adults who experience out-of-hospital cardiac arrest. A science advisory for the public from the Emergency Cardiovascular Care Committee, American Heart Association. Circulation 2008;117(16): 2162–7.
27. Eisenberg MS. Improving survival from out-of-hospital cardiac arrest: back to the basics. Ann Emerg Med 2007;49(3):314–6.
28. Marenco JP, Wang PJ, Link MS, et al. Improving survival from sudden cardiac arrest: the role of the automated external defibrillator. JAMA 2001;285: 1193–200.
29. Cummins RO, Eisenberg M, Bergner L, et al. Sensitivity, accuracy, and safety of an automatic external defibrillator. Lancet 1984;2:318–20.
30. Valenzuela TD, Roe DJ, Nichol G, et al. Outcomes of rapid defibrillation by security officers after cardiac arrest in casinos. N Engl J Med 2000;343:1206–9.
31. Page RL, Joglar JA, Kowal RC, et al. Use of automated external defibrillators by a U.S. airline. N Engl J Med 2000;343:1210–6.
32. van Alem AP, Vrenken RH, de Vos R, et al. Use of automated external defibrillator by first responders in out-of-hospital cardiac arrest: prospective controlled trial. BMJ 2003;327(7427):1312.
33. The public access defibrillation trial investigators. Public access defibrillation and survival after out-of-hospital cardiac arrest. N Engl J Med 2004;351: 637–46.
34. Guidelines 2000 for CPR and Emergency Cardiovascular Care. Part 4: the AED: key link in the chain of survival. The American Heart Association in collaboration with the International Liaison Committee on Resuscitation. Circulation 2000; 102(Suppl 8):60–76.
35. Becker L, Eisenberg M, Fahrenbruch C, et al. Public locations of cardiac arrest: implications for public access defibrillation. Circulation 1998;97(21):2106–9.
36. Gratton M, Lindholm DJ, Campbell JP. Public access defibrillation: Where do we place the AEDs? Prehosp Emerg Care 1999;3(4):303–5.
37. Myerburg RJ, Mitrani R, Interian A Jr, et al. Identification of risk of cardiac arrest and sudden death in athletes. In: Estes NA 3rd, Salem DN, Wang PJ, editors. Sudden cardiac death in the athlete. Armonk (NY): Futura Publishing Co; 1997. p. 25–56.
38. Maron BJ, Gohman TE, Aeppli D. Prevalence of sudden cardiac death during competitive sports activities in Minnesota high school athletes. J Am Coll Cardiol 1998;32(7):1881–4.
39. Liberthson RR. Sudden death from cardiac causes in children and young adults. N Engl J Med 1996; 334(16):1039–44.
40. Topjian AA, Nadkarni VM, Berg RA. Cardiopulmonary resuscitation in children. Curr Opin Crit Care 2009;15(3):203–8.
41. Garza M. An AED in every school: the next step for public access defibrillation. J Exp Med Sci 2003;28: 22–3.
42. Project ADAM. Available at: http://www.chw.org/display/PPF/DocID/26050/router.asp. Accessed September 15, 2009.
43. Litwin PE, Eisenberg MS, Hallstrom AP, et al. The location of collapse and its effect on survival from cardiac arrest. Ann Emerg Med 1987;16(7): 787–91.
44. HAT investigators. Home use of automated external defibrillators for sudden cardiac arrest. N Engl J Med 2008;358:1793–804.

45. Cayten CG. Evaluation. In: Kuehl AE, editor. Prehospital systems and medical oversight. 2nd edition. St. Louis: Mosby Lifeline; 1994. p. 159–67.

46. Culley LL, Clark JJ, Eisenberg MS, et al. Dispatcher-assisted telephone CPR: common delays and time standards for delivery. Ann Emerg Med 1991;20(4):362–6.

47. Abella BS, Sandbo N, Vassilatos P, et al. Chest compression rates during cardiopulmonary resuscitation are suboptimal: a prospective study during in-hospital cardiac arrest. Circulation 2005;111(4): 428–34.

48. Wik L, Kramer-Johansen J, Myklebust H, et al. Quality of cardiopulmonary resuscitation during OHCA. JAMA 2005;293:299–304.

49. Aufderheide TP, Lurie KG. Death by hyperventilation: a common and life-threatening problem during cardiopulmonary resuscitation. Crit Care Med 2004; 32(Suppl 9):S345–51.

50. Aufderheide TP, Pirrallo RG, Yannopoulos D, et al. Incomplete chest wall decompression: a clinical evaluation of CPR performance by EMS personnel and assessment of alternative manual chest compression-decompression techniques. Resuscitation 2005;64(3):353–62.

51. Abella BS, Edelson DP, Kim S, et al. CPR quality improvement during in-hospital cardiac arrest using a real-time audiovisual feedback system. Resuscitation 2007;73(1):54–61.

52. Bobrow BJ, Aufderheide TP, Brady WJ. Maximizing survival from out-of-hospital cardiac arrest. Emerg Med Rep 2008;29(11):121–32.

53. Sunde K, Pytte M, Jacobsen D, et al. Implementation of a standardized treatment protocol for post-resuscitation care after out-of-hospital cardiac arrest. Resuscitation 2007;73:29–39.

54. Langhelle A, Tyvold SS, Lexow K, et al. In-hospital factors associated with improved outcome after out-of hospital cardiac arrest. A comparison between four regions in Norway. Resuscitation 2003;56:247–63.

55. Herlitz J, Engdal J, Svensson L, et al. Major differences in 1-month survival between hospitals in Sweden among initial survivors of out-of-hospital cardiac arrest. Resuscitation 2006;70:404–9.

56. Engdahl J, Abrahamsson P, Bang A, et al. Is hospital care of major importance for outcome after out-of-hospital cardiac arrest? Experience acquired from patients with out-of-hospital cardiac arrest resuscitated by the same emergency medical service and admitted to one of two hospitals over a 16-year period in the municipality of Goteborg. Resuscitation 2000;43:201–11.

57. Liu JM, Yang Q, Pirrallo RG, et al. Hospital variability of out-of-hospital cardiac arrest survival. Prehosp Emerg Care 2008;12(3):339–46.

58. Carr BG, Goyal M, Band RA, et al. A national analysis of the relationship between hospital factors and post-cardiac arrest mortality. Intensive Care Med 2009;35(3):505–11.

59. Carr B, Kahn J, Merchant RM, et al. Inter-hospital variability in post–cardiac arrest mortality. Resuscitation 2009;80:30–4.

60. Hypothermia after Cardiac Arrest Study Group. Mild therapeutic hypothermia to improve the neurologic outcome after cardiac arrest. N Engl J Med 2002; 346(8):549–56.

61. Bernard SA, Gray TW, Buist MD, et al. Treatment of comatose survivors of out-of-hospital cardiac arrest with induced hypothermia. N Engl J Med 2002; 346(8):557–63.

62. Hovdenes J, Laake JH, Aaberge L, et al. Therapeutic hypothermia after out-of-hospital cardiac arrest: experiences with patients treated with percutaneous coronary intervention and cardiogenic shock. Acta Anaesthesiol Scand 2007;51(2):137–42.

63. Nichol G, Karby-Jones R, Salerno C, et al. Systematic review of percutaneous cardiopulmonary bypass for cardiac arrest or cardiogenic shock states. Resuscitation 2006;70:381–94.

64. Spaulding CM, Joly LM, Rosenberg A, et al. Immediate coronary angiography in survivors of out-of-hospital cardiac arrest. N Engl J Med 1997;336: 1629–33.

65. Knafelj R, Radsel P, Ploj T, et al. Primary percutaneous coronary intervention and mild induced hypothermia in comatose survivors of ventricular fibrillation with ST-elevation acute myocardial infarction. Resuscitation 2007;74:227–34.

66. Geocadin RG, Buitrago MM, Torbey MT, et al. Neurologic prognosis and withdrawal of life support after resuscitation from cardiac arrest. Neurology 2006; 67:203–10.

67. Yannopoulos D, Kotsifas K, Aufderheide TP, et al. Cardiac arrest, mild therapeutic hypothermia, and unanticipated cerebral recovery. Neurologist 2007; 13(6):369–75.

68. The AVID investigators. A comparison of antiarrhythmic-drug therapy with implantable defibrillators in patients resuscitated from near-fatal ventricular arrhythmias. N Engl J Med 1997;337:1576–83.

69. Lurie KG, Idris A, Holcomb JB. Level 1 cardiac arrest centers: learning from the trauma surgeons. Acad Emerg Med 2005;12:79–80.

70. Kahn JM, Branas C, Schwab W, et al. Regionalization of medical critical care: What can we learn from the trauma experience? Crit Care Med 2008; 36:3085–9.

71. McNally B, Stokes A, Crouch A, et al. CARES: cardiac arrest registry to enhance survival. Ann Emerg Med 2009; [Epub ahead of print].

72. Eisenberg MS. A plan of action. Resuscitate!: how your community can improve survival from sudden cardiac arrest. Seattle (WA): University of Washington Press; 2009. p. 179–206.

Risk Stratification for Sudden Cardiac Death: The Need to Go Beyond the Left Ventricular Ejection Fraction

Devi Gopinath, MD[a], Otto Costantini, MD[b],*

KEYWORDS
- Sudden cardiac death • Risk stratification
- Non-invasive risk markers • Electrophysiological study
- Left ventricular ejection fraction • Defibrillators

Sudden cardiac death (SCD), death that occurs due to cardiac disease within 1 hour from the onset of symptoms, accounts for as many as 450,000 deaths yearly in the United States, and is responsible for approximately 50% of cardiovascular deaths.[1] It accounts for more deaths than many other common diseases combined (**Fig. 1**). Most, but not all, cases of SCD are related to structural heart disease leading to malignant ventricular tachyarrhythmias.

Over the last 15 years, many clinical trials have established the effectiveness of an implantable cardioverter-defibrillator (ICD) in reducing sudden and total mortality in patients with structural heart disease.[2–5] However, controversy remains about exactly how to identify patients most likely to benefit from an ICD, as well as those who may safely do without an ICD implant. The first primary prevention ICD trial[2,3] used an abnormal electrophysiological study (EPS) in addition to a low left ventricular ejection fraction (LVEF) as high-risk markers for SCD. Although this approach provided a high therapeutic efficacy (four ICDs implanted to save one life), concerns were raised about the residual risk of arrhythmic events in patients with a negative EPS.[6] As a result, more recent ICD trials

selected patients based on the presence of a low LVEF alone. Two of these studies, MADIT II (Multicenter Automatic Difibrillator Implantation Trial II) and SCD HeFT (Sudden Cardiac Death in Heart Failure Trial),[4,5] showed a clear benefit of ICDs in reduction of total mortality, while one showed only a trend toward benefit.[7] With such a strategy, however, the therapeutic efficacy of ICDs is reduced, as at least 15 ICDs need to be implanted to save one life[8] (**Fig. 2**). In addition, recent concerns over device complications, including worsening heart failure, inappropriate shocks, device recalls, the impact on health care costs,[9] and the low number of appropriate shocks (5%–7% per year),[10] has prompted a reexamination of the current guidelines, which recommend ICDs in most patients with LVEF of 0.35 or less.[11]

Ideally, noninvasive electrophysiological markers that more directly reflect arrhythmia substrates may add to the predictive value of a low LVEF and better identify patients for prophylactic ICD implant. Several of these markers have been associated with the risk of SCD, but all have yielded contradictory results or have not been tested prospectively. This review focuses on the most promising tests to date, their clinical significance, and their possible

[a] Heart and Vascular Center, MetroHealth Campus, Case Western Reserve University, 2500 MetroHealth Drive, Cleveland, OH 44109-1998, USA
[b] Heart and Vascular Research Center, MetroHealth Campus, Case Western Reserve University, 2500 MetroHealth Drive, Cleveland, OH 44109-1998, USA
* Corresponding author. Heart and Vascular Research Center, MetroHealth Campus, Case Western Reserve University, 2500 MetroHealth Drive, Cleveland, OH 44109-1998.
E-mail address: ocostantini@metrohealth.org (O. Costantini).

Card Electrophysiol Clin 1 (2009) 51–59
doi:10.1016/j.ccep.2009.08.015
1877-9182/09/$ – see front matter © 2009 Published by Elsevier Inc.

cardiacEP.theclinics.com

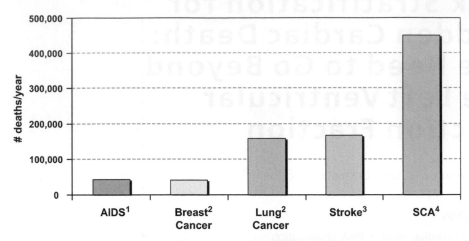

1 U.S. Census Bureau, *Statistical Abstract of the United States: 2001.*

2 American Cancer Society, Inc., *Surveillance Research, Cancer Facts and Figures 2001.*

3 *2002 Heart and Stroke Statistical Update,* American Heart Association.

4 *Circulation.* 2001; 104:2158-2163.

Fig. 1. The impact of sudden cardiac death (SCD). SCD claims more lives than AIDS, breast cancer, lung cancer, and stroke combined. SCA, sudden cardiac arrest.

use in the future, alone or in combination, to improve efficacy and efficiency of risk stratification for SCD compared with a strategy of using a depressed LVEF alone.

HEART-RATE VARIABILITY

It is well established that a significant relationship between the autonomic nervous system and cardiovascular mortality exists. However, the association with SCD is less clear. Heart-rate variability (HRV) parameters measure the influence of the autonomic nervous system on the sinus node and the relative importance of vagal and sympathetic modulation of the heart rate. Due to vagal withdrawal and sympathetic overstimulation, HRV decreases in several disease states, such as diabetes and congestive heart failure, and after myocardial infarction (MI) and heart transplantation.

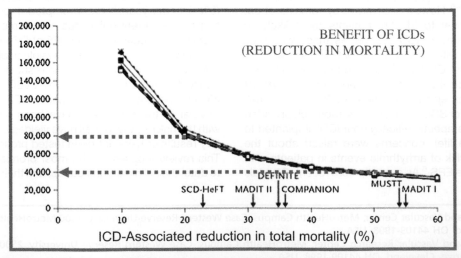

Fig. 2. Reduced cost-effectiveness of ICD. As we moved from such studies as MADIT and MUSTT (Multicenter Unsustained Tachycardia Trial) to such studies as MADIT II and SCD HeFT, ICDs proved less cost-effective as the relative reduction in total mortality decreased. QALY, quality adjusted life year. (*Adapted from* Sanders GD, Hlatky MA, Owens DK. Cost-effectiveness of implantable cardioverter-defibrillators. N Engl J Med 2005;353:1471–80; with permission.)

Quantifying Heart-rate Variability

The variations in heart rate may be evaluated either "short-term" (with a 2-minute ECG strip) or "long-term" (with a 24-hour ambulatory monitor). The two main methods to express HRV are the "time domain" and the "frequency domain." "Time domain" uses continuous measurements of the R-R intervals, while "frequency domain" uses spectral analysis to express the variation in heart rate as a frequency function. Both time domain and frequency measures have been used to predict mortality.

Scientific Evidence

In 1987, Kleiger and colleagues[12] first noted that, after an MI, decreased time-domain measures of HRV were a significant predictor of total mortality after adjusting for other variables. Hartikainen and colleagues[13] showed that, in 575 MI survivors, a depressed HRV, using a time-domain index, and nonsustained ventricular tachycardia were the only predictors of future arrhythmic death. The ATRAMI (Automatic Tone and Reflexes After Myocardial Infarction) study,[14] showed that, after an MI, patients with depressed HRV had a 3.2 relative risk of dying.

Clinical Significance

Although, no clinical trial has used HRV to guide ICD implantation, DINAMIT (Defibrillators In Acute Myocardial Infarction Trial) enrolled patients with a decreased HRV (SD of normal beat to normal beat intervals <70 ms) and LVEF of 0.35 or less to test whether prophylactic implantation of an ICD would reduce total mortality in survivors of a recent MI.[15] There was no difference in overall mortality between the two treatment groups, although a significantly decreased rate of arrhythmic death was noted in the ICD arm. Due to the disappointing results of DINAMIT, and despite the theoretical link to arrhythmogenesis, a low HRV has not been clearly linked to an increased risk of SCD and future studies are needed to establish its role.

SIGNAL AVERAGE ECG

Signal averaging of the CEG improves the signal-to-noise ratio, thus overcoming chest-muscle electrical "noise" and facilitates the detection of low-amplitude late potentials. Late potentials, seen in the terminal portion of the QRS complex, represent postinfarct areas of slow and abnormal ventricular activation, which increase the risk of reentrant malignant ventricular arrhythmias.[16]

Quantifying Signal Average ECG

Most signal processing systems use time-domain analysis, which limits the test to patients without bundle branch block. Frequency-domain analysis can overcome this limitation.[17] Although the definition of an abnormal test varies, a signal average ECG (SAECG) is typically considered abnormal if at least two of the following criteria are fulfilled: (1) a filtered QRS complex of 114 to 120 ms or more, (2) a root mean square voltage of 25 μV or less in the terminal 40 ms of the QRS, and (3) low-amplitude signal ($\leq$40 μV) duration of 40 ms or more.

Scientific Evidence

In a review of 22 prior studies and almost 10,000 patients, Bailey and colleagues[18] examined the evidence linking SAECG to future arrhythmic events after MI. The annual risk of events was 8%. The sensitivity, specificity, and positive predictive value for detecting a tachyarrhythmia within 2 years were 62%, 77%, and 19%, respectively. The CABG-Patch (Coronary Artery Bypass Graft–Patch) trial tested the hypothesis of placing an ICD in 900 patients undergoing coronary artery bypass grafting, with a LVEF of 0.35 or less and an abnormal SAECG.[19] There was no survival benefit in the ICD-treated group.

In a large MUSTT (Multicenter Unsustained Tachycardia Trial) substudy, Gomes and colleagues[20] evaluated the predictive value of an abnormal SAECG (filtered QRS duration $\geq$114 ms) for the primary end point of arrhythmic death in 1268 patients with coronary artery disease (CAD), nonsustained ventricular tachycardia, and LVEF of 0.40 or less. The arrhythmic event rate at 5 years was 28% compared with 17% in patients with a normal filtered QRS (hazard ratio 1.9). Of patients with a combined LVEF of 0.30 or less and an abnormal SAECG, 36% suffered an arrhythmic event, compared with only 13% of those without these abnormalities. Moreover, 44% of patients with this combination had a cardiac death and the total mortality was 50%. Mostly small studies of the predictive value of SAECG in dilated nonischemic cardiomyopathy have yielded mixed, but mostly negative results.

Clinical Significance

The role of SAECG in the risk stratification of patients with CAD appeared very promising up until the negative results of the CABG-Patch trial were published in 1997. However, in CABG-Patch, the arrhythmic death rate was significantly decreased in the ICD group, at the expense of a higher rate of nonarrhythmic death. Furthermore, patients with a negative SAECG were not followed. Therefore, the rates of arrhythmic events between SAECG-positive and SAECG-negative patients cannot be compared. Finally, the revascularization procedure itself might have reduced arrhythmic substrate or increased LVEF, making the results of the trial difficult to interpret. In terms of guiding ICD therapy, the MUSTT substudy shows that an abnormal SAECG can add significantly to the predictive value of an LVEF alone. Given its very high negative predictive value, the SAECG is a test that may add significantly to our ability to predict which patients are at highest and lowest risk of a ventricular tachyarrhythmic event. Its value, however, may be limited to patients with CAD and with a narrow QRS complex.

HEART-RATE TURBULENCE

Heart-rate turbulence (HRT) describes and quantifies the short-term fluctuation in sinus cycle length following a ventricular premature beat (VPB) and its compensatory pause. Schmidt and colleagues[21] discovered that after a VPB, heart rate normally increases for a few beats, and then decreases. Available physiologic investigations confirm that the initial heart-rate acceleration is triggered by transient vagal inhibition in response to the missed baroreflex afferent input caused by hemodynamically inefficient ventricular contraction. A sympathetically mediated overshoot of arterial pressure is responsible for the subsequent heart-rate deceleration through vagal recruitment.[22] Hence, the HRT pattern is blunted in patients with reduced baroreflexes.

Quantifying Heart-rate Turbulence

The physiologic pattern of HRT consists of brief heart-rate acceleration, quantified by the so-called "turbulence onset" (TO), followed by more gradual heart-rate deceleration, quantified by the so-called "turbulence slope" (TS) before the heart rate returns to a preectopic level. In patients with structural heart disease, the acceleration and deceleration are flatter than those in normal control subjects. TO is considered abnormal when the averaged R-R cycle length post-VPB is longer than that pre-VPB and TS is abnormal when the slope is less than 2.5 ms per R-R interval. In the seminal HRT publication by Schmidt and colleagues,[21] the 22 R-R intervals encompassing each VPC (2 before the VPC, 20 after the compensatory pause) were averaged on a 24-hour ambulatory monitor. HRT analysis can also been conducted from implanted cardiac defibrillators and can be induced by intracardiac pacing in the electrophysiology laboratory. Such HRT has been called *induced HRT*. Other less-established parameters to measure HRT exist, but have not been studied enough to know whether they provide superior risk stratification compared with TS and TO.

Scientific Evidence

In the original paper by Schmidt and colleagues,[21] 100 patients with an MI and frequent VPBs had TO and TS measured from 24-hour ambulatory monitors to determine the discriminating threshold between normal and abnormal HRT values (TS = 2.5, TO = 0%). These thresholds were then applied to the 24-hour ambulatory monitors of 1191 patients pooled from two large post-MI clinical trial groups: the European Myocardial Infarction Amiodarone Trial (EMIAT) and the Multicentre Post Infarction Program (MPIP).[23,24] With total mortality as the end point, univariate and multivariate analyses showed that TO and TS were independent predictors of total mortality, in addition to an LVEF of 0.30 or less. In a substudy of the ATRAMI trial, HRT variables increased the risk of ventricular arrhythmias or heart failure death fourfold.[25] Makikallio and colleagues[26] found that abnormal TS was an independent predictor of SCD in approximately 2000 post-MI patients. They reported sensitivity, specificity, positive predictive values, and negative predictive values of 56%, 79%, 6%, 99%, respectively.

Clinical Significance

HRT is attractive because it is a simple and elegant way of measuring cardiac autonomic function, even though compared with other noninvasive risk predictors, the relative risk and positive predictive accuracy of HRT are only modestly better. Barthel and colleagues[27] showed that when abnormal HRT parameters are added to a low LVEF ($\leq$0.30) the 2-year total mortality risk was about 40%. However, in both Barthel's study and in the ATRAMI substudy, the majority of patients had LVEFs of 0.40 or more, and therefore are not candidates for ICD therapy under current guidelines. In fact, in Makikallio's study, HRT was not a significant predictor of SCD in patients with LVEF of 0.35 or less. Therefore, although HRT appears to increase the total mortality risk, its predictive value for SCD has not been adequately established.[28] Furthermore, because HRT can't be measured in patients with atrial fibrillation, in those with no or few VPBs, or in those with too many VPBs, its role in the prediction of SCD in patients with cardiomyopathies is far from established. To date, no prospective clinical studies of ICD therapy have based inclusion on an abnormal HRT.

MICROVOLT T-WAVE ALTERNANS

Microvolt T-wave alternans (MTWA) refers to a beat-to-beat repetitive oscillation in the timing or shape of T waves, which is indiscernible on the surface ECG and predisposes patients to reentrant ventricular tachyarrhythmias and SCD.[29] The pathophysiologic mechanism linking MTWA to arrhythmogenesis initiates when beat-to-beat fluctuations in cellular action potentials occur in diseased myocardial cells. Arrhythmias will develop when adjacent myocardial cells (or regions) alternate in a discordant fashion, leading to heterogeneity (or dispersion) of repolarization, conduction block, and reentry.[30]

Quantifying Microvolt T-wave Alternans

The measurement of MTWA is based on the principle that the magnitude of MTWA increases with increasing heart rate. In a given subject, MTWA develops at a specific heart rate and is usually reproducible and sustained above that heart-rate threshold.[31] In patients with structural heart disease, MTWA develops at slower heart rates than it does in normal subjects. Thus, the heart rate at which MTWA appears is an important determinant of whether a test is normal or abnormal. The test is administered as a submaximal exercise stress ECG, with noise-reducing, multicontact, three-dimensional electrodes to achieve a gradual heart-rate elevation, particularly in the range of 100 to 110 bpm. MTWA cannot be measured in patients with chronic atrial fibrillation or with a paced ventricular rhythm. Comprehensive rules and criteria for interpretation have been published, although challenges in interpretation remain.[31] An indeterminate MTWA test may be caused by such patient factors as nonsustained MTWA or excessive ventricular ectopy, or by such technical factors as too much noise. Kaufman and colleagues[32] have shown that the prognosis of an indeterminate test due to patient factors is at least as bad as that of a positive test. Therefore such indeterminate tests are grouped with the positive tests as "abnormal."

Scientific Evidence

Early studies by Smith and colleagues and Rosenbaum and colleagues[29,33] established MTWA as a marker for vulnerability to clinical arrhythmias. Rosenbaum in 1994 reported, for the first time in humans, that MTWA was an independent predictor of future arrhythmic events and that the predictive value of MTWA was equivalent to that of an EPS. Klingenheben and colleagues[34] showed that MTWA was an important independent predictor

of arrhythmic events in patients with advanced heart failure and LVEF of 0.45 or less. Bloomfield and colleagues[35] prospectively followed 549 patients with LVEF of 0.40 or less with both ischemic and nonischemic cardiomyopathy for an average of 20 months, and reported that patients with an abnormal MTWA test were five times more likely to die or have a sustained ventricular arrhythmia than patients with a negative test. A normal MTWA test had a negative predictive value of 97.5%. Based on the early prospective observational studies, Gehi and colleagues[36] published a meta-analysis assessing the predictive value of MTWA for future arrhythmic events. The positive and negative predictive values of MTWA were 19.3% and 97.2%, respectively, over a mean follow-up time of 21 months. The test was equally predictive in patients with ischemic and nonischemic cardiomyopathy. Recently, our group published results from the Alternans Before Cardioverter Defibrillator (ABCD) trial,[37] a prospective study of 566 patients with CAD, LVEF of 0.40 or less, and a history of nonsustained ventricular tachycardia in which ICD therapy guided by a MTWA-directed strategy was compared with that of an EPS-directed strategy. The predictive values of the two tests for ventricular tachyarrhythmic events or SCD were equivalent. The negative predictive value of the MTWA test was 95%. The highest event rate was in patients who had both a positive EPS and MTWA test (12.6%) and the lowest in patients with both a negative EPS and MTWA test, suggesting a synergistic predictive effect of the two tests. In contrast, the MTWA SCD HeFT substudy[38] showed that an abnormal MTWA does not predict SCD or ventricular tachyarrhythmic events in patients with heart failure and LVEF of 0.35 or less, while the MASTER (Microvolt T-Wave Alternans Testing for Risk Stratification of Post MI Patients) trial[39] showed that an abnormal MTWA does not predict SCD or ventricular tachyarrhythmic events in patients with CAD and an LVEF of 0.30 or less. Much controversy remains about whether the ABCD trial, SCD HeFT substudy, and the MASTER trial should have chosen a total mortality end point rather than a surrogate end point (ie, ICD shocks), as suggested by a recent meta-analysis.[40]

Clinical Significance

Although the majority of early observational trials found a very low total mortality in patients with a negative MTWA test, more recent ones using surrogate end points have shown only a weak or no association with ventricular tachyarrhythmic events or SCD. The early studies had a very low penetration of ICDs, yet the total mortality of MTWA-negative patients was very low. Among MADIT II–like patients, Bloomfield and colleagues[41] showed that MTWA test–negative patients had a total mortality of only 3.8% at 2 years, lower than the 2-year mortality of MADIT II patients protected by an ICD (11%). Also, Chow and colleagues[42] reported that, in patients with ischemic cardiomyopathy, there was no difference in total mortality between patients with a normal MTWA treated with or without an ICD, suggesting that an ICD may not be necessary in those patients. Therefore, the weight of the evidence suggests that in combination with a low LVEF, an MTWA test may help in guiding ICD therapy toward patients at highest risk and possibly away from those at lowest risk. However, randomized trials are needed to prove this hypothesis.

CLINICAL RISK STRATIFICATION

More recently, the role of clinical comorbidities in risk stratification has come to the forefront. Goldenberg and colleagues[43] showed that the benefit of ICDs is highest in patients with one or two high-risk clinical risk factors, but significantly attenuated, or even absent if the clinical risk was either very low or very high. The five clinical risk factors were age more than 70, New York Heart Association classification above 2, serum urea nitrogen greater than 26, atrial fibrillation, and QRS duration

greater than 0.12 ms. An ICD showed no benefit when patients had no risk factors and little benefit in those with three or more risk factors. On the other hand, in patients with one or two risk factors, ICD therapy was associated with a 49% reduction in the risk of death. In a clinical model derived from MUSTT, Buxton and colleagues[44] showed that the risk of death and sudden death are increased by several clinical variables in addition to LVEF and EPS results. Even more importantly, the relation between total and sudden mortality is not linear, and the clinical risk factors tend to increase total mortality more than sudden death.

Clinical Significance

The findings of the Goldenberg study suggest that the benefits of ICD therapy are attenuated in patients with a cardiomyopathy who have either no clinical risk factors or a multitude of them. The former group may be at a very low risk of ventricular tachyarrhythmic events, despite the low LVEF. The latter may have such advanced cardiovascular disease that their high 2-year total mortality (50% in the study) means that an ICD will not prevent death, because the predominant mode of death was nonarrhythmic. By contrast, the benefit of ICD therapy was pronounced (49% mortality reduction) in patients with one or two clinical risk factors. This U-shaped pattern may

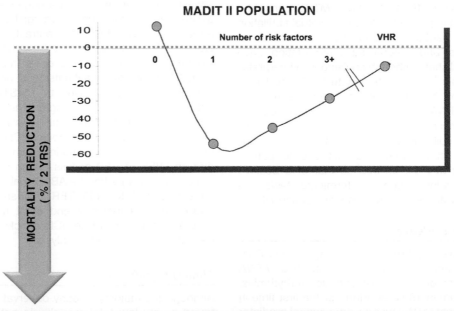

Fig. 3. Effect of clinical risk factors on the benefit of ICDs. The benefit of ICDs is most pronounced in patients with one or two clinical risk factors and much attenuated or nonexistent in patients who are either very low or very high risk (VHR). See text for discussion. (*Data from* Goldenberg I, Vyas AK, Hall WJ, et al. Risk stratification for primary implantation of a cardioverter-defibrillator in patients with ischemic left ventricular dysfunction. J Am Coll Cardiol 2008;51:292–96.)

need to be considered in future trials of risk stratification for SCD (**Fig. 3**).

COMPARISON BETWEEN TESTS

Several studies have attempted to compare the predictive value of noninvasive risk-stratifying tests for the risk of SCD. Gold and colleagues[45] showed that MTWA and EPS were better than a SAECG in predicting death or future ventricular arrhythmias in 215 patients referred to the electrophysiology laboratory. Ikeda and colleagues[46] showed that, in post-MI patients, MTWA and SAECG both predicted future ventricular tachyarrhythmias. Interestingly, the combination of the two had a very high positive (50%) and negative predictive value (99%), suggesting that the tests may be complementary. Hohnloser and colleagues[47] followed 137 patients with dilated cardiomyopathy and compared MTWA, baroreflex sensitivity, heart-rate variability, presence of nonsustained ventricular tachycardia, SAECG, and presence of intraventricular conduction defect. During an average follow-up of 14 months, they found that MTWA was the strongest and the only independent predictor of future ventricular tachyarrhythmias in multivariate analysis. Rashba and colleagues[48] found that MTWA was a better predictor of death or ventricular arrhythmia than EPS in patients with LVEF of 0.40 or less. In patients with a nonischemic cardiomyopathy, Grimm and colleagues[49] found that none of the noninvasive risk stratifiers were helpful in predicting future arrhythmic events.

CURRENT PERSPECTIVE ON RISK STRATIFICATION FOR SUDDEN CARDIAC DEATH AND FUTURE DIRECTIONS

Based on current guidelines and Centers for Medicare and Medicaid Services criteria for reimbursement, ICD implantation is appropriate in most patients based on a low LVEF as the sole stratifier for the risk of SCD. Although this strategy is very safe, it has reduced the cost-effectiveness of ICD therapy and diluted its beneficial effects, as many patients will never experience an appropriate shock. LVEF is a better marker of total mortality than it is of SCD. Finding a better marker of the electrophysiological substrate that underlies complex ventricular arrhythmias remains a challenge, however, as shown by the controversial results of many studies described in this review. Among the tests reviewed, MTWA has been studied most extensively and is currently the most promising noninvasive adjunct to LVEF. Arrhythmic mortality in patients with a negative HRV, HRT, or SAECG is also very low. Whether

patients who test negative to one or all of these risk-stratifying tests are at a low enough risk to safely avoid ICD implant remains to be determined. A strategy using one, two, or more of the other tests, in addition to LVEF, may expose some patients to the risk of SCD without the protection of an ICD. The acceptable risk threshold for deciding which patients should be treated with ICDs is ultimately a societal decision. In the end, the clinician must consider which strategy is most appropriate for each individual patient, depending on comorbidities, potential risk of ICD implant itself, willingness of the patient to undergo implant, and the risk of SCD weighed against the risk of nonsudden or noncardiac death.

It appears improbable that one test will give us the "Holy Grail" for risk stratification of SCD. Rather, as shown by many of the studies above, and in a recent study by Exner and colleagues,[50] future research should aim at using a combination of risk stratifiers to create a SCD "risk score." Randomized ICD intervention trials would then be needed to determine whether such an approach could safely avoid ICD therapy in a very low risk group or identify patients with a more preserved LVEF who are nonetheless at a higher risk for SCD and may benefit from prophylaxis with an ICD.

REFERENCES

1. European Heart Rhythm Association, Heart Rhythm Society, Zipes DP, et al. ACC/AHA/ESC 2006 guidelines for management of patients with ventricular arrhythmias and the prevention of sudden cardiac death. J Am Coll Cardiol 2006;48:e247–346.
2. Moss AJ, Hall WJ, Cannom DS, et al. Improved survival with an implanted defibrillator in patients with coronary disease at high risk for ventricular arrhythmia. N Engl J Med 1996;335:1933–40.
3. Buxton AE, Lee KL, Fisher JD, et al. A randomized study of the prevention of sudden death in patients with coronary artery disease. Multicenter unsustained tachycardia trial investigators. N Engl J Med 1999;341:1882–90.
4. Moss AJ, Zareba W, Hall WJ, et al. Prophylactic implantation of a defibrillator in patients with myocardial infarction and reduced ejection fraction. N Engl J Med 2002;346:877–83.
5. Bardy GH, Lee KL, Mark DB, et al. Amiodarone or an implantable cardioverter-defibrillator for congestive heart failure. N Engl J Med 2005;352:225–37.
6. Buxton AE, Lee KL, DiCarlo L, et al. Electrophysiologic testing to identify patients with coronary artery disease who are at risk for sudden death.

Multicenter unsustained tachycardia trial investigators. N Engl J Med 2000;342:1937–45.

7. Kadish A, Dyer A, Daubert JP, et al. Prophylactic defibrillator implantation in patients with nonischemic dilated cardiomyopathy. N Engl J Med 2004; 350:2151–8.

8. Salukhe TV, Dimopoulos K, Sutton R, et al. Life-years gained from defibrillator implantation: markedly nonlinear increase during 3 years of follow-up and its implications. Circulation 2004;109:1848–53.

9. Sanders GD, Hlatky MA, Owens DK. Cost-effectiveness of implantable cardioverter-defibrillators. N Engl J Med 2005;353:1471–80.

10. Poole JE, Johnson GW, Hellkamp AS, et al. Prognostic importance of defibrillator shocks in patients with heart failure. N Engl J Med 2008;359: 1009–17.

11. Epstein AE, Di Marco JP, Ellenbogen KA, et al. ACC/AHA/HRS 2008 guidelines for device based therapy of cardiac rhythm abnormalities. J Am Coll Cardiol 2008;51:1–62.

12. Kleiger RE, Miller JP, Bigger JT, et al. Decreased heart rate variability and its association with increased mortality after acute myocardial infarction. Am J Cardiol 1987;59:256–62.

13. Hartikainen JE, Malik M, Staunton A, et al. Distinction between arrhythmic and nonarrhythmic death after acute myocardial infarction based on heart rate variability, signal-averaged electrocardiogram, ventricular arrhythmias and left ventricular ejection fraction. J Am Coll Cardiol 1996;28:296–304.

14. Larovere MT, Bigger JT, Marcus FL, et al. Baroreflex sensitivity and heart-rate variability in prediction of total cardiac mortality after myocardial infarction (ATRAMI). Lancet 1998;351:478–84.

15. Hohnloser SH, Kuck KH, Dorian P, et al. Prophylactic use of an implantable cardioverter-defibrillator after acute myocardial infarction (DINAMIT). N Engl J Med 2004;351:2481–8.

16. Simpson MB. Use of signals in the terminal QRS complex to identify patients with recurrent ventricular tachycardia after myocardial infarction. Circulation 1981;64:235–42.

17. Lindsay BD, Markham J, Schechtman KB, et al. Identification of patients with sustained ventricular tachycardia by frequency analysis of signal-averaged electrocardiograms despite the presence of bundle branch block. Circulation 1988;77: 122–30.

18. Bailey JJ, Berson AS, Handelsman H, et al. Utility of current risk stratification tests for predicting major arrhythmic events after myocardial infarction. J Am Coll Cardiol 2001;38:1902–11.

19. Bigger JT Jr. Prophylactic use of implanted cardiac defibrillators in patients at high risk for ventricular arrhythmias after coronary-artery bypass graft surgery. Coronary Artery Bypass Graft (CABG) Patch Trial Investigators. N Engl J Med 1997;337: 1569–75.

20. Gomes JA, Caine ME, Buxton AE. Prediction of long-term outcomes by signal-averaged electrocardiography in patients with unsustained ventricular tachycardia, coronary artery disease, and left ventricular dysfunction. Circulation 2001;104:436–41.

21. Schmidt G, Malik M, Barthel P, et al. Heart-rate turbulence after ventricular premature beats as a predictor of mortality after acute myocardial infarction. Lancet 1999;353:1390–6.

22. Voss A, Baier V, Schumann A, et al. Postextrasystolic regulation patterns of blood pressure and heart rate in patients with idiopathic dilated cardiomyopathy. J Physiol 2002;538:271–8.

23. Julian DG, Gamm AJ, Frangin G, et al. Randomised trial of effect of amiodarone on mortality in patients with left-ventricular dysfunction after recent myocardial infarction EMIAT. Lancet 1997;349:667–74.

24. Bigger JJ, Fleiss JL, Kleiger R, et al. The relationships among ventricular arrhythmias, left ventricular dysfunction, and mortality in the 2 years after myocardial infarction. Circulation 1984;69: 250–8.

25. Ghuran A, Reid F, La Rovere MT, et al. Heart rate turbulence-based predictors of fatal and nonfatal cardiac arrest. The Autonomic Tone and Reflexes After Myocardial Infarction substudy. Am J Cardiol 2002;89:184–90.

26. Makikallio TH, Barthel P, Schneider R, et al. Prediction of sudden cardiac death after acute myocardial infarction: role of Holter monitoring in the modern treatment era. Eur Heart J 2005;26:762–9.

27. Barthel P, Schneider R, Bauer A, et al. Risk stratification after acute myocardial infarction by heart rate turbulence. Circulation 2003;108:1221–6.

28. Francis J, Watanabe MA, Schmidt G. Heart rate turbulence: a new predictor for risk of sudden cardiac death. Ann Noninvasive Electrocardiol 2005;10:102–9.

29. Smith JM, Clancy EA, Valeri CR, et al. Electrical alternans and cardiac electrical instability. Circulation 1988;77:110–21.

30. Pastore JM, Girouard SD, Laurita KR, et al. Mechanism linking T-wave alternans to the genesis of cardiac fibrillation. Circulation 1999;99:1385–94.

31. Bloomfield DM, Hohnloser SH, Cohen RJ. Interpretation and classification of microvolt T wave alternans tests. J Cardiovasc Electrophysiol 2002;13:502–12.

32. Kaufman ES, Bloomfield DM, Steinman RC, et al. "Indeterminate" microvolt T-wave alternans tests predict high risk of death or sustained ventricular arrhythmias in patients with left ventricular dysfunction. J Am Coll Cardiol 2006;48:1399–404.

33. Rosenbaum DS, Jackson LE, Smith JM, et al. Electrical alternans and vulnerability to ventricular arrhythmias. N Engl J Med 1994;330:235–41.

34. Klingenheben T, Zabel M, D'Agostino RB, et al. Predictive value of T-wave alternans for arrhythmic events in patients with congestive heart failure. Lancet 2000;356:651–2.

35. Bloomfield DM, Bigger JT, Steinman RC, et al. Microvolt T-wave alternans and the risk of death or sustained ventricular arrhythmias in patients with left ventricular dysfunction. J Am Coll Cardiol 2006;47:456–63.

36. Gehi AK, Stein RH, Metz LD, et al. Microvolt T-wave alternans for the risk stratification of ventricular tachyarrhythmic events: a meta-analysis. J Am Coll Cardiol 2005;46:75–82.

37. Costantini O, Hohnloser SH, Kirk MK, et al. The Alternans Before Cardioverter Defibrillator (ABCD) trial: strategies using T-wave alternans to improve efficiency of sudden cardiac death prevention. J Am Coll Cardiol 2009;53:471–9.

38. Gold MR, Ip JH, Costantini O, et al. Role of microvolt T-wave alternans in assessment of arrhythmia vulnerability among patients with heart failure and systolic dysfunction: primary results from the T-Wave Alternans Sudden Cardiac Death in Heart Failure trial substudy. Circulation 2008;118:2022–8.

39. Chow T, Kereiakes DJ, Onufer J, et al. Does microvolt T-wave alternans testing predict ventricular tachyarrhythmias in patients with ischemic cardiomyopathy and prophylactic defibrillators? The MASTER (Microvolt T Wave Alternans Testing for Risk Stratification of Post–Myocardial Infarction Patients) trial. J Am Coll Cardiol 2008;52:1607–15.

40. Hohnloser SH, Ikeda T, Cohen RJ. Evidence regarding clinical use of microvolt T-wave alternans. Heart Rhythm 2009;6:S36–44.

41. Bloomfield DM, Steinman RC, Namerow PB, et al. Microvolt T-wave alternans distinguishes between patients likely and patients not likely to benefit from implanted cardiac defibrillator therapy: a solution to the Multicenter Automatic Defibrillator Implantation Trial (MADIT) II conundrum. Circulation 2004; 110:1885–9.

42. Chow T, Kereiakes DJ, Bartone C, et al. Prognostic utility of microvolt T-wave alternans in risk stratification of patients with ischemic cardiomyopathy. J Am Coll Cardiol 2006;47:1820–7.

43. Goldenberg I, Vyas AK, Hall WJ, et al. Risk stratification for primary implantation of a cardioverter-defibrillator in patients with ischemic left ventricular dysfunction. J Am Coll Cardiol 2008;51:288–96.

44. Buxton AE, Lee KL, Hafley GE, et al. Limitations of ejection fraction for prediction of sudden death risk in patients with coronary artery disease: lessons from the MUSTT study. J Am Coll Cardiol 2007;50: 1150–7.

45. Gold MR, Bloomfield DM, Anderson KP, et al. A comparison of T-wave alternans, signal averaged electrocardiography and programmed ventricular stimulation for arrhythmia risk stratification. J Am Coll Cardiol 2000;36:2247–53.

46. Ikeda T, Sakata T, Takami M, et al. Combined assessment of T wave alternans and late potentials used to predict arrhythmic events after myocardial infarction. J Am Coll Cardiol 2000;35: 722–30.

47. Hohnloser SH, Klingenheben T, Bloomfield D, et al. Usefulness of microvolt T-wave alternans for prediction of ventricular tachyarrhythmic events in patients with dilated cardiomyopathy: results from a prospective observational study. J Am Coll Cardiol 2003;41: 2220–4.

48. Rashba EJ, Osman AF, Macmurdy K, et al. Enhanced detection of arrhythmia vulnerability using T wave alternans, left ventricular ejection fraction, and programmed ventricular stimulation: a prospective study in subjects with chronic ischemic heart disease. J Cardiovasc Electrophysiol 2004;15: 170–6.

49. Grimm W, Christ M, Bach J, et al. Noninvasive arrhythmia risk stratification in idiopathic dilated cardiomyopathy: results of the Marburg cardiomyopathy study. Circulation 2003;108:2883–9.

50. Exner DV, Kavanagh KM, Slawnych MP. Noninvasive risk assessment early after a myocardial infarction. The REFINE study. J Am Coll Cardiol 2007;11(50): 2275–84.

End-Stage Renal Disease and Sudden Cardiac Death

Rahul Sakhuja, MD, MPP, MSc[a], Ashok J. Shah, MD[b],
Swapnil Hiremath, MD, MPH[c], Ranjan K. Thakur, MD, MPH, FHRS[d],*

KEYWORDS

- Renal insufficiency • Chronic kidney disease
- Dialysis • Sudden cardiac death • Review
- Therapy • Epidemiology • Predictors

The burden of chronic kidney disease (CKD), defined as diminished glomerular filtration rate (GFR), in the United States is approximately 13% to 16%, with approximately 400,000 patients receiving hemodialysis every year.[1] CKD is classified from stage 1 to 5, with stage 1 representing GFR equal to or greater than 90 mL/min/1.73 m^2 and stage 5 representing end-stage renal disease (ESRD) with GFR equal to or less than 15 mL/min/1.73 m^2 or requiring renal replacement therapy (dialysis or renal transplantation) for survival. Hemodialysis is the modality of renal replacement therapy for the majority of ESRD patients.[1] Over the past 2 decades, the prevalence of CKD has risen dramatically and is expected to continue to increase.[2] By 2030, it is expected that over 2 million patients may be on dialysis.[1]

Patients with ESRD face extraordinarily high mortality rates. In 2006, the death rate for dialysis patients in the United States was almost 8 times higher than that in general population.[1] The 5-year survival remains low (33% for ESRD patients on dialysis) and has improved only marginally (30% a decade ago).[1]

ESRD is an independent predictor of cardiovascular death for a large spectrum of cardiovascular diseases.[3–5] Therefore, it is not surprising that cardiovascular disease is the major cause of death in this population. Cardiovascular causes of death account for 43% of deaths in patients on dialysis. Among patients receiving dialysis, more than 60% of cardiovascular deaths are due to arrhythmias.[6] As such, sudden cardiac death (SCD) accounts for more than 25% of all deaths in dialysis patients, and the rate is increasing.[7] Moreover, survivorship from SCD in patients with ESRD is very poor (Fig. 1). The survival rate for those who undergo cardiopulmonary resuscitation (CPR) is at least 50% lower than the survival rate in the general population.[8–10]

This article reviews the relationship between ESRD, particularly dialysis, and sudden cardiac death (SCD), specifically addressing possible mechanisms, therapies, and prognostic factors.

VENTRICULAR ARRHYTHMIAS AND SUDDEN CARDIAC DEATH IN CHRONIC KIDNEY DISEASE/END-STAGE RENAL DISEASE

Ventricular arrhythmia, particularly ventricular tachycardia degenerating into ventricular fibrillation, is the most common cause of SCD. In a study of 157 patients with SCD captured by 24-hour ambulatory electrocardiographic (EKG)

[a] Interventional Cardiology, Massachusetts General Hospital, 55 Fruit Street, GRB 800, Boston, MA 02114, USA
[b] Cardiac Electrophysiology, Thoracic and Cardiovascular Institute, Sparrow Health System, Michigan State University, 1215 E. Michigan Avenue, Lansing, MI 48912, USA
[c] Division of Nephrology, University of Ottawa, Ottawa Hospital - Civic Campus, 751 Parkdale Avenue, Suite 106, Ottawa, ON K1Y 1J7, Canada
[d] Arrhythmia Service, Thoracic and Cardiovascular Institute, Sparrow Health System, Michigan State University, 405 West Greenlawn, Suite 400, Lansing, MI 48910, USA
* Corresponding author.
E-mail address: thakur@msu.edu (R.K. Thakur).

Card Electrophysiol Clin 1 (2009) 61–77
doi:10.1016/j.ccep.2009.08.006
1877-9182/09/$ – see front matter © 2009 Published by Elsevier Inc.

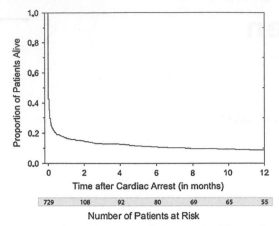

Fig. 1. Kaplan-Meier curve for survival after cardiac arrest in outpatient hemodialysis clinics. (*From* Pun PH, Lehrich RW, Smith SR, et al. Predictors of survival after cardiac arrest in outpatient hemodialysis clinics. Clin J Am Soc Nephrol 2007;2:491–500; with permission.)

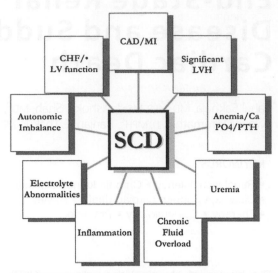

Fig. 2. Causal factors for sudden cardiac death in end stage renal disease. CAD, coronary artery disease; CHF, congestive heart failure; LV, left ventricular; LVH, left ventricular hypertrophy; MI, myocardial infarction; PTH, parathyroid hormone; SCD, sudden cardiac death. (*From* Herzog C, Mangrum J, Passman R. Sudden cardiac death and dialysis patients. Semin Dial 2008;21(4):300–7; with permission.)

monitoring, nearly 85% of deaths were attributed to ventricular arrhythmias.[11] Subsequent data from implantable cardioverter defibrillators (ICDs) have confirmed this finding.

Ventricular arrhythmias are often precipitated by a triggering event in the setting of an altered underlying cardiac substrate. ESRD is associated with alterations in the underlying substrate as well as increased frequency of triggering events. Estimates from small, early studies suggest anywhere from 30% to 90% of patients on dialysis have evidence of ventricular arrhythmias, with variability depending on the definition (eg, premature ventricular complexes versus sustained ventricular arrhythmias).[12–14] Although not all ventricular arrhythmias lead to SCD, ventricular arrhythmias account for nearly 70% of SCD in the peridialysis period.[15] Moreover, in the Antiarrhythmics Versus Implantable Defibrillators (AVID) trial, patients with ventricular tachycardias, even "stable" ventricular tachycardias, were at high risk for SCD. Estimates of sudden cardiac death among dialysis patients are correspondingly extraordinarily high. In addition, the incidence of SCD in dialysis patients increases by approximately 50% on dialysis days.[16]

MECHANISMS OF SUDDEN CARDIAC DEATH IN PATIENTS WITH END-STAGE RENAL FAILURE

The association between ESRD and SCD is multifactorial (**Fig. 2**). The risk factors for ESRD and traditional risk factors for cardiovascular disease, and hence SCD, are similar. In addition, electrolyte abnormalities and their fluctuations likely increase the risk of SCD in ESRD. Many of the risk factors

that predispose the general population to SCD are more prevalent among patients with ESRD.

Renal Milieu

One of the original theories suggested that the increased incidence of cardiac arrhythmias in ESRD is associated with metabolic derangements: dynamic changes in electrolytes (K^+, Ca^{2+}, PO_4^{3-}, HCO_3^-), blood pH, volume status, and blood pressure may increase the risk of SCD in hemodialysis patients compared with the general population. Alterations in electrolyte concentrations associated with ESRD and dialysis may alter the electrical characteristics of myocytes. In turn, this may predispose patients with ESRD to ventricular arrhythmias. Increases in SCD during dialysis and in the hours before hemodialysis at the end of a long weekend interval support these theories.[15,17]

Role of potassium

Hyperkalemia is common among patients with ESRD. In renal failure, the inability to clear potassium leads to its accumulation. In addition, hemodialysis can cause rapid potassium removal and hypokalemia. A significant consequence of alterations in potassium levels is cardiac arrhythmia.[18] Both hyper- and hypokalemia have been associated with ventricular arrhythmias and SCD.[19–21] A large cohort of more than 81,000 patients receiving hemodialysis was followed over 3 years: in this cohort, potassium levels of less than 4.0 or greater than 5.6 mEq/L were associated with increased mortality.[22]

Role of calcium/phosphorus/parathyroid hormone

Calcium phosphate metabolism is altered in hemodialysis. Changes in serum calcium and phosphate levels have been reported to precipitate ventricular arrhythmias.[23,24] A multivariate-adjusted analysis of cause-specific death of more than 12,000 patients demonstrated that hyperphosphatemia, elevated calcium-phosphorus product, and elevated parathyroid hormone were all specifically associated with increased risk of SCD (**Fig. 3**).[25] In particular, para-thyroid hormone dependent myocardial fibrosis in patients with hypertrophy or uremia might contribute to the higher incidence of ventricular arrhythmias.[26–31]

Role of uremia

Uremia has been described as a "pro-arrhythmic" state.[32] Uremia has been shown to cause diffuse intermyocyte fibrosis. Multiple areas of patchy fibrosis create heterogeneous electrophysiologic properties, which underlie reentrant circuits and ventricular tachyarrhythmias.[27,31,33]

Insulin resistance associated with uremia increases the reliance of the myocardium on less efficient fatty acid metabolism, rendering myocytes more prone to cell death.[34,35] In the left ventricular hypertrophy (LVH) variant of uremic cardiomyopathy, a mismatch between myocardial oxygen supply and demand renders patients less tolerant of ischemia and more susceptible to

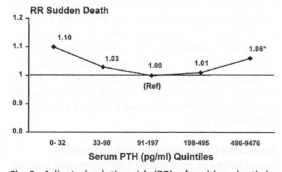

Fig. 3. Adjusted relative risk (RR) of sudden death by serum parathyroid hormone (PTH) levels in quintiles. *P<.05 compared with RR of 1.0. (*From* Ganesh SK, Stack AG, Levin NW, et al. Association of elevated serum PO(4), Ca × PO(4) product, and parathyroid hormone with cardiac mortality risk in chronic hemodialysis patients. J Am Soc Nephrol 2001;12(10):2131–8; with permission.)

arrhythmias.[36] Uremic cardiomyopathy may also manifest with left ventricular dysfunction, which is a predictor of SCD.[37] Finally, uremia increases the risk of SCD through other factors associated with SCD, such as hypertrophy, anemia, and abnormal calcium phosphate handling.[28,30,31]

Role of anemia

Anemia is independently associated with ESRD and SCD. Anemia is associated with increased mortality in patients with ESRD.[38] In addition, anemia is associated with SCD in patients with diastolic heart failure, which is more common in ESRD.[39] However, its specific association with SCD in patients with ESRD remains to be determined. Other possible mechanisms that might mediate this relationship, such as low coronary reserve and myocardial fibrosis.[40]

Acute effects of dialysis

Although ESRD is associated with SCD, the increased risk of SCD around and during hemodialysis suggests that the acute effects of dialysis play a role in SCD. In the setting of reduced coronary flow reserve associated with dialysis patients, hemodynamic alterations accompanying dialysis are more likely to induce ischemia.[41] Moreover, subclinical ischemia might depress left ventricular function.[42] Finally, rapid fluctuations in electrolytes may have arrhythmogenic effects. Some studies suggest that both hemodialysis and peritoneal dialysis are equally arrhythmogenic, whereas others suggest that hemodialysis may be more so.[43–45] Estimates of sudden cardiac death are similar for both peritoneal dialysis and hemodialysis: 58% of cardiac deaths (25% of all deaths) among patients receiving peritoneal dialysis and 64% of cardiac deaths (27% of all deaths) among patients receiving hemodialysis.[9,46]

Overlapping Risk Factors

In addition to risk factors unique to ESRD, traditional risk factors for SCD are highly prevalent in patients with ESRD (**Box 1**).

Myocardial ischemia/infarction

Many studies have shown that renal dysfunction is an independent risk factor for coronary artery disease (CAD).[47] Renal dysfunction predisposes patients to premature development of cardiovascular disease, increases the incidence of myocardial infarction (MI) in patients with CAD, and reduces survival after MI, even among those who undergo revascularization.[48–54] The lower the GFR, the greater the risk.[55] In particular, renal dysfunction is associated with worse outcomes post MI.[56–58]

Box 1
Potential factors increasing the risk of sudden death in dialysis patients

1. Myocardial ischemia/infarction (eg fibrosis, microvessel disease, reduced ischemia tolerance)
2. LVH and hypertension
3. Congestive heart failure
4. Electrolyte shifts (eg pottasium, calcium) and acute volume shifts
5. Abnormal calcium/phosphate metabolism and hyperparathyroidism
6. Sympathetic overactivity and autonomic dysfunction
7. Angiotensin II induced electrical remodeling
8. QT dispersion
9. QT prolonging medications
10. Anemia
11. Uremial-related risk factors (inflammation, oxidative stress)
12. Other (eg obstructive sleep apnea)

Data from Ritz E, Wanner C. The challenge of sudden death in dialysis patients. Clin J Am Soc Nephrol 2008;3(3):920–9.

Ultimately, it is difficult to decipher cause and effect, whether renal disease causes atherosclerotic disease or vice versa. Some attribute the higher incidence of cardiovascular events to "renalism"—the decreased use of proven therapies in patients with ESRD. In fact, patients with ESRD are much less likely to be treated with aspirin, β-blockers, and angiotensin-converting enzyme (ACE) inhibitors relative to non-ESRD patients.[59] Coronary angiograms are performed less frequently in those deemed appropriate for the procedure, probably because of concern about the use of intravenous contrast agents and its nephrotoxic effects.[60]

Nevertheless, ST-segment monitoring has demonstrated increased ischemia during dialysis among patients with ventricular arrhythmias.[13,61] Acute ischemia alters the action potential due to loss of function of the sodium-potassium adenosine triphosphatase pump. The border zone between ischemic and nonischemic tissues, therefore, has heterogeneous electrical properties. This heterogeneity leads to reentrant circuits, triggered by subendocardial Purkinje fibers as well as surges in catecholamines.[33] After the acute phase, collagen deposition and scar formation creates further substrate for reentry; the size of the scar may correlate with the inducibility of ventricular arrhythmias.[62]

Congestive heart failure

Another significant risk factor for SCD is left ventricular systolic dysfunction, especially with clinical heart failure.[37,63] Among a cohort of patients with ESRD, 15% to 28% were reported to have systolic dysfunction at the onset of dialysis.[64,65] Almost one-third of patients starting dialysis have congestive heart failure (CHF).[66] Regardless of the etiology, clinical heart failure increases the risk of SCD up to 5-fold in some studies.[67] Of note, patients with milder heart failure (eg, class II) are more likely to die of SCD than are patients with worse heart failure (eg, class III/IV), who are more likely to die of pump failure and bradyarrhythmias.[68,69] Ultimately, the causes for SCD in patients with CHF are likely varied, particularly among patients with renal dysfunction, for example, neurohormonal activation, sympathetic activation, volume overload, uremia, and associated fibrosis.[40,70]

Left ventricular hypertrophy and hypertension

LVH has long been implicated as a risk factor for SCD. More than 50% of patients with ESRD exhibit LVH, related to factors such as hypertension, anemia, and secondary hyperparathyroidism.[26,64,71,72] The frequency of ventricular arrhythmias is greater in patients with LVH who have renal dysfunction than those who do not.[73,74]

Hypertension occurs in more than 70% of patients with ESRD prior to initiation of dialysis, and is highly prevalent in patients with LVH.[1] Hypertension is also an independent risk factor for SCD.[75,76] In one multivariate model, hypertension was one of the only risk factors for ventricular arrhythmias after adjusting for other factors.[77]

The pathogenesis of SCD among patients with LVH is likely multifactorial.[78] LVH reduces coronary reserve and increases mismatch between myocytes and capillaries, predisposing patients to ischemia.[36,79] Autopsy studies, however, revealed that underlying CAD is not the sole mechanism for SCD.[80] LVH is also associated with increased interstitial fibrosis, particularly in uremic patients.[27] Underlying the hypertrophy is myocardial scar, which may serve as the basis of reentrant arrhythmias.[81,82]

Sympathetic nervous system activation

Renal failure is associated with increased sympathetic activation.[83] The loss of vagal tone associated with renal failure may further increase sympathetic tone.[70] In addition, renalase, which is secreted by the kidneys and catabolizes catecholamines, is reduced in ESRD.[84]

By altering both triggered activity and the underlying substrate the sympathetic nervous system increases the risk of ventricular arrhythmias. Animal studies demonstrated the relationship between sympathetic activation and SCD by showing that cardiac sympathectomy protects against ventricular fibrillation (VF) during coronary occlusion.[85] Patients with ventricular arrhythmias have greater cardiac norepinephrine spillover into plasma, consistent with elevated sympathetic nervous activity.[86] Increased plasma norepinephrine levels in patients with ESRD are associated with increased cardiovascular events.[87] The sympathetic nervous system activates the renin-angiotensin-aldosterone system (RAAS), which can increase myocyte fibrosis.[70,88] Increased sympathetic activation also contributes to hypertension and CHF, which may further increase the risk of SCD.[83]

THERAPY

Therapies focus on preventing SCD in this population, given the poor outcomes, as well as treating those who experience SCD. The dysmetabolic state and decreased renal clearance may alter the efficacy of therapies with proven benefit in patients with normal renal function. The perturbed myocyte transmembrane electrical properties might alter the efficacy of nondrug therapies for prevention and treatment of arrhythmic death in patients with ESRD. Therefore, therapies in patients with ESRD require further study.

Medical Therapy

Changes in delivery of dialysis
Delivery of increased dose of dialysis and use of higher flux membranes has not been shown to increase survival in hemodialysis patients.[89,90] Observational data suggest that the greatest survival is associated with potassium levels between 4.0 and 5.5 mEq/L, it would be difficult to maintain potassium levels in that narrow range with conventional 3-times-a week hemodialysis.[22] Indeed, low-potassium dialysate and intermittent dialysis are associated with cardiac arrhythmias and worse outcomes.[17,91] Low-calcium dialysate similarly predisposes to prolonged QT dispersion, which may predispose to SCD.[43] More frequent and dialysis and alterations in dialysis strategies (ie nocturnal dialysis) are may reduce the arrhythmic potential of dialysis. For example, frequent nocturnal hemodialysis has been shown to improve left ventricular mass compared with conventional hemodialysis,[92] sleep apnea, and baroreflex sensitivity.[93,94] A nonrandomized comparison also suggests that more frequent short daily dialysis may improve survival in hemodialysis patients.[95]

Other medical therapy
Attempts have been made to correct the other metabolic derangements associated with ESRD. Intensive nutritional supplementation has been studied: while increasing prealbumin to more than 30 mg/L was associated with decreased mortality, intradialytic parenteral nutrition was no better than oral nutrition at achieving this.[96] In addition, anemia has been implicated in causing low coronary reserve, predisposing to arrhythmias. However, normalization of anemia with erythropoietin does not reduce, and may increase, cardiovascular events.[97,98] None of these strategies has been shown to reduce overall mortality, and the impact on SCD in particular has not been investigated.

Drug Therapy for Sudden Cardiac Death in Chronic Kidney Disease/End-Stage Renal Disease

β-Blockers, RAAS modulators, antiarrhythmic drugs, and statins have been shown to reduce cardiovascular events in patients with normal renal function. There is some evidence that some of these may be effective in reducing SCD as well.[99]

β-Blockers
β-Blockers have antifibrillatory activity, and have been shown to reduce sudden death in patients with CAD, CHF, and hypertension, all of which are more prevalent in patients with ESRD. In addition, β-blockers have sympathoinhibitory effects, improving heart rate variability and baroreceptor sensitivity.[100–103] However, the data for β-blockers reducing SCD in ESRD are mixed.

Observational studies support the use of β-blockers in chronic dialysis patients, both with and without CHF, even after cardiac arrest.[99,104,105] Carvedilol was associated with a reduction in ventricular tachycardia among patients with hypertension and ischemic heart disease. This result was attributed to modulation of adrenergic tone and prevention of sudden hypokalemia in the first phase of hemodialysis, a potential cause for increased frequency of intra- and postdialytic arrhythmias.[106] There has been only one small, randomized placebo-controlled study of β-blockers in hemodialysis patients. In patients with dilated cardiomyopathy receiving dialysis, there was a greater than 50% reduction in cardiovascular deaths at 2 years in patients receiving carvedilol (**Fig. 4**).[107]

However, a meta-analysis of all observational studies looking at mortality among patients with ICDs in relation to renal function suggested that β-blockers might not be as cardioprotective in the patients receiving dialysis, although not all

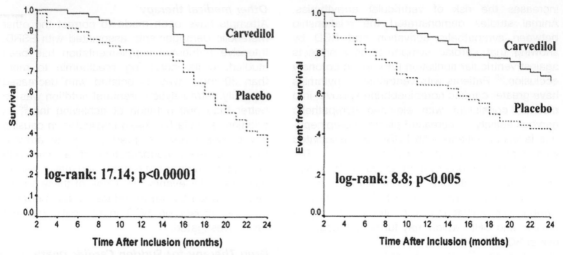

Fig. 4. Kaplan-Meier curves for cardiovascular death (*left*) and for all-cause hospitalization (*right*) during 24-month follow-up cumulative survival rate according to use of carvedilol. (*From* Cice G, Ferrara L, D'Andrea A, et al. Carvedilol increases two-year survival in dialysis patients with dilated cardiomyopathy: a prospective, placebo-controlled trial. J Am Coll Cardiol 2003;41:1438–44; with permission.)

studies in this meta-analysis reported on β-blocker use.[108] Other studies have echoed this concern. One concern regarding the safety of β-blockers in patients on hemodialysis is intradialytic hypotension. Of note, hypotension from β-blockers does not seem to occur more often than with other agents.[109] Moreover, one study suggested that, when carefully managed, β-blockers were not associated with substantial reductions in blood pressure or increases in intradialytic hypotensive episodes, even when using atenolol, which is predominantly renally cleared. However, in this study the average systolic blood pressure was higher at baseline.[110] Another less common concern with β-blockers includes hyperkalemia, mediated by blockade of β_2 receptors, which is more common with non-selective β-blockers.[111,112]

Renin-angiotensin-aldosterone system inhibition

ACE inhibitors, angiotensin receptor blockers (ARBs), and aldosterone antagonists also exhibit antifibrillatory properties. Elevated angiotensin II sensitizes end organs to damaging effects of high sympathetic tone.[113] Moreover, angiotensin II and aldosterone are associated with myocardial hypertrophy and fibrosis, both associated with increased risk for SCD.[88,114,115] It is conceivable that some of the survival benefit of RAAS antagonism is due to a reduction in SCD.

In non-ESRD populations, some trials demonstrate a lower incidence of SCD in patients receiving ACE inhibitors, yet none of the trials report a statistically significant reduction.[116–118]

These post hoc analyses of trials of acute MI or heart failure were underpowered to detect differences in the arrhythmic end points. On the other hand, aldosterone antagonism seems to reduce SCD in patients without ESRD.[119,120]

In renal failure, there are few data on ACE inhibitors/ARBs, despite their proven safety and efficacy in this subgroup.[121] Small studies have reported that independent of their blood pressure effects, ACE inhibitors/ARBs seem to decrease mortality in patients with ESRD on chronic dialysis, even after cardiac arrest.[99,122,123] However, prospective studies in ESRD patients produce varied results. Studies of ACE inhibitors failed to demonstrate a reduction in cardiovascular events or SCD.[124,125] ARBs, on the other hand, may have some benefit. In a small study of 80 patients on chronic hemodialysis, candesartan significantly reduced mortality, including SCD. In the control arm, 4 of 37 patients had severe or fatal arrhythmias versus none of the patients on candesartan (P value not reported).[126] Another small, open-label study also showed a significant improvement in the composite end point of cardiovascular events with the use of ARBs.[127] There are no data on aldosterone antagonism in ESRD, likely due to infrequent use in renal failure patients because of the increased incidence of hyperkalemia observed in patients with normal renal function.

3-Hydroxy-3-methylglutaryl coenzyme A reductase inhibitor

Serum lipids and C-reactive protein (CRP) predict cardiac death in hemodialysis patients.[128,129]

Whereas statins have been shown to reduce cardiovascular death in many high-risk patients. It is unclear whether any reduction in coronary events is due to a reduction in SCD, although there are some data to support an antiarrhythmic effect of statins in patients with normal renal function. In a substudy of the Multicenter Automatic Defibrillator Implantation Trial-II (MADIT-II), patients on statin therapy had a lower rate of ventricular tachycardia (VT)/VF.[130] Moeover, atorvastatin, 80 mg daily, reduced the relative risk of VT/VF recurrence in patients with CAD who have an ICD.[131] Data on the effect of statin therapy on cardiovascular mortality may differ depending on whether the patient is receiving dialysis or not.[132] A Cochrane review of patients with stages 3 to 4 CKD but not on dialysis, suggested a reduction in all-cause and cardiovascular mortality with statin therapy.[133,134] Despite previous observational studies, more recent large randomized trials of statin therapy in patients on dialysis, with or without diabetes, have shown no benefit.[135–137]

Antiarrhythmic drugs
There are no data on the safety and efficacy of antiarrhythmic drugs in patients with renal dysfunction. Regarding safety, there are concerns over the safety of antiarrhythmic agents in the setting of reduced renal clearance. With regard to efficacy, ICDs seem to be superior to antiarrhythmic drugs in patients with normal renal function for both primary and secondary prevention.[138,139] In patients with ischemic cardiomyopathy, β-blockers are the only antiarrhythmic medications shown to prevent SCD.[140] In fact, other antiarrhythmic drugs may even be harmful in some cases.[141,142]

Given the limited role of non–β-blocker antiarrhythmic drugs in SCD in the general population and the concern over the use of these medications in the setting of ESRD, use of these medications in routine clinical practice is limited. Any benefits of antiarrhythmic drugs relative to placebo remain unknown in ESRD patients.

Device Therapy for Sudden Cardiac Death in Chronic Kidney Disease/End-Stage Renal Disease

Implantable defibrillators
None of the trials demonstrating the efficacy of ICDs in primary and secondary prevention included patients with ESRD. Therefore, present understanding of the role of ICDs in dialysis patients is based on very small, single-center observational studies. Even in the absence of data, the number of patients with ESRD receiving ICDs has risen much more rapidly than in the

non-CKD population (**Fig. 5**), though overall use remains limited to 0.6% of patients receiving dialysis.[143] Even among patients who survived a cardiac arrest as well as the subsequent 30 days, only 7.6% received an ICD. This result has prompted some to argue that ICDs are underutilized in the dialysis population.

Only one study has compared survival in dialysis patients with ICDs with those without ICDs for secondary prevention. This retrospective analysis studied a select group of patients from the Medicare database who survived VF/cardiac arrest, were deemed appropriate to receive an ICD within 30 days of admission, were subsequently discharged alive, and survived at least 30 days. Within this select group, ICD implantation was associated with a 42% reduction in risk of mortality using a propensity-adjusted model (**Fig. 6**; $P<.0001$). The 5-year survival was low in both groups (22% in the ICD group vs 12% in the no-ICD group). Of the 288 patients with prior ICDs in this study (who were excluded), 45% survived to discharge, although their long-term survival was unclear.[144] There are no data within the ESRD population evaluating the role of ICDs for primary prevention.

Multiple small studies have studied the impact of ESRD on outcomes in patients with ICD therapy. A recent meta-analysis of 7 observational studies suggested that patients on dialysis receiving an ICD experienced a 2.7 times greater risk of death compared with patients not on dialysis.[108] Thus, despite all of these patients having ICDs, there was still a nearly 3-fold increase in the risk of death over an average of 33 months of follow-up. The most common cause of death was progressive heart failure. Data suggest that whereas dialysis patients receive appropriate shocks for ventricular arrhythmias, their survival is significantly shorter than nondialysis patients.[145] On the other hand,

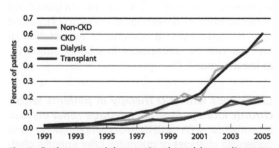

Fig. 5. Patients receiving an implantable cardioverter defibrillator or cardiac resynchronization therapy + defibrillator. CKD, chronic kidney disease. (*From* United States Renal Data System: Cardiovascular special studies, USRDS 2007; with permission.) Available at: http://www.usrds.org/2007/pdf/09_cv_07.pdf.

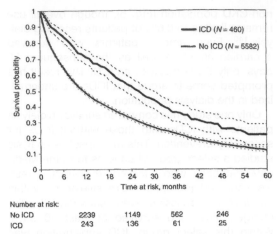

Fig. 6. Estimated unadjusted survival of dialysis patients with and without an implantable cardioverter defibrillator (ICD). P<.0001 by log rank test for comparison of patients with ICD to those without ICD. Dashed lines indicate 95% confidence intervals. (*From* Herzog CA, Li S, Weinhandl ED, et al. Survival of dialysis patients after cardiac arrest and the impact of implantable cardioverter defibrillators. Kidney Int 2005;68(2):818–25; with permission.)

overall the risk of death in patients on dialysis compared with the nondialysis population is 6-fold higher.[1] With this in mind ICDs do seem to narrow the gap. Using a decision analytic model, Amin and colleagues[146] reported that the benefits of ICDs in patients with ESRD might be limited to those younger than 65 years old. The Implantable Cardioverter Defibrillators in Dialysis Patients (ICD2), a pilot study of 200 patients, irrespective of left ventricular ejection fraction, will evaluate ICD versus no ICD in patients 55- to 80-year-old patients receiving dialysis; however, trials with broader inclusion criteria remain necessary.[147] Until then, the indication for ICD and cumulative risk factors for SCD, as well as the anticipated survival, should guide decisions to implant ICDs in patients with ESRD. The most recent guidelines consider primary prevention ICD therapy indicated only in those with "a reasonable expectation of survival with an acceptable functional status for at least 1 year."[148]

Challenges with ICD therapy in patients with chronic kidney disease/end-stage renal disease

In patients with ESRD, ICD implantation and generator changes or upgrades offer specific challenges. Increased bleeding diathesis, anticoagulant and antiplatelet therapies, and malnutrition increase the risk of bleeding.[149] Delayed wound infection is more common than in the general population: the odds were nearly 5 times higher among

those with moderate to severe renal dysfunction.[150] The increased infectious risk is likely related to direct access for pathogens to the blood stream via indwelling catheters as well as increased host susceptibility due to the relatively immunocompromised state.

Moreover, patients continue to have arrhythmic death despite receiving ICD. Patients with ESRD have high defibrillation thresholds; one study found that more than 35% of dialysis patients had high defibrillation thresholds versus less than 10% without CKD.[151] In addition, ICD implantation ipsilateral to dialysis access has been associated with high rates of thrombotic occlusion that may lead to suboptimal dialysis and metabolic derangement, which may in turn lead to subsequent lethal arrhythmia as well as refractoriness to therapy.[152] Meticulous hemostasis and infection control, avoidance of postimplant anticoagulation if possible, placement of intravascular leads on the contralateral side of dialysis access, and high-energy devices are often recommended.

External defibrillators

The incidence of SCD increases during the peridialysis period, and again as the interdialytic interval lengthens (**Fig. 7**).[15,17] One study estimated 0.75 cardiac arrests per center per year.[153] Over 60% of these were due to initial rhythms for which defibrillation would be appropriate.[153] Therefore, there is evidence that automated external defibrillators (AEDs) might prove useful in dialysis centers. There might even be utility in training the social network of a dialysis patient on effective resuscitation, if not providing them with an AED. However, even the use within dialysis centers remains debated. Studies have found varying results regarding the efficacy

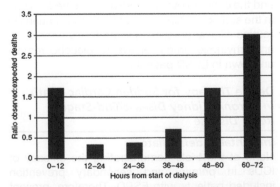

Fig. 7. Ratio of actual to expected number of occurrences of sudden death for each 12-hour interval beginning with the start of hemodialysis. (*From* Bleyer AJ, Hartman J, Brannon PC, et al. Characteristics of sudden death in hemodialysis patients. Kidney Int 2006;69:2268–73; with permission.)

of cardiopulmonary resuscitation and the use of AEDs.[15,154,155] Some of the reduced efficacy of AEDs may be attributable to underutilization.[15]

Coronary revascularization

Given the significance of CAD and myocardial ischemia in SCD, it is not surprising that coronary revascularization is the treatment strategy associated with greatest reduction in risk of SCD post-MI in patients with at least moderate CKD.[156,157] Earlier studies suggested that among patients who are otherwise good operative candidates, surgical revascularization may be a better strategy.[50,52,158] Most studies were small and prior to the routine use of coronary stenting, especially with drug-eluting stents, which are ongoing. Nevertheless, independent of percutaneous or surgical revascularization, 2-year mortality was 48% and 43%, respectively, implying that amelioration of macrovascular coronary disease may be an inadequate clinical strategy.[159]

PREDICTORS

Methods of identifying patients at the highest risk might be helpful in initiating prevention strategies. For example, ensuring compliance with β-blockers and ARBs might be beneficial in high risk patients. Avoiding particular dialysates as well as hyper- or hypokalemia and other electrolyte derangements, or changing the frequency or method of dialysis in this group, may also be considered. However, commonly used predictors of SCD need to be reevaluated in the setting of ESRD. There are sparse data on QT-interval measurements, signal-averaged electrocardiograms, and microvolt T-wave alternans. Biomarkers have not been tested in this particular setting, and there are no data on predictive ability of electrophysiology study in this population.

Electrocardiographic Indicators

Prolonging of the QT interval on EKG corrected for heart rate (QTc) as well as interlead variability, termed "QT dispersion" (QTd), have been associated with ventricular arrythmogenesis.[160,161] Most of the studies on QT intervals in ESRD patients consist of small sample sizes with variable assessment tools and primary outcomes. Several studies have shown acute changes in QTc and QTd during dialysis; however, other studies suggest that these parameters do not reflect repolarization inhomogeneity and electric instability in the setting of ESRD.[40,162–165] Furthermore, few studies have correlated these findings to SCD in ESRD.[42]

The impact of specific electrolyte alterations, such as potassium or calcium levels, on QT parameters in patients with ESRD is also unclear. Studies that have shown an association with prolonged QTc or QTd are contradicted by studies showing no association or change in the QT parameters.[32,40,42] In studies in which electrolyte abnormalities seem to correlate with QT parameters, any attempts to assume causality are often confounded by other factors, such as LVH, which also prolong QTc. In those patients with prolonged QTc or QTd, some studies have similarly found associations with increased risk of SCD but others have not.[160,161,164] From the current data, these tools do not seem to be reliable metrics.

Late potentials on signal-averaged EKG (SAECG) have been associated with increased risk of ventricular arrhythmia in non-ESRD patients.[166] Although late potentials occur more frequently in patients receiving dialysis, it remains debatable whether they predict SCD in this patient population.[167,168]

Heart rate variability reflects autonomic regulation of the cardiovascular system. Diminished heart rate variability reflects an imbalance in the sympathovagal system, and correlates with increased mortality.[169] Patients on hemodialysis demonstrate reduced heart rate variability.[170,171] After multivariate adjustment, heart rate variability also seems to correlate strongly with all-cause and cardiovascular mortality.[172] However, its association with SCD in particular remains to be clearly demonstrated.

Microvolt T-wave alternans

Microscopic fluctuations in the shape and amplitude of the T wave are called microvolt T-wave alternans. The fluctuations have been associated with an increased risk of SCD.[173] However, this has not been well studied in patients with ESRD. In a pilot study of 9 patients on hemodialysis, 7 had abnormal microvolt T-wave alternans studies. Two of 4 patients with normal baseline studies became abnormal after initiating dialysis.[19] This finding corroborates the observation that patients with ESRD are at particularly high risk for SCD. However, microvolt T-wave alternans has not been shown to predict SCD in this population. It remains an interesting, albeit investigational, tool.

Biomarkers

Whereas troponin has been shown to predict both short- and long-term cardiovascular events and mortality in the general population, it has not been specifically shown as a marker for SCD.[174] In fact, there is more evidence for postmortem cardiac troponin in evaluating SCD than antemortem serum troponin.[175–177]

Serum troponins are unaffected by dialysis, but are cleared renally.[178] In asymptomatic patients with ESRD, including those on hemodialysis, elevated serum troponin-T levels retain the ability to predict a high risk of cardiac death.[179,180] The data on the efficacy of troponin-I are more varied.[180–182] The mechanism of death in these studies remains unknown. Troponin levels may be elevated in ESRD patients without other clinical evidence of myocardial ischemia.[183] For example, elevated troponins may reflect LVH and microvascular ischemia. The ability of troponin to predict multiple myocardial pathologies associated with SCD may actually improve its predictive ability.[184] However, the ability of cardiac troponin to predict SCD in the general population, and in the ESRD population, requires further study.

Newer plasma markers that may be associated with SCD have been reported, such as CD5b-9.[185] In addition, biomarkers of inflammation (eg, CRP, interleukin-6), endothelial dysfunction (eg, asymmetric dimethylarginine), sympathetic activation (eg, norepinephrine), oxidative stress (eg, myeloperoxidase), uremia toxins (eg, P-cresol) and other novel biomarkers are being assessed for cardiovascular risk prediction in ESRD. However, these factors have yet to be evaluated in ESRD patients with respect to predicting SCD.[186]

SUMMARY

Patients with ESRD are at a high risk for SCD. SCD is the most common cause of death in this population. As in the general population, ventricular arrhythmias seem to be the most common cause of SCD in ESRD. The increased risk of SCD in ESRD is likely due to factors that are unique to the metabolic derangements associated with this state as well as the increased prevalence of traditional risk factors.

Any effort to prevent or treat SCD in this population requires a multifaceted approach that addresses the hemodynamic, ischemic, metabolic, and structural risk factors within this population. Although still debated, β-blockers and ARBs seem to have the most favorable evidence; however, further studies are still required. Data suggest that statins might have antiarrhythmic properties, but their role in preventing SCD has not been studied. Frequent hemodialysis may be a promising method to reduce peri-dialytic SCD although evidence is still lacking. There are no prospective studies on the use of ICDs in patients with ESRD. Retrospective studies suggest a benefit in a select population, but there is still nearly 3-fold higher odds of death in ICD patients

on dialysis compared with those not receiving dialysis.

Predicting those at the highest risk of death would help to target evaluation and use of therapy. However, many of the current strategies have not been adequately assessed in ESRD. QTc, QTd, and SAECG do not seem useful. Initial data suggest that heart rate variability and microvolt T-wave alternans may have a role.

REFERENCES

1. United States Renal Data System. USRDS 2008 Annual data report, National Institutes of Diabetes and Digestive and Kidney Diseases. Bethesda, MD. Available at: www.usrds.org. Accessed May 19, 2009.
2. Coresh J, Selvin E, Stevens LA, et al. Prevalence of chronic kidney disease in the United States. JAMA 2007;298(17):2038–47.
3. Dries DL, Exner DV, Domanski MJ, et al. The prognostic implications of renal insufficiency in asymptomatic and symptomatic patients with left ventricular systolic dysfunction. J Am Coll Cardiol 2000;35(3):681–9.
4. Hillege HL, Nitsch D, Pfeffer MA, et al. Renal function as a predictor of outcome in a broad spectrum of patients with heart failure. Circulation 2006; 113(5):671–8.
5. Ruilope LM, van Veldhuisen DJ, Ritz E, et al. Renal function: the Cinderella of cardiovascular risk profile. J Am Coll Cardiol 2001;38(7):1782–7.
6. United States Renal Data System. USRDS 2003 Annual data report, National Institutes of Diabetes and Digestive and Kidney Diseases. Bethesda, MD. Accessed May 19, 2009.
7. United States Renal Data System. USRDS 2006 Annual data report, National Institutes of Diabetes and Digestive and Kidney Diseases. Bethesda, MD. Accessed May 19, 2009.
8. Herzog CA. Cardiac arrest in dialysis patients: approaches to alter an abysmal outcome. Kidney Int Suppl 2003;84:S197–200.
9. Herzog CA. Cardiac arrest in dialysis patients: taking a small step. Semin Dial 2004;17(3):184–5.
10. Lai M, Hung K, Huang J, et al. Clinical findings and outcomes of intra-hemodialysis cardiopulmonary resuscitation. Am J Nephrol 1999;19(4):468–73.
11. Bayes de Luna A, Coumel P, Leclercq JF. Ambulatory sudden cardiac death: mechanisms of production of fatal arrhythmia on the basis of data from 157 cases. Am Heart J 1989;117(1):151–9.
12. Erem C, Kulan K, Tuncer C, et al. Cardiac arrhythmias in patients on maintenance hemodialysis. Acta Cardiol 1997;52(1):25–36.
13. Narula AS, Jha V, Bali HK, et al. Cardiac arrhythmias and silent myocardial ischemia during hemodialysis. Ren Fail 2000;22(3):355–68.

14. Sforzini S, Latini R, Mingardi G, et al. Ventricular arrhythmias and four-year mortality in haemodialysis patients. Gruppo Emodialisi e Patologie Cardiovascolari. Lancet 1992;339(8787):212–3.

15. Davis TR, Young BA, Eisenberg MS, et al. Outcome of cardiac arrests attended by emergency medical services staff at community outpatient dialysis centers. Kidney Int 2008;73(8):933–9.

16. Bleyer AJ, Russell GB, Satko SG. Sudden and cardiac death rates in hemodialysis patients. Kidney Int 1999;55(4):1553–9.

17. Bleyer AJ, Hartman J, Brannon PC, et al. Characteristics of sudden death in hemodialysis patients. Kidney Int 2006;69(12):2268–73.

18. Morrison G, Michelson EL, Brown S, et al. Mechanism and prevention of cardiac arrhythmias in chronic hemodialysis patients. Kidney Int 1980; 17(6):811–9.

19. Friedman AN, Groh WJ, Das M. A pilot study in hemodialysis of an electrophysiological tool to measure sudden cardiac death risk. Clin Nephrol 2007;68(3):159–64.

20. Packer M, Lee WH. Provocation of hyper- and hypokalemic sudden death during treatment with and withdrawal of converting-enzyme inhibition in severe chronic congestive heart failure. Am J Cardiol 1986;57(4):347–8.

21. Genovesi S, Valsecchi MG, Rossi E, et al. Sudden death and associated factors in a historical cohort of chronic haemodialysis patients. Nephrol Dial Transplant 2009;24:2529–36.

22. Kovesdy CP, Regidor DL, Mehrotra R, et al. Serum and dialysate potassium concentrations and survival in hemodialysis patients. Clin J Am Soc Nephrol 2007;2(5):999–1007.

23. Akiyama T, Batchelder J, Worsman J, et al. Hypocalcemic torsades de pointes. J Electrocardiol 1989;22(1):89–92.

24. Nemer WF, Teba L, Schiebel F, et al. Cardiac arrest after acute hyperphosphatemia. South Med J 1988; 81(8):1068–9.

25. Ganesh SK, Stack AG, Levin NW, et al. Association of elevated serum PO(4), Ca × PO(4) product, and parathyroid hormone with cardiac mortality risk in chronic hemodialysis patients. J Am Soc Nephrol 2001;12(10):2131–8.

26. London GM, De Vernejoul MC, Fabiani F, et al. Secondary hyperparathyroidism and cardiac hypertrophy in hemodialysis patients. Kidney Int 1987;32(6):900–7.

27. Mall G, Huther W, Schneider J, et al. Diffuse intermyocardiocytic fibrosis in uraemic patients. Nephrol Dial Transplant 1990;5(1):39–44.

28. McGonigle RJ, Fowler MB, Timmis AB, et al. Uremic cardiomyopathy: potential role of vitamin D and parathyroid hormone. Nephron 1984;36(2): 94–100.

29. Ramirez G, Brueggemeyer CD, Newton JL. Cardiac arrhythmias on hemodialysis in chronic renal failure patients. Nephron 1984;36(4):212–8.

30. Ritz E, Rambausek M, Mall G, et al. Cardiac changes in uraemia and their possible relationship to cardiovascular instability on dialysis. Nephrol Dial Transplant 1990;(5 Suppl 1):93–7.

31. Weber KT, Brilla CG, Janicki JS. Myocardial fibrosis: functional significance and regulatory factors. Cardiovasc Res 1993;27(3):341–8.

32. Buemi M, Coppolino G, Bolignano D, et al. Arrhythmias and hemodialysis: role of potassium and new diagnostic tools. Ren Fail 2009;31(1):75–80.

33. Turakhia M, Tseng ZH. Sudden cardiac death: epidemiology, mechanisms, and therapy. Curr Probl Cardiol 2007;32(9):501–46.

34. Ritz E, Koch M. Morbidity and mortality due to hypertension in patients with renal failure. Am J Kidney Dis 1993;21(5 Suppl 2):113–8.

35. Sechi LA, Catena C, Zingaro L, et al. Abnormalities of glucose metabolism in patients with early renal failure. Diabetes 2002;51(4):1226–32.

36. Amann K, Breitbach M, Ritz E, et al. Myocyte/capillary mismatch in the heart of uremic patients. J Am Soc Nephrol 1998;9(6):1018–22.

37. Solomon SD, Zelenkofske S, McMurray JJ, et al. Sudden death in patients with myocardial infarction and left ventricular dysfunction, heart failure, or both. N Engl J Med 2005;352(25):2581–8.

38. Foley RN, Parfrey PS, Harnett JD, et al. The impact of anemia on cardiomyopathy, morbidity, and mortality in end-stage renal disease. Am J Kidney Dis 1996;28(1):53–61.

39. Tada T, Shiba N, Watanabe J, et al. Prognostic value of anemia in predicting sudden death of patients with diastolic heart failure. Int J Cardiol 2008;128(3):419–21.

40. Meier P, Vogt P, Blanc E. Ventricular arrhythmias and sudden cardiac death in end-stage renal disease patients on chronic hemodialysis. Nephron 2001;87(3):199–214.

41. Tok D, Gullu H, Erdogan D, et al. Impaired coronary flow reserve in hemodialysis patients: a transthoracic Doppler echocardiographic study. Nephron Clin Pract 2005;101(4):c200–6.

42. Selby NM, McIntyre CW. The acute cardiac effects of dialysis. Semin Dial 2007;20(3):220–8.

43. Nappi SE, Virtanen VK, Saha HH, et al. QTc dispersion increases during hemodialysis with low-calcium dialysate. Kidney Int 2000;57(5): 2117–22.

44. Redaelli B, Locatelli F, Limido D, et al. Effect of a new model of hemodialysis potassium removal on the control of ventricular arrhythmias. Kidney Int 1996;50(2):609–17.

45. Makaryus AN. Ventricular arrhythmias in dialysis patients. Rev Cardiovasc Med 2006;7(1):17–22.

46. Herzog CA, Mangrum JM, Passman R. Sudden cardiac death and dialysis patients. Semin Dial 2008;21(4):300–7.

47. Weiner DE, Tighiouart H, Amin MG, et al. Chronic kidney disease as a risk factor for cardiovascular disease and all-cause mortality: a pooled analysis of community-based studies. J Am Soc Nephrol 2004;15(5):1307–15.

48. Baigent C, Burbury K, Wheeler D. Premature cardiovascular disease in chronic renal failure. Lancet 2000;356(9224):147–52.

49. Trespalacios FC, Taylor AJ, Agodoa LY, et al. Incident acute coronary syndromes in chronic dialysis patients in the United States. Kidney Int 2002;62(5): 1799–805.

50. Reddan DN, Szczech LA, Tuttle RH, et al. Chronic kidney disease, mortality, and treatment strategies among patients with clinically significant coronary artery disease. J Am Soc Nephrol 2003;14(9): 2373–80.

51. Sadeghi HM, Stone GW, Grines CL, et al. Impact of renal insufficiency in patients undergoing primary angioplasty for acute myocardial infarction. Circulation 2003;108(22):2769–75.

52. Szczech LA, Reddan DN, Owen WF, et al. Differential survival after coronary revascularization procedures among patients with renal insufficiency. Kidney Int 2001;60(1):292–9.

53. West AJ, Dixon SR, Kahn JK, et al. Effectiveness of primary angioplasty for acute myocardial infarction in patients on dialysis. Am J Cardiol 2004;93(4): 468–70.

54. Zakeri R, Freemantle N, Barnett V, et al. Relation between mild renal dysfunction and outcomes after coronary artery bypass grafting. Circulation 2005; 112(9 Suppl):I270–5.

55. Go AS, Chertow GM, Fan D, et al. Chronic kidney disease and the risks of death, cardiovascular events, and hospitalization. N Engl J Med 2004; 351(13):1296–305.

56. Shlipak MG, Heidenreich PA, Noguchi H, et al. Association of renal insufficiency with treatment and outcomes after myocardial infarction in elderly patients. Ann Intern Med 2002;137(7):555–62.

57. Anavekar NS, McMurray JJ, Velazquez EJ, et al. Relation between renal dysfunction and cardiovascular outcomes after myocardial infarction. N Engl J Med 2004;351(13):1285–95.

58. Herzog CA, Ma JZ, Collins AJ. Poor long-term survival after acute myocardial infarction among patients on long-term dialysis. N Engl J Med 1998;339(12):799–805.

59. Berger AK, Duval S, Krumholz HM. Aspirin, beta-blocker, and angiotensin-converting enzyme inhibitor therapy in patients with end-stage renal disease and an acute myocardial infarction. J Am Coll Cardiol 2003;42(2):201–8.

60. Chertow GM, Normand SL, McNeil BJ. "Renalism": inappropriately low rates of coronary angiography in elderly individuals with renal insufficiency. J Am Soc Nephrol 2004;15(9):2462–8.

61. Mohi-ud-din K, Bali HK, Banerjee S, et al. Silent myocardial ischemia and high-grade ventricular arrhythmias in patients on maintenance hemodialysis. Ren Fail 2005;27(2):171–5.

62. Nazarian S, Bluemke DA, Lardo AC, et al. Magnetic resonance assessment of the substrate for inducible ventricular tachycardia in nonischemic cardiomyopathy. Circulation 2005;112(18):2821–5.

63. Bigger JT Jr, Fleiss JL, Kleiger R, et al. The relationships among ventricular arrhythmias, left ventricular dysfunction, and mortality in the 2 years after myocardial infarction. Circulation 1984;69(2):250–8.

64. Foley RN, Parfrey PS, Harnett JD, et al. Clinical and echocardiographic disease in patients starting end-stage renal disease therapy. Kidney Int 1995; 47(1):186–92.

65. Mangrum AJ, Lin D, Dimarco JP, et al. Sudden cardiac death and left ventricular function in renal dialysis patients. Heart Rhythm 2006;3:S154.

66. Harnett JD, Foley RN, Kent GM, et al. Congestive heart failure in dialysis patients: prevalence, incidence, prognosis and risk factors. Kidney Int 1995;47(3):884–90.

67. Kannel WB, Wilson PW, D'Agostino RB, et al. Sudden coronary death in women. Am Heart J 1998;136(2):205–12.

68. Effect of metoprolol CR/XL in chronic heart failure: Metoprolol CR/XL randomised intervention trial in congestive heart failure (MERIT-HF). Lancet 1999; 353(9169):2001–7.

69. Luu M, Stevenson WG, Stevenson LW, et al. Diverse mechanisms of unexpected cardiac arrest in advanced heart failure. Circulation 1989;80(6): 1675–80.

70. Remppis A, Ritz E. Cardiac problems in the dialysis patient: beyond coronary disease. Semin Dial 2008;21(4):319–25.

71. Mann JF. What are the short-term and long-term consequences of anaemia in CRF patients? Nephrol Dial Transplant 1999;(14 Suppl 2):29–36.

72. Mehta BR, Ireland MA, Shiu MF. Echocardiographic evaluation of cardiac size and function in dialysis patients. Clin Nephrol 1983;20(2):61–6.

73. Messerli FH, Ventura HO, Elizardi DJ, et al. Hypertension and sudden death. Increased ventricular ectopic activity in left ventricular hypertrophy. Am J Med 1984;77(1):18–22.

74. Silberberg JS, Barre PE, Prichard SS, et al. Impact of left ventricular hypertrophy on survival in end-stage renal disease. Kidney Int 1989;36(2):286–90.

75. Harnett JD, Parfrey PS, Griffiths SM, et al. Left ventricular hypertrophy in end-stage renal disease. Nephron 1988;48(2):107–15.

76. McLenachan JM, Henderson E, Morris KI, et al. Ventricular arrhythmias in patients with hypertensive left ventricular hypertrophy. N Engl J Med 1987;317(13):787–92.

77. De Lima JJ, Lopes HF, Grupi CJ, et al. Blood pressure influences the occurrence of complex ventricular arrhythmia in hemodialysis patients. Hypertension 1995;26(6 Pt 2):1200–3.

78. Gross ML, Ritz E. Hypertrophy and fibrosis in the cardiomyopathy of uremia—beyond coronary heart disease. Semin Dial 2008;21(4):308–18.

79. Marcus ML, Koyanagi S, Harrison DG, et al. Abnormalities in the coronary circulation that occur as a consequence of cardiac hypertrophy. Am J Med 1983;75(3):62–6.

80. Burke AP, Farb A, Liang YH, et al. Effect of hypertension and cardiac hypertrophy on coronary artery morphology in sudden cardiac death. Circulation 1996;94(12):3138–45.

81. Moon JC, McKenna WJ, McCrohon JA, et al. Toward clinical risk assessment in hypertrophic cardiomyopathy with gadolinium cardiovascular magnetic resonance. J Am Coll Cardiol 2003;41(9):1561–7.

82. Spirito P, Bellone P, Harris KM, et al. Magnitude of left ventricular hypertrophy and risk of sudden death in hypertrophic cardiomyopathy. N Engl J Med 2000;342(24):1778–85.

83. Schlaich MP, Socratous F, Hennebry S, et al. Sympathetic activation in chronic renal failure. J Am Soc Nephrol 2009;20(5):933–9.

84. Xu J, Li G, Wang P, et al. Renalase is a novel, soluble monoamine oxidase that regulates cardiac function and blood pressure. J Clin Invest 2005;115(5):1275–80.

85. Harris AS, Estandia A, Tillotson RF. Ventricular ectopic rhythms and ventricular fibrillation following cardiac sympathectomy and coronary occlusion. Am J Physiol 1951;165(3):505–12.

86. Meredith IT, Broughton A, Jennings GL, et al. Evidence of a selective increase in cardiac sympathetic activity in patients with sustained ventricular arrhythmias. N Engl J Med 1991;325(9):618–24.

87. Zoccali C, Mallamaci F, Parlongo S, et al. Plasma norepinephrine predicts survival and incident cardiovascular events in patients with end-stage renal disease. Circulation 2002;105(11):1354–9.

88. Kawano H, Do YS, Kawano Y, et al. Angiotensin II has multiple profibrotic effects in human cardiac fibroblasts. Circulation 2000;101(10):1130–7.

89. Eknoyan GM, Beck GJ, Cheung AK, et al. Effect of dialysis dose and membrane flux in maintenance hemodialysis. N Engl J Med 2002;347:2010–9.

90. Locatelli F, Martin-Malo A, Hannedouche T, et al. Membrane Permeability Outcome (MPO) Study Group. Effect of membrane permeability on survival of hemodialysis patients. J Am Soc Nephrol 2009;20(3):645–54.

91. Karnik JA, Young BS, Lew NL, et al. Cardiac arrest and sudden death in dialysis units. Kidney Int 2001;60(1):350–7.

92. Culleton BF, Walsh M, Scott W, et al. Effect of frequent nocturnal hemodialysis vs conventional hemodialysis on left ventricular mass and quality of life: a randomized controlled trial. JAMA 2007;298(11):1291–9.

93. Beecroft JM, Duffin J, Pierratos A, et al. Decreased chemosensitivity and improvement of sleep apnea by nocturnal hemodialysis. Sleep Med 2009;10(1):47–54.

94. Chan CT, Shen XS, Picton P, et al. Nocturnal home hemodialysis improves baroreflex effectiveness index of end-stage renal disease patients. J Hypertens 2008;26(9):1795–800.

95. Kjellstrand CM, Buoncristiani U, Ting G, et al. Short daily haemodialysis: survival in 415 patients treated for 1006 patient-years. Nephrol Dial Transplant 2008;23(10):3283–9.

96. Cano NJ, Fouque D, Roth H, et al. Intradialytic parenteral nutrition does not improve survival in malnourished hemodialysis patients: a 2-year multicenter, prospective, randomized study. J Am Soc Nephrol 2007;18(9):2583–91.

97. Drueke TB, Locatelli F, Clyne N, et al. Normalization of hemoglobin level in patients with chronic kidney disease and anemia. N Engl J Med 2006;355(20):2071–84.

98. Singh AK, Szczech L, Tang KL, et al. Correction of anemia with epoetin alfa in chronic kidney disease. N Engl J Med 2006;355(20):2085–98.

99. Pun PH, Lehrich RW, Smith SR, et al. Predictors of survival after cardiac arrest in outpatient hemodialysis clinics. Clin J Am Soc Nephrol 2007;2(3):491–500.

100. Azevedo ER, Kubo T, Mak S, et al. Nonselective versus selective beta-adrenergic receptor blockade in congestive heart failure: differential effects on sympathetic activity. Circulation 2001;104(18):2194–9.

101. Mortara A, La Rovere MT, Pinna GD, et al. Nonselective beta-adrenergic blocking agent, carvedilol, improves arterial baroflex gain and heart rate variability in patients with stable chronic heart failure. J Am Coll Cardiol 2000;36(5):1612–8.

102. Piccirillo G, Luparini RL, Celli V, et al. Effects of carvedilol on heart rate and blood pressure variability in subjects with chronic heart failure. Am J Cardiol 2000;86(12):1392–5, A1396.

103. Ryden L, Ariniego R, Arnman K, et al. A double-blind trial of metoprolol in acute myocardial infarction. Effects on ventricular tachyarrhythmias. N Engl J Med 1983;308(11):614–8.

104. Abbott KC, Trespalacios FC, Agodoa LY, et al. Beta-blocker use in long-term dialysis patients: association with hospitalized heart failure and mortality. Arch Intern Med 2004;164(22):2465–71.

105. Ritz E, Dikow R, Adamzcak M, et al. Congestive heart failure due to systolic dysfunction: the Cinderella of cardiovascular management in dialysis patients. Semin Dial 2002;15(3):135–40.

106. Cice G, Tagliamonte E, Ferrara L, et al. [Complex ventricular arrhythmias and carvedilol: efficacy in hemodialyzed uremic patients]. Cardiologia 1998; 43(6):597–604 [in Italian].

107. Cice G, Ferrara L, D'Andrea A, et al. Carvedilol increases two-year survival in dialysis patients with dilated cardiomyopathy: a prospective, placebo-controlled trial. J Am Coll Cardiol 2003; 41(9):1438–44.

108. Sakhuja R, Keebler M, Lai TS, et al. Meta-analysis of mortality in dialysis patients with an implantable cardioverter defibrillator. Am J Cardiol 2009;103(5): 735–41.

109. de Fremont JF, Coevoet B, Andrejak M, et al. Effects of antihypertensive drugs on dialysis-resistant hypertension, plasma renin and dopamine betahydroxylase activities, metabolic risk factors and calcium phosphate homeostasis: comparison of metoprolol, alphamethyldopa and clonidine in a cross-over trial. Clin Nephrol 1979;12(5): 198–205.

110. Agarwal R. Supervised atenolol therapy in the management of hemodialysis hypertension. Kidney Int 1999;55(4):1528–35.

111. Hamad A, Salameh M, Zihlif M, et al. Life-threatening hyperkalemia after intravenous labetolol injection for hypertensive emergency in a hemodialysis patient. Am J Nephrol 2001;21(3):241–4.

112. Nowicki M, Miszczak-Kuban J. Nonselective beta-adrenergic blockade augments fasting hyperkalemia in hemodialysis patients. Nephron 2002; 91(2):222–7.

113. Ligtenberg G, Blankestijn PJ, Oey PL, et al. Reduction of sympathetic hyperactivity by enalapril in patients with chronic renal failure. N Engl J Med 1999;340(17):1321–8.

114. Dohi Y, Ohashi M, Sugiyama M, et al. Candesartan reduces oxidative stress and inflammation in patients with essential hypertension. Hypertens Res 2003;26(9):691–7.

115. Sun Y, Zhang J, Lu L, et al. Aldosterone-induced inflammation in the rat heart: role of oxidative stress. Am J Pathol 2002;161(5):1773–81.

116. Kober L, Torp-Pedersen C, Carlsen JE, et al. A clinical trial of the angiotensin-converting-enzyme inhibitor trandolapril in patients with left ventricular dysfunction after myocardial infarction. Trandolapril Cardiac Evaluation (TRACE) Study Group. N Engl J Med 1995;333(25):1670–6.

117. Pfeffer MA, Braunwald E, Moye LA, et al. Effect of captopril on mortality and morbidity in patients with left ventricular dysfunction after myocardial infarction. Results of the survival and ventricular enlargement trial. The SAVE Investigators. N Engl J Med 1992;327(10):669–77.

118. Swedberg K, Held P, Kjekshus J, et al. Effects of the early administration of enalapril on mortality in patients with acute myocardial infarction. Results of the Cooperative New Scandinavian Enalapril Survival Study II (CONSENSUS II). N Engl J Med 1992;327(10):678–84.

119. Pitt B, Remme W, Zannad F, et al. Eplerenone, a selective aldosterone blocker, in patients with left ventricular dysfunction after myocardial infarction. N Engl J Med 2003;348(14):1309–21.

120. Pitt B, Zannad F, Remme WJ, et al. The effect of spironolactone on morbidity and mortality in patients with severe heart failure. Randomized Aldactone Evaluation Study Investigators. N Engl J Med 1999;341(10):709–17.

121. Hou FF, Zhang X, Zhang GH, et al. Efficacy and safety of benazepril for advanced chronic renal insufficiency. N Engl J Med 2006;354(2):131–40.

122. Fang W, Oreopoulos DG, Bargman JM. Use of ACE inhibitors or angiotensin receptor blockers and survival in patients on peritoneal dialysis. Nephrol Dial Transplant 2008;23(11):3704–10.

123. Efrati S, Zaidenstein R, Dishy V, et al. ACE inhibitors and survival of hemodialysis patients. Am J Kidney Dis 2002;40(5):1023–9.

124. Hsia J, Jablonski KA, Rice MM, et al. Sudden cardiac death in patients with stable coronary artery disease and preserved left ventricular systolic function. Am J Cardiol 2008;101(4):457–61.

125. Zannad F, Kessler M, Lehert P, et al. Prevention of cardiovascular events in end-stage renal disease: results of a randomized trial of fosinopril and implications for future studies. Kidney Int 2006;70(7): 1318–24.

126. Takahashi A, Takase H, Toriyama T, et al. Candesartan, an angiotensin II type-1 receptor blocker, reduces cardiovascular events in patients on chronic haemodialysis—a randomized study. Nephrol Dial Transplant 2006;21(9):2507–12.

127. Suzuki H, Kanno Y, Sugahara S, et al. Effect of angiotensin receptor blockers on cardiovascular events in patients undergoing hemodialysis: an open-label randomized controlled trial. Am J Kidney Dis 2008;52(3):501–6.

128. Tschope W, Koch M, Thomas B, et al. Serum lipids predict cardiac death in diabetic patients on maintenance hemodialysis. Results of a prospective study. The German Study Group Diabetes and Uremia. Nephron 1993;64(3):354–8.

129. Yeun JY, Levine RA, Mantadilok V, et al. C-reactive protein predicts all-cause and cardiovascular mortality in hemodialysis patients. Am J Kidney Dis 2000;35(3):469–76.

130. De Sutter J, Tavernier R, De Buyzere M, et al. Lipid lowering drugs and recurrences of life-threatening

ventricular arrhythmias in high-risk patients. J Am Coll Cardiol 2000;36(3):766–72.

131. De Sutter J. Intensive lipid-lowering therapy and ventricular arrhythmias in patients with coronary artery disease and internal cardioverter defibrillators. Boston: Heart Rhythm Society (MA); 2006. Accessed June 1, 2009.

132. Thavendiranathan P, Bagai A, Brookhart MA, et al. Primary prevention of cardiovascular diseases with statin therapy: a meta-analysis of randomized controlled trials. Arch Intern Med 2006;166(21): 2307–13.

133. Navaneethan SD, Pansini F, Perkovic V, et al. HMG CoA reductase inhibitors (statins) for people with chronic kidney disease not requiring dialysis. Cochrane Database Syst Rev 2009;(2):CD007784.

134. Tonelli M, Isles C, Curhan GC, et al. Effect of pravastatin on cardiovascular events in people with chronic kidney disease. Circulation 2004;110(12): 1557–63.

135. Fellstrom BC, Jardine AG, Schmieder RE, et al. Rosuvastatin and cardiovascular events in patients undergoing hemodialysis. N Engl J Med 2009; 360(14):1395–407.

136. Seliger SL, Weiss NS, Gillen DL, et al. HMG-CoA reductase inhibitors are associated with reduced mortality in ESRD patients. Kidney Int 2002;61(1): 297–304.

137. Wanner C, Krane V, Marz W, et al. Atorvastatin in patients with type 2 diabetes mellitus undergoing hemodialysis. N Engl J Med 2005;353(3):238–48.

138. Lee DS, Green LD, Liu PP, et al. Effectiveness of implantable defibrillators for preventing arrhythmic events and death: a meta-analysis. J Am Coll Cardiol 2003;41(9):1573–82.

139. Desai AS, Fang JC, Maisel WH, et al. Implantable defibrillators for the prevention of mortality in patients with nonischemic cardiomyopathy: a meta-analysis of randomized controlled trials. JAMA 2004;292(23):2874–9.

140. Yusuf S, Peto R, Lewis J, et al. Beta blockade during and after myocardial infarction: an overview of the randomized trials. Prog Cardiovasc Dis 1985;27(5):335–71.

141. The Cardiac Arrhythmia Suppression Trial (CAST) Investigators Preliminary report: effect of encainide and flecainide on mortality in a randomized trial of arrhythmia suppression after myocardial infarction. N Engl J Med 1989;321(6):406–12.

142. Bardy GH, Lee KL, Mark DB, et al. Amiodarone or an implantable cardioverter-defibrillator for congestive heart failure. N Engl J Med 2005; 352(3):225–37.

143. United States Renal Data System. USRDS 2007 Annual data report, National Institutes of Diabetes and Digestive and Kidney Diseases. Bethesda, MD. Accessed May 19, 2009.

144. Herzog CA, Li S, Weinhandl ED, et al. Survival of dialysis patients after cardiac arrest and the impact of implantable cardioverter defibrillators. Kidney Int 2005;68(2):818–25.

145. Robin J, Weinberg K, Tiongson J, et al. Renal dialysis as a risk factor for appropriate therapies and mortality in implantable cardioverter-defibrillator recipients. Heart Rhythm 2006;3(10):1196–201.

146. Amin MS, Fox AD, Kalahasty G, et al. Benefit of primary prevention implantable cardioverter-defibrillators in the setting of chronic kidney disease: a decision model analysis. J Cardiovasc Electrophysiol 2008;19:1275–80.

147. de Bie MK, Lekkerkerker JC, van Dam B, et al. Prevention of sudden cardiac death: rationale and design of the implantable cardioverter defibrillators in dialysis patients (ICD2) trial—a prospective pilot study. Curr Med Res Opin 2008;24(8):2151–7.

148. Epstein AE, DiMarco JP, Ellenbogen KA, et al. ACC/AHA/HRS 2008 Guidelines for Device-based therapy of cardiac rhythm abnormalities: a report of the American College of Cardiology/American Heart Association Task Force on Practice Guidelines (Writing Committee to Revise the ACC/AHA/ NASPE 2002 Guideline Update for Implantation of Cardiac Pacemakers and Antiarrhythmia Devices) developed in collaboration with the American Association for Thoracic Surgery and Society of Thoracic Surgeons. J Am Coll Cardiol 2008; 51(21):e1–62.

149. Dasgupta A, Montalvo J, Medendorp S, et al. Increased complication rates of cardiac rhythm management devices in ESRD patients. Am J Kidney Dis 2007;49(5):656–63.

150. Bloom H, Heeke B, Leon A, et al. Renal insufficiency and the risk of infection from pacemaker or defibrillator surgery. Pacing Clin Electrophysiol 2006;29(2):142–5.

151. Wase A, Basit A, Nazir R, et al. Impact of chronic kidney disease upon survival among implantable cardioverter-defibrillator recipients. J Interv Card Electrophysiol 2004;11(3):199–204.

152. Teruya TH, Abou-Zamzam AM Jr, Limm W, et al. Symptomatic subclavian vein stenosis and occlusion in hemodialysis patients with transvenous pacemakers. Ann Vasc Surg 2003;17(5):526–9.

153. Becker L, Eisenberg M, Fahrenbruch C, et al. Cardiac arrest in medical and dental practices: implications for automated external defibrillators. Arch Intern Med 2001;161(12):1509–12.

154. Lafrance JP, Nolin L, Senecal L, et al. Predictors and outcome of cardiopulmonary resuscitation (CPR) calls in a large haemodialysis unit over a seven-year period. Nephrol Dial Transplant 2006;21(4):1006–12.

155. Lehrich RW, Pun PH, Tanenbaum ND, et al. Automated external defibrillators and survival from

cardiac arrest in the outpatient hemodialysis clinic. J Am Soc Nephrol 2007;18(1):312–20.

156. Makikallio TH, Barthel P, Schneider R, et al. Frequency of sudden cardiac death among acute myocardial infarction survivors with optimized medical and revascularization therapy. Am J Cardiol 2006;97(4):480–4.

157. Johnston N, Jernberg T, Lagerqvist B, et al. Early invasive treatment benefits patients with renal dysfunction in unstable coronary artery disease. Am Heart J 2006;152(6):1052–8.

158. Franga DL, Kratz JM, Crumbley AJ, et al. Early and long-term results of coronary artery bypass grafting in dialysis patients. Ann Thorac Surg 2000; 70(3):813–8 [discussion: 819].

159. Herzog CA, Strief JW, Collins AJ, et al. Cause-specific mortality of dialysis patients after coronary revascularization: why don't dialysis patients have better survival after coronary intervention? Nephrol Dial Transplant 2008;23(8):2629–33.

160. Day CP, McComb JM, Campbell RW. QT dispersion: an indication of arrhythmia risk in patients with long QT intervals. Br Heart J 1990;63(6): 342–4.

161. Schwartz PJ, Wolf S. QT interval prolongation as predictor of sudden death in patients with myocardial infarction. Circulation 1978;57(6):1074–7.

162. Coumel P, Maison-Blanche P, Badilini F. Dispersion of ventricular repolarization: reality? Illusion? Significance? Circulation 1998;97(25):2491–3.

163. Cupisti A, Galetta F, Caprioli R, et al. Potassium removal increases the QTc interval dispersion during hemodialysis. Nephron 1999;82(2):122–6.

164. Gussak HM, Gellens ME, Gussak I, et al. Q-T interval dispersion and its arrhythmogenic potential in hemodialyzed patients: methodological aspects. Nephron 1999;82(3):278.

165. Lorincz I, Matyus J, Zilahi Z, et al. QT dispersion in patients with end-stage renal failure and during hemodialysis. J Am Soc Nephrol 1999;10(6): 1297–302.

166. Lindsay BD, Ambos HD, Schechtman KB, et al. Noninvasive detection of patients with ischemic and nonischemic heart disease prone to ventricular fibrillation. J Am Coll Cardiol 1990;16(7):1656–64.

167. Morales MA, Gremigni C, Dattolo P, et al. Signal-averaged ECG abnormalities in haemodialysis patients. Role of dialysis. Nephrol Dial Transplant 1998;13(3):668–73.

168. Roithinger FX, Punzengruber C, Rossoll M, et al. Ventricular late potentials in haemodialysis patients and the risk of sudden death. Nephrol Dial Transplant 1992;7(10):1013–8.

169. La Rovere MT, Bigger JT Jr, Marcus FI, et al. Baroreflex sensitivity and heart-rate variability in prediction of total cardiac mortality after myocardial infarction. ATRAMI (Autonomic Tone and Reflexes

After Myocardial Infarction) Investigators. Lancet Feb 14 1998;351(9101):478–84.

170. Kurata C, Uehara A, Sugi T, et al. Cardiac autonomic neuropathy in patients with chronic renal failure on hemodialysis. Nephron 2000;84(4):312–9.

171. Rubinger D, Revis N, Pollak A, et al. Predictors of haemodynamic instability and heart rate variability during haemodialysis. Nephrol Dial Transplant 2004;19(8):2053–60.

172. Oikawa K, Ishihara R, Maeda T, et al. Prognostic value of heart rate variability in patients with renal failure on hemodialysis. Int J Cardiol 2009;131(3):370–7.

173. Gehi AK, Stein RH, Metz LD, et al. Microvolt T-wave alternans for the risk stratification of ventricular tachyarrhythmic events: a meta-analysis. J Am Coll Cardiol 2005;46(1):75–82.

174. Galvani M, Ottani F, Ferrini D, et al. Prognostic influence of elevated values of cardiac troponin I in patients with unstable angina. Circulation 1997; 95(8):2053–9.

175. Kontos MC, Anderson FP, Alimard R, et al. Ability of troponin I to predict cardiac events in patients admitted from the emergency department. J Am Coll Cardiol 2000;36(6):1818–23.

176. Ellingsen CL, Hetland O. Serum concentrations of cardiac troponin T in sudden death. Am J Forensic Med Pathol 2004;25(3):213–5.

177. Khalifa AB, Najjar M, Addad F, et al. Cardiac troponin T (cTn T) and the postmortem diagnosis of sudden death. Am J Forensic Med Pathol 2006;27(2):175–7.

178. Donnino MW, Karriem-Norwood V, Rivers EP, et al. Prevalence of elevated troponin I in end-stage renal disease patients receiving hemodialysis. Acad Emerg Med 2004;11(9):979–81.

179. deFilippi C, Wasserman S, Rosanio S, et al. Cardiac troponin T and C-reactive protein for predicting prognosis, coronary atherosclerosis, and cardiomyopathy in patients undergoing long-term hemodialysis. JAMA 2003;290(3):353–9.

180. Khan NA, Hemmelgarn BR, Tonelli M, et al. Prognostic value of troponin T and I among asymptomatic patients with end-stage renal disease: a meta-analysis. Circulation 2005;112(20):3088–96.

181. Porter GA, Norton T, Bennett WB. Troponin T, A predictor of death in chronic haemodialysis patients. Eur Heart J 1998;(19 Suppl N):N34–7.

182. Roppolo LP, Fitzgerald R, Dillow J, et al. A comparison of troponin T and troponin I as predictors of cardiac events in patients undergoing chronic dialysis at a Veteran's Hospital: a pilot study. J Am Coll Cardiol 1999;34(2):448–54.

183. deFilippi CR, Thorn EM, Aggarwal M, et al. Frequency and cause of cardiac troponin T elevation in chronic hemodialysis patients from study of cardiovascular magnetic resonance. Am J Cardiol 2007;100(5):885–9.

184. Mallamaci F, Zoccali C, Parlongo S, et al. Diagnostic value of troponin T for alterations in left ventricular mass and function in dialysis patients. Kidney Int 2002;62(5):1884–90.
185. Campobasso CP, Dell'Erba AS, Addante A, et al. Sudden cardiac death and myocardial ischemia indicators: a comparative study of four immunohistochemical markers. Am J Forensic Med Pathol 2008;29(2):154–61.
186. Stenvinkel P, Carrero JJ, Axelsson J, et al. Emerging biomarkers for evaluating cardiovascular risk in the chronic kidney disease patient: how do new pieces fit into the uremic puzzle? Clin J Am Soc Nephrol 2008;3(2):505–21.

Implantable Cardioverter Defibrillator in Patients with Coronary Artery Disease

Ilan Goldenberg, MD, Arthur J. Moss, MD*

KEYWORDS
- Implantable cardioverter defibrillator
- Coronary artery disease • Sudden cardiac death
- Primary prevention • Secondary prevention

Sudden cardiac death (SCD) is responsible for more than 400,000 deaths annually in the United States, overwhelmingly as a result of ventricular fibrillation. Coronary artery disease (CAD) is the most common cause of SCD, accounting for more than 80% of cases of SCD, whereas nonischemic cardiomyopathy and hereditary causes including hypertrophic cardiomyopathy, congenital long QT syndrome, the Brugada syndrome, and arrhythmogenic right ventricular dysplasia contribute for a lower proportion of SCD cases.[1] The risk of SCD varies between 20% and 30% among patients with depressed left ventricular (LV) systolic function. Furthermore, SCD risk increases in a nearly exponential manner as ejection fraction (EF) falls below 30%.[2,3] In addition to the severity of LV dysfunction, the degree of functional impairment as evaluated by New York Heart Association (NYHA) functional classification has also been shown to be a powerful independent predictor of SCD.[4,5] Although the absolute number of sudden deaths is greatest for patients with NYHA functional class IV symptoms, SCD accounts for only 35% of all-cause mortality in this group of patients. Conversely, SCD accounts for 64% of deaths among patients with compensated NYHA functional class II heart failure symptoms.[4,5] Thus, patients with mildly symptomatic (ie,

well-compensated) heart failure should not be viewed as being at low risk for sudden death. In the past 2 decades, data from major clinical trials have consistently demonstrated that most antiarrhythmic drugs do not reduce the risk of SCD in adult patients with acquired heart disease.[6–11] Accordingly, device-based therapy was developed as an alternative means to reduce arrhythmic mortality in high-risk cardiac patients. The first implanted defibrillator was designed by Drs Michel Mirowski, Morton Mower, and associates, who miniaturized the components of the external defibrillator into a device small enough to be implanted in humans and coupled it with a unique sensing algorithm to discriminate between normal rhythm and ventricular fibrillation. After documenting the safety and efficacy of automatic internal cardiac defibrillation in animals, they reported clinical success in three patients in 1980.[12] This success ushered in a series of randomized trials documenting the improved survival of high-risk cardiac patients with an implantable cardiac defibrillator (ICD).

In this review, we outline current indications for ICD therapy for the primary and secondary prevention of SCD in CAD patients, emphasizing data from major clinical trials regarding the efficacy and limitations of the ICD in this group of patients.

This manuscript was requested by Dr Ranjan K. Thakur, editor of *Cardiac Electrophysiology Clinics*.
Heart Research Follow-up Program, Cardiology Division, Department of Medicine, University of Rochester School of Medicine and Dentistry, Box 653, 601 Elmwood Avenue, Rochester, NY 14642-8653, USA
* Corresponding author.
E-mail address: heartajm@heart.rochester.edu (A.J. Moss).

Card Electrophysiol Clin 1 (2009) 79–93
doi:10.1016/j.ccep.2009.08.008
1877-9182/09/$ – see front matter © 2009 Published by Elsevier Inc.

cardiacEP.theclinics.com

CLINICAL TRIALS

Defibrillator therapy was initially studied for the secondary prevention of arrhythmic mortality in patients who had experienced life-threatening ventricular tachyarrhythmias owing to the relatively high recurrence rate of potentially fatal dysrhythmias in this population.[13–15] Subsequently, asymptomatic patients with left ventricular dysfunction and without additional risk factors were also shown to be at high risk for arrhythmic death.[16,17] These data have led to a series of major prospective randomized trials that evaluated the role of primary prevention with an ICD in high-risk cardiac patients.[18–28] A summary of prospective randomized secondary and primary prevention ICD trials that enrolled patients with CAD is presented in **Tables 1** and **2**, respectively, and the highlights of these trials are discussed in the following sections.

Secondary Prevention Implantable Cardiac Defibrillator Trials

Most patients enrolled in the three major trials that evaluated the benefit of ICD therapy for the secondary prevention of SCD had established CAD. In this population, despite differences in sample size that affected statistical significance, the studies demonstrated a similar magnitude of survival benefit with an ICD among patients who have experienced life-threatening cardiac arrhythmias (**Table 1**). The Antiarrhythmics versus Implantable Defibrillators (AVID) Trial[13] enrolled 1016 subjects who were resuscitated from near-fatal ventricular tachycardia (VT) or ventricular fibrillation (VF), experienced sustained VT with syncope, or experienced symptomatic sustained VT with an ejection fraction (EF) of 40% or less. Eighty-one percent of study patients had established CAD, and the ICD therapy was shown to be associated with a significant 29% reduction in the risk of all-cause mortality in this population. The Canadian Implantable Defibrillator Study (CIDS) Trial[14] randomized 659 patients with resuscitated VF or VT or with unmonitored syncope to treatment with an ICD or amiodarone. Similar to AVID, 82% of the CIDS population had established CAD. Defibrillator therapy in the study was associated with a nonsignificant 20% reduction in the risk of all-cause mortality ($P = .14$), and a marginally significant 33% reduction in the risk of SCD ($P = .09$). The relatively small Cardiac Arrest Study Hamburg (CASH)[15] comprised 288 survivors of cardiac arrest who were randomized to ICD or antiarrhythmic-drug therapy (amiodarone, metoprolol, or propafenone). Three-quarters of enrolled patients had CAD, and ICD therapy in the CASH

population was associated with a (nonsignificant) 23% reduction in total mortality as compared with antiarrhythmic therapy with amiodarone or metoprolol. Random assignment to propafenone was stopped early in the trial because of excess mortality.

A meta-analysis of the three secondary prevention ICD trials, performed by Connolly and colleagues,[29] demonstrated a significant 28% ($P = .006$) reduction in the risk of death with an ICD that was attributable almost entirely to a 50% reduction in arrhythmic death. Notably, the same meta-analysis showed that the benefit of secondary prevention with an ICD is apparent mainly in low-EF (<35%) patients.[29]

Primary Prevention Implantable Cardiac Defibrillator Trials

Of the eight randomized clinical trials that evaluated the efficacy of device therapy in patients who did not experience a prior episode of life-threatening ventricular tachyarrhymia,[18,22–28] six studies enrolled patients who had LV dysfunction associated with CAD.[22–27] Notably, a survival benefit was observed in the four major primary prevention trials that enrolled CAD patients in whom the ICD was not implanted in proximity to an acute coronary event or coronary revascularization, whereas the benefit of the ICD was not evident when the device was implanted in high-risk CAD patients who experienced recent myocardial infarction (MI) or among those in whom the device was implanted at the time of coronary artery bypass graft (CABG) surgery (**Table 2**).

The Multicenter Automatic Defibrillator Implantation Trial (MADIT) was the first major randomized primary prevention ICD trial testing the hypothesis that prophylactic ICD implantation would be associated with a survival benefit in a subset of post-MI patients with LV dysfunction, considered to be at high risk for ventricular tachyarrhythmias.[22] The study enrolled 196 prior-MI patients with EF of 35% or less, NYHA heart failure class I-III, a documented episode of asymptomatic unsustained ventricular tachycardia, and inducible, nonsuppressible, ventricular tachyarrhythmia on electrophysiologic study. Mortality rates after 27 months of follow-up were 16% and 39% in the respective ICD and conventional therapy groups, corresponding to a significant 54% ($P = .009$) reduction in the risk of death with an ICD. Subsequently, the Multicenter Automatic Defibrillator Implantation Trial-II (MADIT-II)[23] evaluated ICD efficacy among low-EF patients without the requirement of further risk stratification. The study randomized 1232 prior-MI

Table 1
Clinical features and results from major secondary prevention ICD trials

| | | | Clinical Features | | | | Results | |
| | | | | | | | Crude Death | Risk Reduction |
Study	Sample Size	Design	Patients	Age (Y)	Ischemic Cause (%)	EF (%)	Rate (%)	with ICD
Secondary prevention								
AVID[13]	1016	ICD vs antiarrhythmic drugs	Resuscitated from near-fatal VF or post-cardioversion from sustained VT.	65	81	32	Non-ICD: 24 ICD: 16	28% (P = .02)
CIDS[14]	659	ICD vs amiodarone	Resuscitated VF or VT or with unmonitored syncope	63	82	33	Non-ICD: 30 ICD: 25	20% (P = .14)
CASH[15]	288	ICD vs amiodarone vs metoprolol	Survivors of cardiac arrest secondary to documented ventricular arrhythmias.	58	73	46	Non-ICD: 44 ICD: 36	23% (P = .08)

Abbreviations: CAD, coronary artery disease; CABG, coronary artery bypass graft surgery; CRT-D, cardiac-resynchronization therapy with pacemaker-defibrillator; EF, ejection fraction; ICD, implantable cardioverter defibrillator; I & NICM, ischemic and nonischemic cardiomyopathy; NSVT, nonsustained ventricular tachycardia; OPT, optimal pharmacologic therapy; PVC, premature ventricular contraction; SAECG, signal-averaged electrocardiogram; VF, ventricular fibrillation; VT, ventricular tachycardia.

Table 2
Clinical features and results from major primary prevention ICD trials that enrolled patients with coronary artery disease

		Clinical Features					Results	
Study	Sample Size	Design	Patients	Age (Y)	Ischemic Cause (%)	EF (%)	Crude Death Rate (%)	Risk Reduction with ICD
MADIT[22]	196	ICD vs antiarrhythmic drugs	Previous MI, EF ≤ 0.35, NSVT, EPS+	63	100	26	Non-ICD: 39 ICD: 12	54% (P = .0.01)
MADIT-II[23]	1232	ICD vs OPT	Prior MI, EF ≤ 0.30	64	100	26	Non-ICD: 20 ICD: 14	31% (P = .02)
CABG-Patch[24]	900	ICD vs no antiarrhythmic drugs	CAD, abnormal SAECG, CABG surgery	64	100	27	Non-ICD: 5 ICD: 4	None
DINAMIT[25]	674	ICD vs OPT	NICM, EF ≤ 0.35, NSVT or 10 PVC/24 h	62	100	28	Non-ICD: 17 ICD: 19	None
COMPANION[26]	1520	CRT vs CRT-D vs OPT	I & NICM, EF ≤ 0.35, QRS>120 ms	67	55	21	Medical: 25 CRT: 21 CRT-D: 18	40% (P<.001)
SCD-HeFT[27]	2521	ICD vs OPT vs Amiodarone	I & NICM, EF ≤ 0.35	60	52	25	Placebo: 29 Amiodarone: 28 ICD: 22	23% (P = .007)

Abbreviations: CAD, coronary artery disease; CABG, coronary artery bypass graft surgery; CRT-D, cardiac-resynchronization therapy with pacemaker-defibrillator; EF, ejection fraction; EPS, electrophysiologic study; ICD, implantable cardioverter defibrillator; I & NICM, ischemic and nonischemic cardiomyopathy; MI, myocardial infarction; NSVT, nonsustained ventricular tachycardia; OPT, optimal pharmacologic therapy; PVC, premature ventricular contraction; SAECG, signal-averaged electrocardiogram.

patients with EF of 30% or less and NYHA class I-III to ICD or conventional medical therapy. During an average follow-up of 20 months, mortality rates were significantly lower in the ICD group (**Fig. 1**), corresponding to a significant 31% reduction in the risk of death with an ICD (P = .016). In contrast, the Coronary Artery Bypass Graft (CABG)-Patch Trial,[24] did not demonstrate a significant survival benefit for prophylactic ICD implantation in patients undergoing elective CABG who had an EF of 35% or less and abnormalities on signal-averaged electrocardiograms. Similarly, in the Defibrillator in Acute Myocardial Infarction Trial (DINAMIT),[25] there was no survival benefit with an ICD in early post-MI patients (6–40 days) with reduced LV (EF ≤ 35%) and impaired cardiac autonomic function (manifested as depressed heart-rate variability or an elevated average 24-hour heart rate on Holter monitoring).

The Comparison of Medical Therapy, Pacing, and Defibrillation in Heart Failure (COMPANION) Trial[26] compared optimized medical therapy, optimized medical therapy with cardiac resynchronization therapy (CRT), and optimized medical therapy with CRT combined with a defibrillator (CRT-D) in patients with LV dysfunction (EF ≤ 35%) and a prolonged QRS duration (≥ 120 msec). More than 50% of enrolled patients had established CAD. During a mean follow-up period of 16 months, crude mortality rate was 25% in the optimized medical therapy group, 21% in the CRT group, and 18% in the CRT-D group. CRT-D was associated with a somewhat greater survival benefit than was CRT without defibrillator backup. The benefit of CRT-D in the study was consistent in patients with ischemic and nonischemic cardiomyopathy.[26] In the Sudden Cardiac Death in Heart Failure Trial (SCD-HeFT),[27] 2521

ischemic and nonischemic cardiomyopathy patients with NYHA class II or III and EF of 35% or less were randomized to optimized heart failure therapy, optimized heart failure therapy with the addition of amiodarone, or medical treatment with the addition of a shock-only single-lead ICD. At 5-year follow-up, mortality rates were similar in the placebo and amiodarone groups, whereas ICD therapy was associated with an overall significant 23% reduction in the risk of death as compared with placebo. The benefit of the ICD in SCD-HeFT was consistent in enrolled patients who had either ischemic or nonischemic cardiomyopathy (**Fig. 2**A and B, respectively).

Data from a meta-analysis of 10 primary prevention ICD trials,[19] that also included the nonrandomized ICD comparison in the Multicenter Unsustained Tachycardia Trial [MUSTT][20] and 2 smaller studies that assessed the benefit of the ICD in patients with nonischemic cardiomyopathy,[21,28] demonstrated a significant overall survival benefit with an ICD as a primary prevention strategy in patients with LV dysfunction. All-cause mortality rates were shown to be lower among the 3530 randomized to ICD therapy (18.5%) as compared with the 3723 patients randomized to non-ICD therapy (26.4%), corresponding to a 25% relative reduction in all-cause mortality with the ICD (P = .003).[19]

American College of Cardiology/American Heart Association/Heart Rhythm Society (ACC/AHA/HRS) Practice Guidelines

A summary of the main recommendations for primary and secondary implantation of an ICD is provided in **Table 3**. Notably, primary prevention guidelines do not distinguish between ischemic

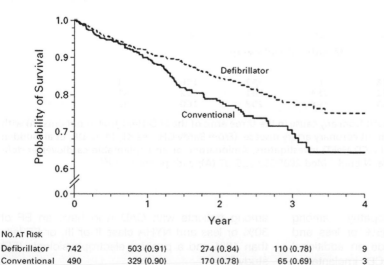

No. at Risk

Defibrillator	742	503 (0.91)	274 (0.84)	110 (0.78)	9
Conventional	490	329 (0.90)	170 (0.78)	65 (0.69)	3

Fig. 1. Kaplan-Meier estimates of the probability of survival in the ICD-allocated group and the conventional medical therapy group of MADIT-II. The difference in survival between the two groups was significant (nominal P = .007, by the log-rank test). (*From* Moss AJ, Zareba W, Hall WJ, et al. Prophylactic implantation of a defibrillator in patients with myocardial infarction and reduced ejection fraction. N Engl J Med 1997;337:1569–75; with permission).[23]

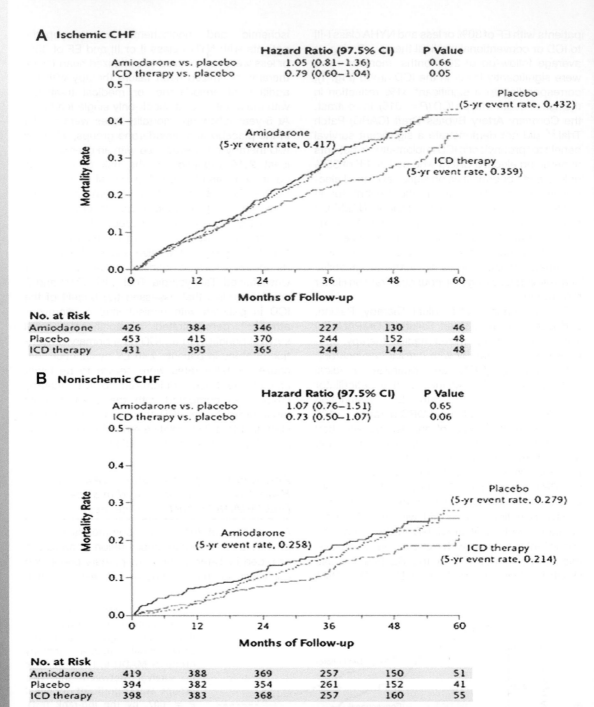

Fig. 2. Kaplan-Meier estimates of death from any cause in the three arms of the SCD-HeFT trial in patients (*A*) with coronary artery disease; and (*B*) without coronary artery disease. (*From* Bardy GH, Lee KL, Mark DB, et al. Sudden Cardiac Death in Heart Failure Trial (SCD-HeFT) Investigators. Amiodarone or an implantable cardioverter-defibrillator for congestive heart failure. N Engl J Med 2005;352:225–37 (A); with permission.)[27]

and nonischemic cardiomyopathy among patients who have an EF of 35% or less and NYHA class II or III, but include an additional recommendation for primary ICD implantation among patients with CAD who have an EF of 30% or less and NYHA class II or III, or EF less than 40% and a positive electrophysiologic (EP) study.[30]

Table 3
Current recommendations for implantable cardioverter defibrillator implantation for the primary and secondary prevention of sudden cardiac death[30]

Class	Recommendation	Level of Evidence
Secondary prevention		
I	Prior cardiac arrest due to VF or VT not due to a transient or reversible cause	A
I	Spontaneous sustained VT in association with structural heart disease	B
I	Syncope of undetermined origin with clinically relevant, hemodynamically significant sustained VT or VF induced at EP study	B
IIa	Unexplained syncope, significant LV dysfunction, nonischemic DCM.	C
IIa	Sustained VT and normal or near-normal ventricular function	C
Primary prevention		
I	Ischemic- (>40 days post-MI) or non-ischemic- patients with EF ≤35%; NYHA class II to III	A
I	>40 days post-MI, LVEF<30%, NYHA Class I.	A
I	Prior MI + Nonsustained VT, LVEF <40%, inducible VF or sustained VT at EP study	B

Abbreviations: DCM, dilated cardiomyopathy; EP, electrophysiologic; LVEF, left ventricular ejection fraction; MI, myocardial infarction; NYHA, New York Heart Association; VF, ventricular fibrillation; VT, ventricular tachycardia.

Data from ACC/AHA/HRS 2008 Guidelines for Device-Based Therapy of Cardiac Rhythm Abnormalities. A Report of the American College of Cardiology/American Heart Association Task Force on Practice Guidelines (Writing Committee to Revise the ACC/AHA/NASPE 2002 Guideline Update for Implantation of Cardiac Pacemakers and Antiarrhythmia Devices). Circulation 2008;117:e350–408.

PRIMARY PREVENTION WITH AN IMPLANTABLE CARDIAC DEFIBRILLATOR IN RISK SUBSETS OF PATIENTS WITH CORONARY ARTERY DISEASE

Subgroup analyses in MADIT-II did not identify significant differences in ICD efficacy in patients subsets categorized by age,[31] sex,[32] NYHA class, or QRS duration.[23] However, data from recent ICD trials suggest considerable risk heterogeneity in the low-EF population, with a relatively small rate of appropriate ICD therapy after implantation (25% to 30% in SCD-HeFT[27] and MADIT-II[33]). Thus, it appears that a proportion of currently implanted patients may not derive benefit from the device during long-term follow-up. Data from studies that assessed ICD efficacy in risk subsets of MADIT-II patients are summarized in **Table 4**, with the main clinical implications from these analyses discussed as follows.

Time Dependence of Implantable Cardiac Defibrillator Benefit After Coronary Revascularization and Acute Coronary Events

Myocardial ischemia has been suggested to be an important trigger for development of ventricular tachyarrhythmias.[34] Therefore, coronary revascularization may attenuate subsequent SCD risk and thereby affect ICD efficacy. Data from the Studies of Left Ventricular Dysfunction (SOLVD) trials have shown that in patients with an EF of 35% or less, prior CABG was independently associated with a significant 25% reduction in risk of death and a 46% reduction in risk of SCD.[35] These findings may explain the lack of improved survival with an ICD in the CABG-Patch patients in whom an ICD was implanted prophylactically at the time of CABG.[24] Notably, subanalysis of CABG-Patch revealed that most of the deaths (71%) in the study were nonarrhythmic in nature,[36] further suggesting that recent coronary revascularization attenuates the risk of arrhythmic mortality in patients with ischemic LV dysfunction. We have similarly observed in the MADIT-II population that the mode of death among patients enrolled during the early postcoronary revascularization period was dominated by nonarrhythmic mortality (83%), whereas after this early time period the proportion of deaths that were not sudden in nature was reduced to 40%.[37] Accordingly, MADIT-II patients who were enrolled for more than 6 months following coronary revascularization enjoyed a significant survival benefit as a result of the ICD (hazard ratio (HR) = 0.64; P = .01), whereas no survival benefit was found in the low-risk group of patients who were enrolled for 6 months or less following revascularization

Table 4
Data from Multicenter Automatic Defibrillator Implantation Trial-II regarding implantable cardioverter
defibrillator efficacy in risk subsets of patients with coronary artery disease

Subgroup	HR	95% Confidence Interval	P Value
Gender[32]			
Female	0.57	0.28–1.18	.132
Male	0.66	0.48–0.91	.011
Age[31]			
≥75 years	0.56	0.29–1.08	.08
<75 years	0.63	0.45–0.88	.01
Time from coronary revascularization[37]			
≤6 months	1.10	0.40–3.0	.86
>6 months	0.64	0.46–0.89	.009
Time from MI[39]			
<18 months	0.97	0.51–1.81	.92
≥18 months	0.55	0.39–0.78	.001
Renal function[40]			
eGFR <35 mL/min/1.73 m^2	0.95	0.23–4.00	.62
eGFR ≥35 mL/min/1.73 m^2	0.34	0.20–0.56	<.001
Systolic blood pressure[43]			
>130 mm Hg	1.04	0.55–1.97	.89
≥130 mm Hg	0.61	0.45–0.83	.002

Abbreviations: eGFR, estimated glomerular filtration rate; MI, myocardial infarction.

(HR = 1.19; *P* = .76) (**Table 4**; **Fig. 3**). A recent subanalysis of CAD patients enrolled in SCD-HeFT demonstrated consistent findings.[38] The study demonstrated a trend toward improved survival with an ICD in patients who had their CABG more than 2 years before randomization (HR = 0.71; 95% confidence interval [CI] 0.49–1.04]) that was not observed in patients who had their CABG 2 years or less before randomization

(HR = 1.40; 95% CI 0.61–3.24). Thus, it appears that the lack of defibrillator benefit when a device is implanted in proximity to a coronary revascularization procedure in the three trials was related to the fact that most deaths during this time period were nonarrhythmic in nature.

A similar time-dependent effect on ICD benefit was shown following an acute coronary event. The DINAMIT trial suggested that the reduction

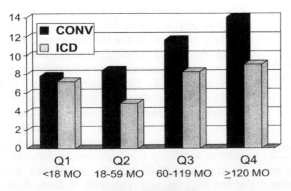

MORTALITY RATE

CONV (n) 125 118 112 105
ICD (n)   175 165 172 187

TIME FROM MI

Fig. 3. Two-year Kaplan-Meier estimates of all-cause mortality in the two treatment groups of MADIT-II by time from coronary revascularization (time periods: ≤6 months; 7–36 months, 36–60 months; and >60 months). (*From* Goldenberg I, Moss AJ, McNitt S, et al, for the Multicenter Automatic Defibrillator Implantation Trial II Investigators. Time-Dependence of Defibrillator Benefit after Coronary Revascularization in the Multicenter Automatic Defibrillator Implantation Trial-II. Am Coll Cardiol 2006;47:1811–7 (B); with permission.)[37]

in the risk of arrhythmic death with an ICD in the high-risk early post-MI period may be transformed into subsequent nonarrhythmic mortality, resulting in a neutral effect of the ICD on survival during this time period.[25] Subsequently, Wilber and colleagues,[39] in a subgroup analysis from MADIT-II, further evaluated the effect of time from MI on ICD efficacy. The study showed that in stable post-MI patients more than 1 month after the acute event, mortality risk is increased as a function of time from MI, resulting in enhanced ICD benefit for more than 18 months post-MI (**Table 4**; **Fig. 4**). The findings from the two trials suggest attenuated ICD efficacy in the high-risk (early <1 month) and low-risk (stable 1–18 months) post-MI subgroups, with enhanced defibrillator efficacy in intermediate-risk patients who experienced more remote MI.

Competing Risk of Arrhythmic and Nonarrhythmic Mortality in Patients with Coronary Artery Disease with an Implantable Cardiac Defibrillator

We have recently assessed ICD efficacy among patients enrolled in MADIT-II who had varying

degrees of renal dysfunction.[40] Our data demonstrate that the benefit of the ICD in CAD patients with chronic kidney disease is not uniform (**Table 4**; **Fig. 5**). Thus, although patients with mild to moderate renal dysfunction experienced a pronounced reduction in the risk of all-cause mortality (32% reduction; $P = .01$) and SCD (66% reduction; $P<.001$), those with more advanced kidney disease (estimated glomerular filtration rate [eGFR] <35 mL/min/1.73 m^2) did not derive a significant benefit from primary device implantation (all-cause mortality: HR = 1.09 [$P = .84$], SCD: HR = 0.95 [$P = .95$]). A possible explanation for these findings relates to the fact that nonarrhythmic mortality was the predominant mode of death among ICD-treated patients with advanced renal dysfunction, accounting for 65% of observed mortality cases. These findings suggest that the competing risks of arrhythmic and nonarrhythmic mortality may limit ICD efficacy in patients with advanced kidney disease.

The competing risk between arrhythmic and nonarrhythmic events among patients with an ICD was also demonstrated in two recent studies that assessed the risk of heart failure events among patients with an ICD.[41,42] In MADIT-II,

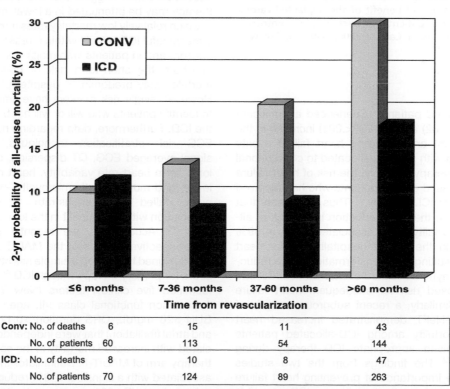

Fig. 4. Mortality rates (per 100 person-years of follow-up) in MADIT-II patients randomized to conventional (CONV) medical therapy patients (*black bars*) and ICD therapy, grouped by time from MI in quartiles (Q). MI, myocardial infarction. (*From* Wilber DJ, Zareba W, Hall WJ, et al. Time dependence of mortality risk and defibrillator benefit after myocardial infarction. Circulation 2004;109:1082–4 (B); with permission.)[39]

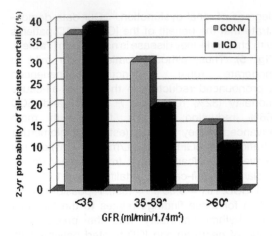

Conv:	No. of deaths	14	49	44
	No. of patients	39	160	286
ICD:	No. of deaths	16	44	49
	No. of patients	41	227	470

Fig. 5. Two-year Kaplan-Meier estimates of the cumulative probability of all-cause mortality in the two treatment groups of MADIT-II by eGFR category. *P<.05. ICD, implanted cardioverter defibrillator; GFR, glomerular filtration rate. (*From* Goldenberg I, Moss AJ, McNitt S, et al. for the Multicenter Automatic Defibrillator Implantation Trial-II Investigators. Relations among renal function, risk of sudden cardiac death, and benefit of the implanted cardiac defibrillator in patients with ischemic left ventricular dysfunction. Am J Cardiol 2006;98:485–90 (B); with permission.)[40]

ICD-allocated patients experienced a significant 39% (P = .02) and 58% (P<.001) increase in the risk for first and recurrent heart failure events compared with patients allocated to conventional medical therapy. Notably, the risk of heart failure was increased among patients who had received appropriate ICD therapy.[41] Thus, it appears that in MADIT-II, the 31% reduction in the risk of all-cause mortality was associated with a 39% increase in the risk of hospitalization for heart failure, resulting in a transformation of the reduction in arrhythmia-related events with an ICD into an increased risk for subsequent heart failure events. Similarly, a recent subgroup analysis of the SCD-HeFT demonstrated increased heart failure mortality among ICD-allocated patients who received appropriate ICD therapy during the trial.[42] The findings from the two studies stress the importance of preventing heart failure progression in patients with an ICD, possibly through the combined usage of optimized adjunctive medical therapy or resynchronization therapy.

Implantable Cardiac Defibrillator Benefit in Patients with a Low Risk for Arrhythmic Mortality

A recent subanalysis from MADIT-II demonstrated an inverse relationship between blood pressure levels (both systolic and diastolic) and the risk of sudden cardiac mortality,[43] resulting in attenuated ICD efficacy in the lower-risk, upper systolic (>130 mm Hg) and diastolic (≥80 mm Hg) blood pressure values, and enhanced efficacy among patients with lower blood pressure values who have a higher risk of SCD (**Table 4**; Goldenberg and colleagues[43]). These findings suggest that noninvasive hemodynamic parameters may be useful to identify a lower-risk subset of patients with ischemic cardiomyopathy, in whom the benefit of the ICD is more limited because of a relatively lower risk for arrhythmic death.

Suggested Clinical Approach to Risk Stratification for Primary Implantable Cardiac Defibrillator Implantation in Patients with Coronary Artery Disease with Left Ventricular Dysfunction

The subanalyses from the major ICD trials described earlier suggest that the benefit of ICD therapy may be attenuated in a lower-risk subset, in which relatively low mortality rates may preclude a meaningful ICD benefit within a reasonable time horizon, and in patients with major comorbidities, in whom the short-term risk of nonarrhythmic mortality may predominate despite ICD therapy. However, single risk markers have limited ability to identify patients who will or will not benefit from the ICD. Furthermore, data regarding noninvasive ECG risk stratification techniques, including signal-averaged ECG, QT dispersion, short- and long- term heart rate variability, heart rate turbulence, and more recently microvolt T-wave alternans, failed to demonstrate a consistent association with ICD benefit in the low-EF population.[44,45] Accordingly, we recently performed a retrospective analysis of the MADIT-II trial that was designed to develop a simple risk stratification score for primary therapy with an ICD.[46] The study identified five clinical factors (New York Heart Association functional class >II, age >70 years, BUN >26 mg/dL, QRS duration >0.12 seconds, and atrial fibrillation) that were independently associated with increased mortality in the conventional therapy arm of MADIT-II. Defibrillator therapy was associated with a significant 49% reduction in the risk of death (P<.001) among patients with 1 or more risk factors (n = 786), whereas no ICD benefit was identified in about a third of the study population (n = 345) who had 0 risk factors (HR = 0.96;

$P = .91$), and in a prespecified subset of very high risk patients with comorbidities and advanced renal dysfunction (HR = 1.00; $P>.99$). These data suggest a U-shaped pattern for ICD efficacy in the low-EF population (**Fig. 6**), with pronounced benefit in intermediate-risk patients and attenuated efficacy in lower- and higher-risk subsets.

Consistent with our clinical risk stratification findings, we recently used long-term mortality data in the MADIT-II population, and developed a similar risk score that can be used to assess the long-term risk of death among ICD-treated patients with ischemic LV dysfunction (**Fig. 7**; Cygankiewicz and colleagues[47]).

OTHER CONSIDERATIONS
Inappropriate Implantable Cardiac Defibrillator Therapies

In MADIT II, 11.5% of implanted patients experienced inappropriate ICD shocks, which constituted 31.2% of total shocks.[48] Predictors of inappropriate ICD shocks in the trial included smoking, atrial fibrillation, diastolic hypertension, and prior appropriate shocks. Notably, inappropriate therapies in MADIT-II were shown to be associated with increased probability of death, further stressing the importance of efforts to reduce their occurrence.

Quality of Life

Patients' psychological responses to implantation of a defibrillator are highly variable. In the AVID trial, patients who reported shocks during follow-up also reported reductions in their physical functioning and mental well-being and increased anxiety.[49] In MADIT-II, appropriate ICD shocks were associated with a significant reduction in physical functioning at 1 year, but not in mental well-being,[50] whereas a recent subanalysis of the SCD-HeFT trial showed that single-lead

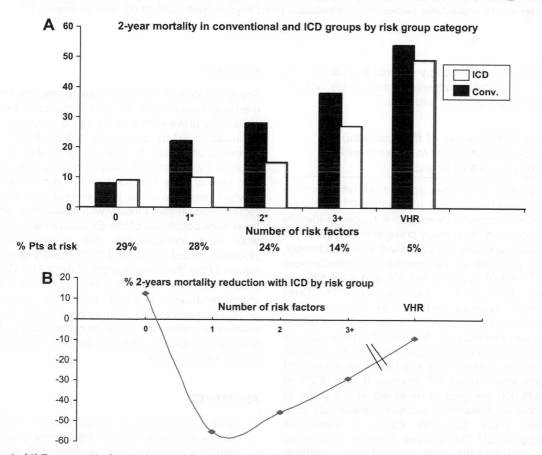

Fig. 6. (A) Two-year Kaplan-Meier mortality rates in the ICD and conventional therapy groups; and (B) the corresponding 2-year mortality rate reduction with an ICD, by risk score and in VHR patients. *$P < .05$ for the comparison between the conventional therapy and ICD groups. VHR, very high risk defined as serum creatinine ≥2.5 mg/dL or blood urea nitrogen ≥50 mg/dL. (From Goldenberg I, Vyas AK, Hall, WJ, et al. MADIT-II Investigators. Risk stratification for primary implantation of a cardioverter-defibrillator in patients with ischemic left ventricular dysfunction. J Am Coll Cardiol 2008;51:288–96 (B); with permission.)[46]

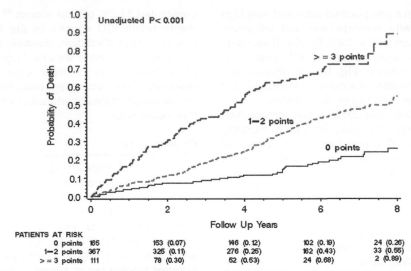

Fig. 7. Long-term mortality in ICD-treated patients in MADIT-II by risk factor counts (age, NYHA class, nonsinus rhythm, QRS duration, diabetes mellitus). (*From* Cygankiewicz I, Gillespie J, Zareba W, et al. MADIT II Investigators. Predictors of long-term mortality in Multicenter Automatic Defibrillator Implantation Trial II (MADIT II) patients with implantable cardioverter-defibrillators. Heart Rhythm 2009;6:468–73 (B); with permission.)[47]

shock-only ICD therapy was not associated with any detectable adverse quality-of-life effects during 30 months of follow-up.[51]

Cost-Effectiveness of the Implantable Cardiac Defibrillator in Patients with Coronary Artery Disease

Several recent studies reported cost-effectiveness estimates for MADIT-II–type patients.[52,53] Sanders and colleagues[52] developed a model to identify the costs in the primary prevention trials in which ICD therapy was associated with a survival benefit, and reported an incremental cost-effectiveness ratio (iCER) between $68,300 and $101,500 per year-of-life-saved in this population. The Duke study[53] showed lifetime and 12-year iCERs between $50,500 and $79,900 per year-of-life-saved, respectively, for MADIT-II-type patients who were followed at Duke University. By contrast, a recent analysis that was based on actual cost data from MADIT-II[54] reported a high iCER of $235,000 per year-of-life-saved at 3.5 years of follow-up. Secondary analyses of these data identified more favorable iCERs in higher-risk subgroups.[54] This analysis, however, was based on cost data that were obtained over a relatively short follow-up time. Thus, long-term data are required for a more comprehensive assessment of the cost-effectiveness of primary prevention with an ICD in patients with ischemic left ventricular dysfunction.

SUMMARY

The application of implantable device therapy has markedly increased in the past 2 decades, from secondary prevention with an ICD in survivors of a cardiac arrest to primary prevention of SCD in asymptomatic patients with ischemic and nonischemic LV dysfunction. Based on major randomized clinical trials that have shown a consistent survival benefit with an ICD, current guidelines recommend primary therapy with an ICD to a relatively large population of low-EF patients with CAD who have considerable risk heterogeneity. However, recent data from MADIT-II suggest limitations of the life-saving benefit of the ICD in CAD in very low subsets and high-risk subgroups with major comorbidity in whom arrhythmic mortality does not predominate. Ongoing research may continue to refine risk stratification and delineate groups who derive enhanced long-term survival benefit from the ICD.

REFERENCES

1. Lloyd-Jones D, Adams R, Carnethon M, et al. Heart disease and stroke statistics–2009 update: a report from the American Heart Association Statistics Committee and Stroke Statistics Subcommittee. Circulation 2009;119:480–6.
2. The Multicentre Postinfarction Research Group. Risk stratification and survival after myocardial infarction. N Engl J Med 1983;309:331–6.

3. Bigger JT Jr, Fleiss JL, Kleiger R, et al. The relationships among ventricular arrhythmias, left ventricular dysfunction, and mortality in the 2 years after myocardial infarction. Circulation 1984;69:250–8.

4. Luu M, Stevenson WG, Stevenson LW, et al. Diverse mechanisms of unexpected cardiac arrest in advanced heart failure. Circulation 1989;80: 1675–80.

5. Huikuri A, Castellanos, Myerburg RJ. Sudden death due to cardiac arrhythmias. N Engl J Med 2001;345: 1473–82.

6. Echt DS, Liebson PR, Mitchell LB, et al. Mortality and morbidity in patients receiving encainide, flecainide, or placebo. N Engl J Med 1991;324:781–8.

7. Waldo AL, Camm AJ, deRuyter H, et al. Effect of d-sotalol on mortality in patients with left ventricular dysfunction after recent and remote myocardial infarction. Lancet 1996;348:7–12.

8. Singh SN, Fletcher RD, Fisher SG, et al. Amiodarone in patients with congestive heart failure and asymptomatic ventricular arrhythmia. N Engl J Med 1995; 333:77–82.

9. Doval HC, Nul DR, Grancelli HO, et al. Randomized trial of low-dose amiodarone in severe congestive heart failure. Grupo de Estudio de la Sobrevida en la Insuficiencia Cardiaca en Argentina (GESICA). Lancet 1994;344:493–8.

10. Julian DG, Camm AJ, Frangin G, et al. Randomised trial of effect of amiodarone on mortality in patients with left-ventricular dysfunction after recent myocardial infarction: EMIAT. Lancet 1997;349:667–74.

11. Cairns JA, Connolly SJ, Roberts R, et al. Randomised trial of outcome after myocardial infarction in patients with frequent or repetitive premature depolarisations: CAMIAT. Lancet 1997;349:675–82.

12. Mirowski M, Reid PR, Mower MM, et al. Termination of malignant ventricular arrhythmias with an implanted automatic defibrillator in human beings. N Engl J Med 1980;303:322–4.

13. The AVID investigators. A comparison of antiarrhythmic drug therapy with implantable defibrillators in patients resuscitated from near fatal ventricular arrhythmias. N Engl J Med 1997;337:1576–83.

14. Connolly SJ, Gent M, Roberts RS, et al. Canadian Implantable Defibrillator Study (CIDS): a randomized trial of the implantable cardioverter defibrillator against amiodarone. Circulation 2000;101: 1297–302.

15. Kuck KH, Cappato R, Siebels J, et al. Randomized comparison of antiarrhythmic drug therapy with implantable defibrillators in patients resuscitated from cardiac arrest: the Cardiac Arrest Study Hamburg (CASH). Circulation 2000;102:748–54.

16. Buxton AE, Marchlinski FE, Waxman HL, et al. Prognostic factors in nonsustained ventricular tachycardia. Am J Cardiol 1984;53:1275–9.

17. Wilber DJ, Olshansky B, Moran JF, et al. Electrophysiological testing and nonsustained ventricular tachycardia: use and limitations in patients with coronary artery disease and impaired ventricular function. Circulation 1990;82:350–8.

18. Kadish A, Dyer A, Daubert JP, et al. Prophylactic defibrillator implantation in patients with nonischemic dilated cardiomyopathy. N Engl J Med 2004; 350:2151–8.

19. Nanthakumar K, Epstein AE, Kay GN, et al. Prophylactic implantable cardioverter-defibrillator therapy in patients with left ventricular systolic dysfunction a pooled analysis of 10 primary prevention trials. J Am Coll Cardiol 2004;44: 2166–72.

20. Buxton AE, Lee KL, Fisher JD, et al. A randomized study of the prevention of sudden death in patients with coronary artery disease. N Engl J Med 1999; 341:1882–90.

21. Bansch D, Antz M, Boczor S, et al. Primary prevention of sudden cardiac death in idiopathic dilated cardiomyopathy: the Cardiomyopathy Trial (CAT). Circulation 2002;105:1453–8.

22. Moss AJ, Hall WJ, Cannom DS, et al. Improved survival with an implanted defibrillator in patients with coronary disease at high risk for ventricular arrhythmia. Multicenter Automatic Defibrillator Implantation Trial Investigators. N Engl J Med 1996;335:1933–40.

23. Moss AJ, Zareba W, Hall WJ, et al. Prophylactic implantation of a defibrillator in patients with myocardial infarction and reduced ejection fraction. N Engl J Med 2002;346:877–83.

24. Bigger JT Jr. Prophylactic use of implanted cardiac defibrillators in patients at high risk for ventricular arrhythmias after coronary-artery bypass graft surgery. Coronary Artery Bypass Graft (CABG) Patch Trial Investigators. N Engl J Med 1997;337: 1569–75.

25. Hohnloser SH, Kuck KH, Dorian P, et al. Prophylactic use of an implantable cardioverter-defibrillator after acute myocardial infarction. N Engl J Med 2004; 351:2481–8.

26. Bristow MR, Saxon LA, Boehmer J, et al. Cardiac-resynchronization therapy with or without an implantable defibrillator in advanced chronic heart failure. N Engl J Med 2004;350:2140–50.

27. Bardy GH, Lee KL, Mark DB, et al. Sudden Cardiac Death in Heart Failure Trial (SCD-HeFT) Investigators. Amiodarone or an implantable cardioverter-defibrillator for congestive heart failure. N Engl J Med 2005;352:225–37.

28. Strickberger SA, Hummel JD, Bartlett TG, et al. Amiodarone versus implantable cardioverter-defibrillator: randomized trial in patients with nonischemic dilated cardiomyopathy and asymptomatic

nonsustained ventricular tachycardia—AMIOVIRT. J Am Coll Cardiol 2003;41:1707–12.

29. Connolly SJ, Hallstrom AP, Cappato R, et al. Meta-analysis of the implantable cardioverter defibrillator secondary prevention trials: AVID, CASH and CIDS studies. Eur Heart J 2000;21:2071–8.

30. Epstein AE, Dimarco JP, Ellenbogen KA, et al. ACC/AHA/HRS 2008 Guidelines for Device-Based Therapy of Cardiac Rhythm Abnormalities. A Report of the American College of Cardiology/American Heart Association Task Force on Practice Guidelines (Writing Committee to Revise the ACC/AHA/NASPE 2002 Guideline Update for Implantation of Cardiac Pacemakers and Antiarrhythmia Devices). Circulation 2008;117:e350–408.

31. Huang DT, Sesselberg HW, McNitt S, et al. Improved survival associated with prophylactic implantable defibrillators in elderly patients with prior myocardial infarction and depressed ventricular function: a MADIT-II substudy. J Cardiovasc Electrophysiol 2007;18:833–8.

32. Zareba W, Moss AJ, Jackson Hall W, et al. Clinical course and implantable cardioverter defibrillator therapy in postinfarction women with severe left ventricular dysfunction. J Cardiovasc Electrophysiol 2005;16:1265–70.

33. Daubert JP, Zareba W, Hall WJ, et al. Predictive value of ventricular arrhythmia inducibility for subsequent ventricular tachycardia or ventricular fibrillation in Multicenter Automatic Defibrillator Implantation Trial (MADIT) II patients. J Am Coll Cardiol 2006;47:98–107.

34. O'Rourke RA. Role of myocardial revascularization in sudden cardiac death. Circulation 1992;85: I112–7.

35. Veenhuyzen GD, Singh SN, McAreavey D, et al. Prior coronary artery bypass surgery and risk of death among patients with ischemic left ventricular dysfunction. Circulation 2001;104:1489–93.

36. Bigger JT Jr. Whang W, Rottman JN, et al. Mechanisms of death in the CABG Patch trial: a randomized trial of implantable cardiac defibrillator prophylaxis in patients at high risk of death after coronary artery bypass graft surgery. Circulation 1999;99:1416–21.

37. Goldenberg I, Moss AJ, McNitt S, et al. Time-dependence of defibrillator benefit after coronary revascularization in the Multicenter Automatic Defibrillator Implantation Trial-II. J Am Coll Cardiol 2006;47: 1811–7.

38. Al-Khatib SM, Hellkamp AS, Lee KL, et al. Implantable cardioverter defibrillator therapy in patients with prior coronary revascularization in the Sudden Cardiac Death in Heart Failure Trial (SCD-HeFT). J Cardiovasc Electrophysiol 2008;10:1059–65.

39. Wilber DJ, Zareba W, Hall WJ, et al. Time dependence of mortality risk and defibrillator benefit after myocardial infarction. Circulation 2004;109: 1082–4.

40. Goldenberg I, Moss AJ, McNitt S, et al. Relations among renal function, risk of sudden cardiac death, and benefit of the implanted cardiac defibrillator in patients with ischemic left ventricular dysfunction. Am J Cardiol 2006;98:485–90.

41. Goldenberg I, Moss AJ, Hall WJ, et al. Causes and consequences of heart failure after prophylactic implantation of a defibrillator in the MADIT-II Trial. Circulation 2006;113:2810–7.

42. Poole JE, Johnson GW, Hellkamp AS, et al. Prognostic importance of defibrillator shocks in patients with heart failure. N Engl J Med 2008; 359:1058–9.

43. Goldenberg I, Moss AJ, McNitt S, et al. Inverse relationship of blood pressure levels to sudden cardiac mortality and benefit of the implantable cardioverter-defibrillator in patients with ischemic left ventricular dysfunction. J Am Coll Cardiol 2007;49:1427–33.

44. Goldberger JJ, Cain ME, Hohnloser SH, et al. American Heart Association; American College of Cardiology Foundation; Heart Rhythm Society. American Heart Association/American College of Cardiology Foundation/Heart Rhythm Society scientific statement on noninvasive risk stratification techniques for identifying patients at risk for sudden cardiac death: a scientific statement from the American Heart Association Council on Clinical Cardiology Committee on Electrocardiography and Arrhythmias and Council on Epidemiology and Prevention. Circulation 2008;118:1497–518.

45. Gold MR, Ip JH, Costantini O, et al. Role of microvolt T-wave alternans in assessment of arrhythmia vulnerability among patients with heart failure and systolic dysfunction: primary results from the T-wave alternans sudden cardiac death in heart failure trial substudy. Circulation 2008;118(20): 2022–8.

46. Goldenberg I, Vyas AK, Hall WJ, et al. Risk stratification for primary implantation of a cardioverter-defibrillator in patients with ischemic left ventricular dysfunction. J Am Coll Cardiol 2008;51: 288–96.

47. Cygankiewicz I, Gillespie J, Zareba W, et al. Predictors of long-term mortality in Multicenter Automatic Defibrillator Implantation Trial II (MADIT II) patients with implantable cardioverter-defibrillators. Heart Rhythm 2009;6:468–73.

48. Daubert JP, Zareba W, Cannom DS, et al. Inappropriate implantable cardioverter-defibrillator shocks in MADIT II: frequency, mechanisms, predictors, and survival impact. J Am Coll Cardiol 2008;51: 1357–65.

49. Schron EB, Exner DV, Yao Q, et al. Quality of life in the Antiarrhythmics Versus Implantable Defibrillators

trial: impact of therapy and influence of adverse symptoms and defibrillator shocks. Circulation 2002;105:589–94.

50. Piotrowicz K, Noyes K, Lyness JM, et al. Physical functioning and mental well-being in association with health outcome in patients enrolled in the Multicenter Automatic Defibrillator Implantation Trial. Eur Heart J 2007;28:601–7.

51. Mark DB, Anstrom KJ, Sun JL, et al. Quality of life with defibrillator therapy or amiodarone in heart failure. N Engl J Med 2008;359:999–1008.

52. Sanders GD, Hlatky MA, Owens DK. Cost-effectiveness of implantable cardioverter-defibrillators. N Engl J Med 2005;353:1471–80.

53. Al-Khatib SM, Anstrom KJ, Eisenstein EL, et al. Clinical and economic implications of the Multicenter Automatic Defibrillator Implantation Trial-II. Ann Intern Med 2005;142:593–600.

54. Zwanziger J, Hall WJ, Dick AW, et al. The cost effectiveness of implantable cardioverter-defibrillators: results from the Multicenter Automatic Defibrillator Implantation Trial (MADIT)-II. J Am Coll Cardiol 2006;47:2310–8.

Implantable Cardioverter Defibrillator Therapy for Primary Prevention of Sudden Cardiac Death—An Argument for Guideline Adherence

Eric N. Prystowsky, MD, FACC, FAHA, FHRS[a,b,]*,
Richard I. Fogel, MD, FACC, FHRS[a],
Benzy J. Padanilam, MD[a], David Rardon, MD, FACC[a]

KEYWORDS
- Sudden cardiac death • Implantable defibrillator
- Congestive heart failure
- Cardiac resynchronization therapy • Guidelines

Sudden cardiac death (SCD) is considered the most common cause of death in adults in the United States. In a report from the Centers for Disease Control and Prevention,[1] 452,340 of 728,743 (63.4%) cardiac deaths were considered SCD. Coronary artery disease (CAD) is the most common pathologic finding in patients who die suddenly.[2] Adabag and colleagues[3] reevaluated the risk of SCD after myocardial infarction (MI) in a population-based surveillance study in Olmstead County, Minnesota. Follow-up was obtained in 2997 hospital survivors of MI between 1979 and 2005. During a median follow-up of 4.7 years, 282 of 1160 deaths (24%) were attributed to SCD. These investigators noted a cumulative incidence of 1.2% SCD in the first month after MI but a rate of 1.2% per year thereafter. The risk of SCD appeared to increase in patients with an occurrence of heart failure (HF) during follow-up. These investigators concluded that the risk of SCD following MI has declined significantly over the past 3 decades in community practice in their area of the country. These investigators found a particularly high incidence of SCD in the first month after MI. Solomon and colleagues[4] similarly reported in patients with a left ventricular ejection fraction (LVEF) of 30% or less a rather high risk in this early period after MI.

The cause of SCD in patients with CAD is not always clear. Some patients may die from an acute ischemic event that may precipitate ventricular fibrillation (VF), whereas other patients may develop sustained ventricular tachycardia (VT) in an area of the scar from the previous MI and unrelated to any acute ischemic event. The addition of HF through multiple mechanisms can make the electrophysiologic milieu more unstable and more prone to the emergence of life-threatening ventricular arrhythmias.

[a] Clinical Electrophysiology Laboratory, St Vincent Hospital, The Care Group, 8333 Naab Road, Suite 400, Indianapolis, IN 46062, USA
[b] Duke University Medical Center, Durham, North Carolina, USA
* Corresponding author. Clinical Electrophysiology Laboratory, St Vincent Hospital, The Care Group, 8333 Naab Road, Suite 400, Indianapolis, IN 46260.
E-mail address: eprystow@thecaregroup.com (E.N. Prystowsky).

Card Electrophysiol Clin 1 (2009) 95–103
doi:10.1016/j.ccep.2009.08.011
1877-9182/09/$ – see front matter © 2009 Published by Elsevier Inc.

To investigate the incidence of acute coronary artery occlusion among patients with sudden cardiac arrest outside of the hospital, Spaulding and colleagues[5] performed coronary angiography immediately after hospitalization in 84 consecutive survivors of out-of-hospital cardiac arrest. Sixty patients had significant CAD. Of these, 40 (48%) had coronary artery occlusion. The investigators commented that the high prevalence of occlusion of coronary arteries in their study substantiated the role of rupture of atherosclerotic plaques as the trigger of acute coronary syndromes and subsequent cardiac arrest.

Plaque morphology in men with CAD who died suddenly was evaluated by Burke and colleagues[6] in an autopsy study. In 59 of 113 patients, acute coronary thrombi were noted. Plaque rupture occurred in 41 patients and plaque erosions occurred in 18 patients. In a related study, Burke and colleagues[7] analyzed plaque rupture in SCD as related to death during exertion versus rest. SCD happened in 25 of 141 men during emotional stress or strenuous physical activity. There was an important difference in plaque rupture noted in those patients with SCD during exertion (17 of 25, 68%) versus those dying at rest (27 of 116, 23%).

A take-home message from the studies on CAD and SCD noted above is that the mechanisms that cause SCD in patients with CAD are complex, not only at the myocardial tissue level, but also within the coronary arteries. Furthermore, of all the interventions we can do to minimize sudden death, the most important is to eliminate CAD, which should always be the ultimate goal. That said, this will certainly not happen in the foreseeable future, and it is key to identify patients at risk for sudden death and apply evidence-based medicine to minimize its occurrence. For individuals at risk for the development of CAD, appropriate use of medications and lifestyle changes should be undertaken. For patients who have suffered an MI, analysis of their risk for SCD should be undertaken and those who require an implantable cardioverter defibrillator (ICD) should have this discussed with their physician. The data supporting primary prevention of SCD in patients with CAD and other conditions are presented later.

DEVELOPMENT OF THE IMPLANTABLE CARDIOVERTER DEFIBRILLATOR

In the early 1980s an electrophysiology study was performed by one of the authors (ENP) on a man in his 30s who had a nonischemic dilated cardiomyopathy and documented sustained VT. In that era, we routinely performed serial electrophysiologic-pharmacologic testing with antiarrhythmic drugs to determine the best therapy for patients to prevent recurrence of VT or SCD; there was no ICD option then. We were able to find the drug that prevented induction of sustained VT and he was discharged taking it. We learned months later that the patient died suddenly, leaving his wife without a husband and their young children without a father. Such circumstances are a clear reminder of the inadequacies of drug therapy and methods to judge efficacy. Fortunately, an answer was just around the corner.

Dr. Michele Mirowski invented the ICD.[8] He described the key elements of it in a 1970 publication. The first system design incorporated a single transvenous lead positioned in the right ventricle and a patch on the anterior chest wall with defibrillation achieved using 30 to 50 J.[8] In a subsequent study, Mirowski and colleagues[9] confirmed the concept of internal defibrillation in a study of 25 animals. In 1980, Mirowski and colleagues[10] gained approval to study the initial automatic implantable defibrillator and the first implant took place on February 4, 1980, at Johns Hopkins Hospital. The initial device had no programming capability, no telemetry, and it was committed to deliver a shock regardless of whether tachycardia persisted. In 1985, the Food and Drug Administration initially approved the ICD for patient care.

During the next 2 decades, there were two major areas of research regarding the ICD. The first involved a continuing series of technological improvements in both the ICD generator and lead system. Monophasic wave-form shocks gave way to biphasic energy delivery, and surgical placement of leads was supplanted by transvenous lead systems. The devices became both smaller and more advanced. Pari passu with the technological advances came a series of randomized controlled trials to delineate much better which patients were the best candidates to receive an ICD for primary prevention of SCD. The next section provides details of the key randomized trials.

IMPLANTABLE CARDIOVERTER DEFIBRILLATOR PRIMARY PREVENTION RANDOMIZED CONTROLLED TRIALS
Multicenter Automatic Defibrillator Implantation Trial

The Multicenter Automatic Defibrillator Implantation Trial (MADIT) study included patients with a prior MI, LVEF of 35% or less, spontaneous non-sustained VT, and inducible VT at electrophysiologic study that was not suppressed with intravenous procainamide.[11] Patients were randomized to receive an ICD or what was considered conventional medical therapy at that time, mostly amiodarone. The trial was prematurely terminated after a follow-up of 27 months because the ICD group had a 54% reduction in mortality compared with patients in the conventional medical treatment group. The mean LVEF was 25% in the conventional group and 27% in the ICD group.

Multicenter Unsustained Tachycardia Trial

The Multicenter Unsustained Tachycardia Trial (MUSTT) investigated the hypothesis that electrophysiologic testing to guide antiarrhythmic therapy could reduce the risk of cardiac arrest and sudden death.[12,13] Patients eligible for the trial had CAD with nonsustained VT and LVEF of 40% or less. As mentioned previously, a standard practice among electrophysiologists was to perform serial electrophysiologic-pharmacologic testing to evaluate the effectiveness of antiarrhythmic drug therapy in patients who had inducible VT or VF. MUSTT evaluated the concept of serial electrophysiologic testing as a means to guide therapy to reduce sudden death and cardiac arrest. Patients were included who had inducible sustained monomorphic VT with one to three extrastimuli or sustained polymorphic VT/VF with two or fewer extrastimuli. Patients were randomized to receive either no specific antiarrhythmic treatment or to receive electrophysiologically guided therapy. Antiarrhythmic agents were randomized in the trial and an ICD could be implanted if drugs proved ineffective. There were 704 patients who agreed to randomization. The mean LVEF was 30% for the electrophysiologically guided treatment group and 29% for the no antiarrhythmic therapy group. The median follow-up was 39 months. At 2 years, the overall mortality was 22% for patients randomized to electrophysiologically guided treatment and 28% for patients in the control group. At 5 years, the overall mortality was 42% for patients randomized to electrophysiologically guided treatment compared with 48% for those in the control group. Cardiac arrest or arrhythmic deaths at 2 years was 18% in the control group and 12% in those randomized to electrophysiologically guided therapy. Cardiac arrest or arrhythmic deaths at 5 years was 32% in the control group compared and 25% in those randomized to electrophysiologically guided therapy. The benefit of electrophysiologically guided therapy in MUSTT was related to those patients receiving an ICD and unrelated to antiarrhythmic drug therapy.[14] For patients who received an ICD, the 5-year cardiac arrest/arrhythmic death rate was 9% compared with 37% for patients who received antiarrhythmic drugs. Furthermore, the overall 5-year mortality rate was 55% for those who received antiarrhythmic drugs compared with only 24% for patients who had an ICD.

MUSTT taught us two important things. First, it demonstrated for the first time that the concept of serial electrophysiologic-pharmacologic testing was not useful in predicting long-term outcomes in patients with inducible sustained VT or VF. Thus, this methodology appropriately fell out of favor after the publication of MUSTT. Second, along with MADIT, it showed that ICD treatment in patients with CAD, reduced LVEF, and inducible sustained VT can dramatically reduce mortality.

Multicenter Automatic Defibrillator Implantation Trial–II

The Multicenter Automatic Defibrillator Implantation Trial–II (MADIT-II) employed a simple enrollment criteria:[15] Patients had to have had an MI at least 1 month before and have an LVEF of 30% or less. There were 1232 patients who were randomized to receive an ICD or conventional medical therapy. The mean LVEF was 23% for both groups. The overall mortality rates during an average follow-up of 20 months was 19.8% in the conventional therapy group compared with 14.2% in the ICD group. This led to a 31% relative risk reduction in all-cause mortality with the ICD. This finding was not as robust as the 54% relative risk reductions in all-cause mortality with MUSTT and 60% relative risk reductions in all-cause mortality with MADIT. Regardless, these results were statistically significant.

An 8-year analysis of MADIT-II was presented by Goldenberg[16] at the Heart Rhythm Society late-breaking trial session in May 2009. There appeared to be a total 8-year benefit of 37%. He stated that in the current 8-year analysis, the life-year saved analysis increased to 1.2, suggesting an absolute number of $50,000 per year of life saved or possibly lower. In a related analysis, Dr Goldenberg noted that the number needed to treat with ICD therapy to save one life was initially reported at 17 but during the 8 years of follow-up this was reduced to 6.

These as yet unpublished data suggest we need to evaluate primary prevention ICD therapy with a longer viewing lens. In other words, these patients appear to have a progressive risk for sudden death and over time it is likely that increasing numbers will remain alive because of their ICD.

Sudden Cardiac Death in Heart Failure Trial

The Sudden Cardiac Death in Heart Failure Trial (SCD-HeFT) randomized 2521 patients with either ischemic or nonischemic cardiomyopathy who had an LVEF of 35% or less and New York Heart Association class II or III HF to one of three treatment strategies: conventional therapy for HF plus placebo; conventional therapy plus amiodarone; and conventional therapy plus an ICD.[17] During a mean follow-up of 45.5 months, there was no difference in survival between patients receiving standard therapy alone and those receiving standard therapy and amiodarone. However, there was 23% lower all-cause mortality in patients who received conventional therapy plus an ICD. The absolute reduction in mortality was 7.2% after 5 years in the overall patient population. The median LVEF was 24% for the ICD group, 25% for the placebo group, and 25% for the amiodarone group. This study produced two key observations. First, the benefit of the ICD was present for both patients with ischemic and nonischemic myopathy and HF. Second, amiodarone did not afford any survival benefit in these patients.

The results of the amiodarone arm of this study were quite important. Before SCD-HeFT, there was a continuing debate, though supported by very little data, that amiodarone might be useful for reducing mortality in patients with systolic HF. The results of SCD-HeFT clearly demonstrated that amiodarone not only failed to improve survival, but that it was quite inferior to an ICD for this indication. This shut the door (for good, it is hoped) on a more-than-2–decade debate over this issue.

Trials Demonstrating No Difference in All-Cause Mortality

Coronary artery bypass graft–patch study
The Coronary Artery Bypass Graft–Patch (CABG-Patch) study included patients undergoing elective bypass graft surgery who had an LVEF of 35% or less and an abnormal signal-averaged electrocardiogram.[18] Adding the abnormal signal-averaged electrocardiogram supposedly targeted those patients with an anatomic substrate more prone to the development of sustained VT or VF. There were 900 patients randomly assigned to receive an ICD or not at the time of surgery. The mean LVEF was 27% for both groups. The primary end point was overall mortality, and during an average follow-up of 32 months no evidence of improved survival was documented in patients who received an ICD.

Defibrillators in non-ischemic cardiomyopathy treatment evaluations
The Defibrillators in Non-Ischemic Cardiomyopathy Treatment Evaluations (DEFINITE) trial evaluated the usefulness of an ICD to reduce mortality in patients who only had nonischemic cardiomyopathy.[19] Additional inclusion criteria were LVEF of 35% or less, history of symptomatic HF, and the presence of either nonsustained VT or more than 10 premature ventricular complexes per hour. The prespecified primary end point was death from any cause. Sudden death from arrhythmia was a prespecified secondary end point. There were 458 patients randomized to standard medical therapy or standard medical therapy plus an ICD. The mean LVEF was 22% for standard therapy and 21% for the ICD group. During a mean follow-up of 29 months, there was no difference between groups in the overall mortality, but patients in the ICD group did have a significant reduction in the risk of SCD from arrhythmia.

In our opinion, DEFINITE was underpowered to demonstrate its primary end point but its results in SCD reduction are consistent with that noted in SCD-HeFT.

Cardiomyopathy trial
The Cardiomyopathy Trial (CAT) enrolled patients with nonischemic cardiomyopathy who had LVEF of 30% or less and New York Heart Association class II or III for HF symptoms.[20] The primary end point was all-cause mortality at 1 year. This was a small trial enrolling only 104 patients randomized to ICD or medical therapy. The mean LVEF was 24% in the ICD group and 25% in the control group. At a mean follow-up of 5.5 years, there was no difference between groups in all-cause mortality.

Defibrillators in acute myocardial infarction trial
The Defibrillators in Acute Myocardial Infarction Trial (DINAMIT) was designed to test whether survivors of a recent MI would derive a survival benefit from an ICD.[21] Entry criteria included patients 6 to 40 days after MI, LVEF of 35% or less, New York Heart Association class I to III for HF, and a noninvasive measure of perceived increased risk for sudden death. The noninvasive indicators were either abnormal heart rate variability or elevated heart rate on a 24-hour ECG recording. There were 674 patients randomized to conventional therapy versus conventional therapy and an ICD. The primary end point was all-cause mortality. During an average follow-up of 30 months, there was no difference in overall mortality between groups. Interestingly, the group that received an ICD had a 58% relative risk reduction of arrhythmic death. Quite surprisingly, there was an increase in nonarrhythmic cardiovascular mortality in patients who received an ICD. The

sum total of these data led to a neutral result in all-cause mortality.

DINAMIT seems to put the clinician between a rock and a hard place. As mentioned earlier, studies have demonstrated a relatively high risk for sudden death in the first month after MI in patients with substantial reduction of LVEF.[3,4] It is not surprising that an apparent arrhythmic survival benefit occurred with the ICD, but a worsening survival in nonarrhythmic cardiovascular mortality was unexpected. Whether one is simply saving patients destined to die from other means is not clear and future studies will, we hope, shed light on the best method to treat this important group of patients. For the moment, no data support use of an ICD as primary prevention in a DINAMIT patient population.

Cardiac Resynchronization Trials

Comparison of medical therapy pacing defibrillation in heart failure

The Comparison of Medical Therapy Pacing Defibrillation in Heart Failure (COMPANION) trial evaluated cardiac resynchronization therapy (CRT) and, in part, its effects on improving survival.[22] Entry criteria included New York Heart Association class III or IV for HF in either ischemic or nonischemic cardiomyopathy, a LVEF of 35% or less, a QRS interval of 120 ms or more, a PR interval of more than 150 ms, and sinus rhythm. There were three treatment strategies: optimal pharmacologic therapy; optimal pharmacologic therapy plus CRT pacemaker (CRT-P); and optimal pharmacologic therapy plus CRT defibrillator (CRT-D). The primary end point was a composite of death from any cause or hospitalization for any cause, and a secondary end point was death from any cause. A total of 1520 patients participated in this trial. The LVEF was 22% for pharmacologic therapy, 20% for CRT-P, and 22% for CRT-D. Both CRT-P and CRT-D when compared with the optimal pharmacologic treatment group decreased the risk of the primary end point with the hazard ratio of approximately 0.8. The CRT-D treatment arm significantly reduced by 36% the risk of the secondary end point of death from any cause. The CRT-P group approached but did not reach statistical significance with a reduction of 24%.

Cardiac resynchronization–heart failure trial

The Cardiac Resynchronization–Heart Failure trial included patients who had New York Heart Association class III or IV HF with an LVEF of 35% or less and a QRS duration of at least 120 ms.[23] Patients were randomized to standard pharmacologic therapy or such therapy plus a CRT-P. The primary end point was death from any cause or unplanned hospitalization for a major cardiovascular event, and the principle secondary end point was death from any cause. There were 813 patients enrolled and followed for a mean of 29 months. The median LVEF was 25% for both groups. The CRT-P group demonstrated a significant advantage in the primary end point: 39% of patients with CRT-P compared with 55% in the pharmacologic treatment group, with a hazard ratio of 0.63. Also, CRT-P reduced mortality and SCD occurred in 29 of the 82 patient deaths in the CRT-P group.

CRT is a unique therapy for a group of patients who are markedly symptomatic from their HF and meet other indications for resynchronization therapy. It appears that CRT can reduce mortality even without a defibrillator, but there is an added advantage with the CRT-D that can further reduce mortality in such patients.

GUIDELINES FOR PRIMARY PREVENTION IMPLANTABLE CARDIOVERTER DEFIBRILLATOR IMPLANTATION

Wherever possible, guideline recommendations for ICD implantation are based on randomized controlled trials, but in some cases they are generated from a review of published data and expert consensus. The most recent guidelines, published in 2008,[24] are from the American College of Cardiology, the American Heart Association, and the Heart Rhythm Society, and serve as an update of the previously published guidelines. Recommendations are listed with the level of evidence supporting it. A class I indication suggests there is evidence and/or general agreement that a given procedure or therapy is beneficial, useful, and effective. Class II is divided into IIA and IIB. Class IIA is for conditions in which there is conflicting evidence and/or a divergence of opinion about the usefulness or efficacy of a procedure or treatment, but the weight of evidence or opinion is in favor of the usefulness/efficacy. Class IIB suggests the usefulness or efficacy is less well established by evidence and/or opinion. Class III is reserved for conditions in which there is general agreement that a procedure or treatment is not useful or effective and may even be harmful.

The level of evidence to support a classification recommendation is designated A, B, or C. Level A consists of data from multiple randomized clinical trials or meta-analyses. Level B evidence comes from a single randomized trial or from nonrandomized studies. Finally, level C evidence, which is the most common level of evidence available for many recommendations, is a consensus opinion of the guideline writers.

Class I Recommendations for Primary Prevention Implantable Cardioverter Defibrillator Therapy

Box 1 summarizes the class I recommendations for primary prevention ICD treatment. Note that these data are derived from the randomized clinical trials discussed in the previous section. The first indication is for patients who have LVEF less than 35%, who have had a previous MI, whose latest MI was at least 40 days before, and who have New York Heart Association class II or III HF symptoms. This recommendation has level A evidence. The second recommendation is for patients who have had a previous MI, whose last MI was at least 40 days before, who have LVEF less than 30%, and who have New York Heart Association class I HF symptoms. This recommendation also carries level A evidence. The third recommendation for patients who have had a previous MI relates back to the MUSTT and MADIT studies. Patients with nonsustained VT, LVEF less than 40%, inducible sustained VT or VF at electrophysiologic study are included. There is level B evidence for this indication. The fourth recommendation is for patients who have a nonischemic dilated cardiomyopathy with a LVEF of 35% or less and New York Heart Association class II or III HF symptoms; this carries a level B evidence.

Class II Recommendations for Primary Prevention Implantable Cardioverter Defibrillator Therapy

Many and varied types of pathophysiologic states can lead to sudden death and can occur too infrequently to allow robust data to be collected in a large randomized clinical trial. Many such examples are listed under the class IIA ICD indications (**Boxes 2** and **3**) Note that several genetic syndromes with normal myocardial function are included in this level of recommendation (eg, long-QT syndrome, Brugada syndrome, and catecholaminergic polymorphic VT). In the absence of a major arrhythmic event, it is often difficult to determine which of these patients are the best candidates for an ICD. One should remember that these individuals are often young and therefore will require multiple ICD generator changes over their lifetimes and likely one or more lead revisions.

In our experience, cardiac sarcoidosis is a particularly pernicious disease.[25] These patients are known to die suddenly, often with only minimal cardiac dysfunction. The disease can be progressive and unpredictable. For example, many years ago, we prescribed a dual-chamber pacemaker to a patient with cardiac sarcoidosis who had documented high-grade atrioventricular block with syncope. Approximately 9 months later, the

---

Box 1
Class I indications for primary prevention for ICD therapy

Prior MI; LVEF less than 35%; New York Heart Association II/III; more than 40 days post-MI

Prior MI; LVEF less than 30%; New York Heart Association I; more than 40 days post-MI

Prior MI; LVEF less than 40%; nonsustained VT; inducible sustained VT or VF at electrophysiologic study

Nonischemic dilated cardiomyopathy; LVEF less than 35%; New York Heart Association II/III

From Epstein AE, DiMarco JP, Ellenbogen KA, et al. ACC/AHA/HRS 2008 guidelines for device-based therapy of cardiac rhythm abnormalities. J Am Coll Cardiol 2008;51:1–62, DOI:10.1016/jacc.2008.02.032; with permission.

Box 2
Class IIA recommendations for primary prevention ICD therapy in patients with no history of sustained VT/VF

Nonischemic dilated cardiomyopathy, significant left ventricular dysfunction, unexplained syncope

Hypertrophic cardiomyopathy with more than one major risk factor for SCD

Arrhythmogenic right ventricular dysplasia/cardiomyopathy with more than one risk factor for SCD

Long-QT syndrome with syncope and/or VT with beta-blockers

Non-hospitalized patients awaiting transplantation

Brugada syndrome with syncope or VT without cardiac arrest

Catecholaminergic polymorphic VT with syncope while receiving beta-blockers

Cardiac sarcoidosis

Giant cell myocarditis

Chagas disease

From Epstein AE, DiMarco JP, Ellenbogen KA et al. ACC/AHA/HRS 2008 guidelines for device-based therapy of cardiac rhythm abnormalities. J Am Coll Cardiol 2008;51:1–62, DOI:10.1016/jacc.2008.02.032; with permission.

Box 3
Class IIB recommendations for primary prevention ICD therapy in patients with no history of sustained VT/VF

Nonischemic dilated cardiomyopathy; LVEF less than 35%; New York Heart Association I

Long-QT syndrome with risk factors for SCD

Advanced structural heart disease and syncope without etiology

Familial cardiomyopathy associated with SCD

Left ventricular noncompaction

From Epstein AE, DiMarco JP, Ellenbogen KA et al. ACC/AHA/HRS 2008 guidelines for device-based therapy of cardiac rhythm abnormalities. J Am Coll Cardiol 2008;51:1–62, DOI:10.1016/jacc.2008.02.032; with permission.

patient had recurrent syncope and now had long runs of monomorphic VT requiring antiarrhythmic drug suppression and subsequent upgrade of the pacemaker to a dual-chamber ICD. It should be noted that the patient initially underwent electrophysiologic testing, at which time no arrhythmias were induced. We have a rather low threshold for implanting an ICD in patients with documented cardiac sarcoidosis.

The clinical situations listed in **Box 3** concern class IIB indications. A decision to implant an ICD in such individuals requires even more "soul searching" because the data to support such a decision are much less robust.

GUIDELINE ADHERENCE?

The development of professional society guidelines is a high-level process involving a group of experts who review the literature in detail to make evidence-based treatment recommendations for the medical community. It seems axiomatic that this long and expensive process is performed with the end goal of improvement in patient care. Therefore, a reasonable person would naturally conclude that physicians encountering patients meeting class I indications for a primary prevention ICD would have a detailed discussion of this issue with their patient and the result in many instances would be an ICD implant. Unfortunately, and all too frequently, this process is not undertaken. Current estimates are that about 20% of patients with a class I indication for a primary prevention ICD have received one and, in many cases, the discussion probably did not take place at all. Shah and colleagues[26] evaluated adherence to guidelines for ICD therapy in

patients with HF who were recently hospitalized. In patients who met class I indications for ICD therapy, the overall percent who received an ICD was 20% with a range among hospitals from 0% to 80%, and a mean rate of implantation of 17%. Even more disturbing is the unconscionable inequality in ICD use among women and black patients, who are underrepresented in this therapy.[27,28] A straw-man argument has been previously forwarded that suggested there were not enough implanting physicians to allow appropriate numbers of patients to receive ICD therapy. Curtis and colleagues[29] recently showed that many nonelectrophysiologists are currently implanting ICD systems, although electrophysiologists had a lower risk of procedural complications. In essence, the shortage of cardiologists trained in ICD implantation cannot account for the marked underutilization of primary prevention ICD therapy.

PERSONAL COMMENTARY

Having witnessed the development of the ICD and the subsequent successful completion of multiple randomized clinical trials demonstrating beyond doubt its effectiveness in reducing sudden death, we are discouraged to see cardiologists largely ignoring the guideline recommendations for primary prevention ICD implantation. The vast majority of patients who meet class I indications for an ICD most likely have a cardiologist involved in their care who is responsible for discussing this issue with the patient. Reasons not to prescribe an ICD are likely multifactorial. Some physicians may think it is better to wait until a patient has an episode of sustained VT or cardiac arrest and then target this obviously high-risk person for ICD therapy. However, in most places in the United States, the rate of successful resuscitation from a cardiac arrest is less than 10%, and home-use automated external defibrillators for relatively high-risk patients have not proven to be very successful.[30] Another point often espoused is that ICDs are expensive and the health care dollar could be more appropriately spent on other things (eg, childhood vaccination programs). ICDs are expensive but this therapy is well within the accepted costs among other cardiovascular treatments we routinely use. To our knowledge, there are no data to suggest increased ICD use would preclude patients receiving other therapies.

A legitimate issue raised by many thoughtful proponents of ICD therapy is the limitations of using an LVEF to decide who is the best candidate for ICD treatment.[31] Indeed, more work needs to be done to define the best candidates for ICDs.

Until those data are available, it is important to follow the evidence-based recommendations from multiple randomized controlled trials and offer ICD therapy to patients who meet class I indications. Finally, some of the advocates for less ICD use often complain of both too many inappropriate and too few appropriate ICD therapies. It is unfortunate that many implanting physicians do not take the time to individualize programming for each patient, which in our experience reduces ICD therapies for events other than VT or VF to less than 5%. Regarding "too few" shocks, this claim relates to the fact that the majority of patients who receive an ICD do not have therapy during the life of the first device implanted. While true, as of yet we do not have a method to define more precisely those patients in the overall high-risk group who are most likely to receive potentially life-saving therapy from the ICD within the first few years of implant. Just because the patient never required therapy from the initial ICD does not mean the patient should not have received the ICD in the first place. That is, when an ICD does not provide therapy, the physician may incorrectly conclude that the ICD was "not needed." In contrast, the physician does not draw the same conclusion when a patient receiving a statin or angiotensin-converting enzyme inhibitor does not die, even though the physician has no idea if the therapy was beneficial.

We hope that soon more physicians will discuss the need for a primary prevention ICD in appropriate patients. Not all patients who meet criteria will be good candidates for an ICD and certainly some patients will decide against an ICD for their own reasons. Such an approach will undoubtedly help reduce the incidence of SCD.

REFERENCES

1. Anonymous. State-specific mortality from sudden cardiac death—United States, 1999. MMWR Morb Mortal Wkly Rep 2002;51:123–6.
2. Cannom DS, Prystowsky EN. Management of ventricular arrhythmias: detection, drugs, and devices. JAMA 1999;281:172–9.
3. Adabag AS, Therneau TM, Gersh BJ, et al. Sudden cardiac death after myocardial infarction. JAMA 2008;300:2022–9.
4. Solomon SD, Zelenkofske S, McMurray JJ, et al. Sudden death in patients with myocardial infarction and left ventricular dysfunction, heart failure, or both. N Engl J Med 2005;352:2581–8.
5. Spaulding CM, Joly LM, Rosenberg A, et al. Immediate coronary angiography in survivors of out-of-hospital cardiac arrest. N Engl J Med 1997;336: 1629–33.
6. Burke AP, Farb A, Malcom GT, et al. Coronary risk factors and plaque morphology in men with coronary disease who died suddenly. N Engl J Med 1997;336:1276–82.
7. Burke AP, Farb A, Malcom GT, et al. Plaque rupture and sudden death related to exertion in men with coronary artery disease. JAMA 1999;281:921–6.
8. Cannom DS, Prystowsky EN. Evolution of implantable cardioverter defibrillator. J Cardiovasc Electrophysiol 2004;15:375–85.
9. Mirowski M, Mower MM, Lanfer A, et al. A chronically implanted system for automatic defibrillation in active conscious dogs: experimental model for treatment of sudden death from ventricular fibrillation. Circulation 1978;58:90–4.
10. Mirowski M, Reid PR, Mower MM, et al. Termination of malignant ventricular arrhythmias with an implanted automatic defibrillator in human beings. N Engl J Med 1980;303:322–4.
11. Moss AJ, Hall WJ, Cannom DS, et al. Improved survival with an implanted defibrillator in patients with coronary disease at high risk for ventricular arrhythmia. N Engl J Med 1996;335:1933–40.
12. Buxton AE, Lee KL, Fisher JD, et al. A randomized study of the prevention of sudden death in patients with coronary artery disease. N Engl J Med 1999; 341:1882–90.
13. Buxton AE, Lee KL, DiCarlo L, et al. Electrophysiologic testing to identify patients with coronary artery disease who are at risk for sudden death. N Engl J Med 2000;342:1937–45.
14. Lee KL, Hafley G, Fisher JD, et al. Effect of implantable defibrillators on arrhythmic events and mortality in the multicenter unsustained tachycardia trial. Circulation 2002;106:233–8.
15. Moss AJ, Zareba W, Hall WJ, et al. Prophylactic implantation of a defibrillator in patients with myocardial infarction and reduced ejection fraction. N Engl J Med 2002;346:877–83.
16. Goldenberg I. Late breaking trial presentation. Heart Rhythm Society; 2009.
17. Bardy GH, Lee KL, Mark DB, et al. Amiodarone or an implantable cardioverter-defibrillator for congestive heart failure. N Engl J Med 2005; 352:225–37.
18. Bigger JT, Coronary Artery Bypass Graft (CABG) Patch Trial Investigators. Prophylactic use of implanted cardiac defibrillators in patients at high risk for ventricular arrhythmias after coronary artery bypass graft surgery. N Engl J Med 1997;337: 1569–75.
19. Kadish A, Dyer A, Daubert SP, et al. Prophylactic defibrillator implantation in patients with nonischemic dilated cardiomyopathy. N Engl J Med 2004; 350:2151–8.
20. Bänsch D, Antz M, Boczor S, et al. Primary prevention of sudden cardiac death in idiopathic dilated

cardiomyopathy: the Cardiomyopathy Trial (CAT). Circulation 2002;105:1453–8.

21. Hohnloser S, Kuck KH, Dorian P, et al. Prophylactic use of an implantable cardioverter-defibrillator after acute myocardial infarction. N Engl J Med 2004; 351:2481–8.

22. Bristow MR, Saxon LA, Boehmer J, et al. Cardiac-resynchronization therapy with or without an implantable defibrillator in advanced chronic heart failure. N Engl J Med 2004;350:2140–50.

23. Cleland JG, Daubert JC, Erdmann E, et al. The effect of cardiac resynchronization on morbidity and mortality in heart failure. N Engl J Med 2005;352: 1539–49.

24. Epstein AE, DiMarco JP, Ellenbogen KA, et al. ACC/AHA/HRS 2008 Guidelines for device-based therapy of cardiac rhythm abnormalities. J Am Coll Cardiol 2008;51:1–62, DOI:10.1016/jacc.2008.02.032.

25. Kim JS, Judson MA, Donnino R, et al. Cardiac sarcoidosis. Am Heart J 2009;157:9–21.

26. Shah B, Hernandez AF, Liang Li, et al. Hospital variation and characteristics of implantable cardioverter-defibrillator use in patients with heart failure. J Am Coll Cardiol 2009;53:416–22.

27. Curtis LH, Al-Khatib SM, Shea AM, et al. Sex differences in the use of implantable cardioverter-defibrillators for primary and secondary prevention of sudden cardiac death. JAMA 2007;298:1517–24.

28. Hernandez AF, Fonarow GC, Liang L, et al. Sex and racial difference in the use of implantable cardioverter-defibrillators among patients hospitalized with heart failure. JAMA 2007;298:1525–32.

29. Curtis JP, Luebbert JJ, Wang Y, et al. Association of physician certification and outcomes among patients receiving an implantable cardioverter-defibrillator. JAMA 2009;301:1661–70.

30. Bardy GH, Lee KL, Mark DB, et al. Home use of automated external defibrillators for sudden cardiac arrest. N Engl J Med 2008;358:1793–804.

31. Buxton AE, Lee KL, Hafley GE, et al. Limitations of ejection fraction for prediction of sudden death risk in patients with coronary artery disease: lessons from the MUSTT Study. J Am Coll Cardiol 2007;50: 1150–7.

Implantable Cardioverter-Defibrillator Therapy for Primary Prevention of Sudden Cardiac Death: An Argument for Restraint

Roderick Tung, MD[a,b,]*, Mark E. Josephson, MD[c]

KEYWORDS

- Defibrillator • Ventricular tachycardia
- Sudden death • Primary prevention • Proarrhythmia
- Cost-effectiveness

After publication of secondary prevention trials for sudden cardiac death in the mid 1990s, evaluation of implantable cardioverter-defibrillator (ICD) therapy in the lower risk, primary prevention populations were undertaken. These trials resulted in upgrading the role of ICD from a restricted "last resort" treatment to a broad-reaching preemptive strategy. The outcomes from ICD trials for primary prevention in the postmyocardial infarction setting[1,2] and in patients with nonischemic cardiomyopathy[3,4] led to the quick adoption of these data into guidelines, and they have remained in the most recent guidelines update.[5] Although it is estimated that a total of 220,000 patients undergo ICD implantation per year, only 10% to 20% of these patients experience life-saving therapy; this leaves up to 90% of the targeted population as "nonresponders," without deriving clinical benefit, while incurring all of the risks from ICD implantation.

A class I indication is defined as an evidence-based recommendation wherein the benefits of therapy clearly outweigh the risks, and therefore

becomes synonymous with the "standard of care."[5] Although ICD therapy is frequently marketed and sold as an "insurance policy," this analogy is not applicable when the policy, or therapy, has potential for harm. ICD implantation comes with attendant costs, and the principle of nonmaleficence necessitates weighing any life-saving benefit against the potential for unnecessary shocks, procedural complications, infection, device malfunction, manufacturer recalls, and proarrhythmia.

In this article, the authors: (1) review the landmark primary prevention trials to assess the incidence of sudden death and the absolute magnitude of benefit derived from ICD therapy; (2) examine the discrepancy between trial patients and real-world implementation of ICD therapy; (3) present the potential for risks incurred from ICD implantation; and (4) examine the natural history of patients who receive appropriate ICD therapy and the durability of ICD benefit with respect to cost-effective analyses, to support the authors' position that ICD therapy should not be routinely

[a] UCLA Cardiac Arrhythmia Center, Los Angeles, CA, USA
[b] Ronald Reagan UCLA Medical Center, David Geffen School of Medicine at UCLA, 10833 Le Conte Avenue, BH 307 CHS, Los Angeles, CA 90095, USA
[c] Beth Israel Deaconess Medical Center, Boston, MA, USA
* Corresponding author.
E-mail address: rtung@mednet.ucla.edu (R. Tung).

Card Electrophysiol Clin 1 (2009) 105–116
doi:10.1016/j.ccep.2009.08.001
1877-9182/09/$ – see front matter © 2009 Published by Elsevier Inc.

used for the primary prevention of sudden cardiac death.

PRIMARY PREVENTION IN THE POSTMYOCARDIAL INFARCTION SETTING

The MADIT trial (Multicenter Automatic Defibrillator Implantation Trial) enrolled 196 patients with prior myocardial infarction (>3 weeks), ejection fraction (EF) less than 35%, with inducible sustained ventricular tachycardia, which could not be suppressed with procainamide.[1] Although ICD therapy improved survival by 23% over conventional therapy (74% amiodarone use) at 5 years, more of these deaths were spared from nonarrhythmic, noncardiac, and unknown causes (n = 14) than from arrhythmic death (n = 10), when compared with conventional therapy. As classifying the mode of death is fraught with potential inaccuracies, this implausible improvement in mortality may have been the result of statistical aberration due to small sample size.

The results of MADIT are not generalizable to current medical practice for several reasons. Although β-blockers (8% conventional vs 26% ICD at discharge) and angiotensin-converting enzyme (ACE) inhibitors (55% conventional vs 60% ICD at discharge) were used more frequently in ICD patients at 1 month, the overall low rate of medication administration is not in compliance with current postmyocardial infarction treatment guidelines. Data from patients who were screened and excluded were not available, therefore the denominator for this highly selected population remains unknown. In addition, there are no data on those patients who were suppressible with procainamide. Lastly, induction of sustained ventricular arrhythmias and procainamide suppression is rarely, if ever, performed in current practice, and this feature may have been important for identifying patients more likely to experience adverse events (mortality rate 39%). For this reason, it is difficult to categorize the MADIT population as a primary prevention group as these patients had spontaneous, nonsustained ventricular tachycardia with inducible drug-refractory sustained ventricular tachycardia (VT). This event rate in the control arm was higher than those seen in secondary prevention trials (25.3% in AVID [Antiarrhythmics Versus Implantable Defibrillators] vs 32% in MADIT, at 2 years).

The larger MADIT II study, enrolling 1232 patients with coronary artery disease and EF less than 30%, demonstrated a 5.6% absolute mortality benefit (19.8% vs 14.2%, number needed to treat for 20% reduction) at 20 months in patients receiving ICD.[2] This difference, the smallest difference seen in any ICD trial demonstrating statistically significant benefit, was likely attenuated by a lower risk population enrolled without spontaneous ventricular arrhythmias or mandated electrophysiology study (approximately 10% lower event rate compared with MADIT). In addition, the equivalent high rate of β-blockade in both arms (70%) and low rates of amiodarone therapy (13% ICD vs 10% control) were likely factors that drove the event rates lower.

Several insights often overlooked in MADIT II deserve mention. When examining the subgroup analysis, patients with QRS less than 150 ms and EF greater than 25% did not derive benefit (95% confidence interval [CI] >1.0), suggesting that a sicker subpopulation within MADIT may be most optimal for selection. Goldenberg and colleagues[6] performed a proportional hazards regression analysis of the MADIT II population to evaluate the impact of age, renal function, functional class, QRS duration, and atrial fibrillation on ICD efficacy. These investigators reported a U-shaped curve for ICD efficacy, showing that patients with the lowest and highest risk scores had attenuated benefit from ICD therapy.

An unexpected 5% absolute increase in hospitalizations for new or worsened congestive heart failure was seen in the ICD group (19.9% vs 14.9%). Of note, this 5% trend in increased heart failure (P = .09) is the exact reverse of the mortality rates and absolute overall benefit. This observation confirmed some of the initial suspicion that right ventricular pacing and ICD discharges may have deleterious effects on myocardial function. Furthermore, depriving a patient of sudden death may shift the mode of death to pump failure, which has the potential to be more costly and morbid.

Similar phenomena were observed in the Defibrillator in Acute Myocardial Infarction Trial (DINAMIT), which examined the role of ICD in 674 patients with an EF of less than 35% and impaired autonomic tone, 6 to 40 days post acute myocardial infarction.[7] The prevention of arrhythmic death with ICD (hazard ratio [HR] 0.42, CI 0.22–0.83, P = .009) was counterbalanced by excess death from nonarrhythmic causes (HR 1.75, CI 1.11–2.76, P = .02). The potential for causal harm from ICD shocks was again suggested by a substudy that showed the increased risk from nonarrhythmic death to be confined only to those that received ICD discharges.

Due to the lack of mortality benefit seen immediately after myocardial infarction, the current guidelines specify a 40-day blanking period during which ICD implantation is contraindicated. The findings of DINAMIT contradict the inferences from the VALIANT study (VALsartan In Acute myocardial iNfarcTion),[8] which showed that patients with reduced systolic function were at highest risk for sudden cardiac death in the first 30 days after myocardial infarction. Although guidelines have adopted a 40-day blanking period from DINAMIT, a gap in data exists from the immediate to chronic setting, as the majority of patients in MADIT I and MADIT II were enrolled outside of 6 months after myocardial infarction (75% and 88%, respectively). The mean interval from index myocardial infarction in MADIT II was 6.7 years. A bimodal distribution of risk was suggested by the time-dependent benefit of ICD in MADIT II, which found benefit only for remote events outside of 18 months that persisted up to 15 years after index myocardial infarction.[9] The optimal timing of defibrillator implantation after myocardial infarction currently remains unknown.

NONSIGNIFICANCE OF IMPLANTABLE CARDIOVERTER-DEFIBRILLATOR THERAPY IN PATIENTS WITH NONISCHEMIC CARDIOMYOPATHY

Despite the inclusion of the nonischemic etiologies into class I ICD primary prevention recommendations, not a single trial has demonstrated a statistically significant mortality benefit from ICD in this group. The Cardiomyopathy Trial (CAT; EF <30%, n = 104) and Amiodarone Versus Implantable Cardioverter Defibrillator Trial (AMIOVIRT; EF <35% with nonsustained VT, n = 103) were both terminated prematurely due to futility.[10,11]

The largest and only prospective trial of exclusively nonischemic patients was the Defibrillators in Nonischemic Cardiomyopathy Treatment Evaluation (DEFINITE), which randomized 458 patients with EF less than 36% and nonsustained VT to standard medical therapy or single-chamber ICD.[3] The primary end point of all-cause mortality failed to reach statistical significance at 29 months (14.1% control vs 7.2%, P = .08). The rate of sudden cardiac death was 6.6%, which was more than half the incidence of appropriate ICD therapy. The low event rates in this study of relatively small sample size may also be attributed to the low usage of amiodarone in the control group, and high equitable rates of β-blocker (85%) and ACE inhibitor (95%) as background therapy.

The Sudden Cardiac Death Heart Failure Trial (SCD-HeFT) was the largest primary prevention defibrillator trial to date, with a combination of ischemic (52%) and nonischemic (48%) etiologies: 2521 patients with EF less than 35%, class II to III heart failure randomized to conventional medical therapy, amiodarone, or ICD therapy.[4] Compared with placebo, ICD reduced all-cause mortality

from 29% to 22% at 45 months (P = .007). The 2-year mortality rate was approximately 20%, similar to the MADIT II population. Prespecified subgroup analysis was performed by New York Heart Association (NYHA) class and etiology, but due to 6 interim analyses of the data, the level of significance was determined to be a more stringent (P<0.023). Neither ischemic nor nonischemic subgroups met statistical significance (P = .05 and .06, respectively). Of note, benefit from ICD was seen only in NYHA class II patients (HR 0.54, CI 0.4–0.74, P<.001) and amiodarone was harmful when compared with placebo in patients with NYHA class III (1.44, CI 1.05–1.97, P = .01).

In accordance with statistical dictum, subgroup analysis should be hypothesis generating, rather than leading to practice guidelines. The nonsignificant benefit in the nonischemic cardiomyopathy subgroup analysis was implemented into Heart Rhythm Society guidelines, and lack of benefit in NYHA III patients was left out. The inconclusive nature of the aforementioned data calls the class I, level B estimate of certainty into question for this population.

ISSUES IN TRIAL METHODOLOGY

β-Blocker use, which has been demonstrated to reduce arrhythmic and all-cause mortality in the postmyocardial infarction and chronic systolic dysfunction settings, can have an effect on the outcome of ICD trials. First, greater use of β-blockade decreases overall event rates, thereby diminishing the power of a study to demonstrate benefit from ICD therapy if the sample size is not increased. Furthermore, if patients randomized to ICD were disproportionately treated with higher rates of β-blockade, overall benefit seemingly from ICD would be accentuated. Indeed, this was the case in 3 of the 4 trials that have proven significant survival benefit with ICD, including SCD-HeFT and MADIT (Table 1). In the recently published long-term follow-up of MADIT II, the rate of β-blockade was significantly lower in those that experienced mortality (53%) compared with those who survived (71%) at 63 months follow-up P<.001.

With the exception of SCD-HeFT, trial patients randomized to "control" received antiarrhythmic drug therapy. Although significant differences between randomized groups may be attributed to the superiority of the active treatment tested, the possibility of an inferior performance in the "control" arm, worse than that of placebo, must not be overlooked. Although there was a prevailing sentiment that randomizing patients to placebo was unethical, not a single randomized

Table 1
Influence of β-blocker use disparities on ICD trial outcomes

Significant Mortality Benefit Demonstrated	ICD (%)	Control (%)	Nonsignificant Differences Shown	ICD	Control
AVID (n = 1,016)[a]	42	16	Coronary artery bypass grafting patch (n = 900)	19	16
MADIT (n = 196)[a]	26	8	CAT (n = 104)	4	4
MADIT II (n = 1232)	70	70	AMIOVIRT (n = 103)	53	50
SCD-HeFT (n = 2521)[a]	82	79	DEFINITE (n = 450)	85	85
			DINAMIT (n = 674)	87	86
			CIDS (n = 659)[a,b]	37	21
			CASH[a]	0	96

[a] Statistical significance between groups.
[b] Treatment differences may be confounded by higher usage of sotalol and class I drugs in ICD group.

prospective trial has demonstrated improved overall mortality from antiarrhythmic therapy. In fact, several concerning signals that suggest increased mortality from antiarrhythmic therapy when compared with placebo have been seen in recent trials.

The potential for harm from antiarrhythmic therapy has been well documented historically from trials like CAST (Cardiac Arrhythmia Suppression Trial) and SWORD (Survival with Oral D-Sotalol).[12,13] The propafenone active treatment arm had to be discontinued in CASH (Cardiac Arrest Study Hamburg) due to a 61% increase in mortality at 11 months.[14] In MADIT, patients in the control group had a 10% higher mortality rate if they were taking amiodarone at 1 month (36% amiodarone vs 26% no amiodarone).

In 2 trials of ICD with "placebo" controls, antiarrhythmic therapy performed worse than standard therapy. In SCD-HeFT, amiodarone was significantly worse than placebo (HR 1.44, CI 1.05–1.97, $P = .01$) in the prespecified NYHA class III patients. However, this trend was not seen in the overall study. In MUSTT (Multicenter Unsustained Tachycardia Trial), patients who were randomized to electrophysiologic-guided antiarrhythmic therapy had worse outcomes than those who were randomized to no antiarrhythmic therapy. No formal comparison was commented on, despite a 10% absolute increased incidence of death at 5 years.

REAL-WORLD VERSUS TRIAL PATIENTS: GENERALIZABILITY GAP

There are at least 2 degrees of separation that contribute to the difficulty in generalizing and applying ICD clinical trial data into the real world.

First, there is the discordance between the inclusion criteria of a study and the actual population that is enrolled. As an example, the average enrolled EF was 7% and 11% less than the enrollment cutoff in MADIT II and SCD-HeFT, respectively, although published guidelines are strictly based on inclusion criteria.[15]

Second, the discrepancy between the actual enrolled population and the patient characteristics seen in the real world further amplifies a generalizability gap. An increasing number of noncardiac comorbidities has the potential to blunt or negate the benefit of ICD therapy due to competing risks for death. Patients with noncardiac comorbidities, including advanced age, diabetes mellitus, peripheral vascular disease, renal disease, and pulmonary disease, tend to be underrepresented in clinical trials. The potential futility of ICD efficacy in patients with chronic and end-stage renal disease has been suggested by multiple retrospective cohort analyses.[16–19] Indeed, there exists a discrepancy in the real world between eligibility and implantation rates, and justifiably so.

Although they remain at highest risk for sudden cardiac death, comprising more than 65% of 465,000 out-of-hospital deaths in 1999,[20] routine implantation in elderly patients (>70 years) who would otherwise qualify for ICD is debatable. Patients older than 75 years were underrepresented in the landmark trials and patients older than 80 were specifically excluded in MADIT (mean age 62 ± 9 years). The median age of patients in SCD-HeFT was 61 and patients older than 65 years did not benefit from ICD therapy. The mean age in MADIT II was 64 ± 10, and only 16% of patients enrolled were older than 75 years. A meta-analysis of secondary prevention trials showed that patients older than 75 did not benefit from ICD implantation (HR 1.06, CI 0.69–1.64, all-cause mortality).[21] Single-center ICD registries have demonstrated steep increases in both cardiac and noncardiac mortality in patients older than 75 years.[22,23] Advanced age clearly presents multiple competing risks for death, and age was also a significant independent predictor of mortality in the long-term follow-up of MADIT II.

However, the real-world extrapolation of data has resulted in 1 out of 6 Medicare ICD implants in patients older than 80 years, with a mean age of 70. The recently published ACT registry (Advancements in ICD Therapy) showed that more than 40% of patients undergoing primary prevention ICD implantation were older than 70 years, with 12% older than 80.[24] This upward drift in age representation in the real world not substantiated by trial data is concerning, not only on scientific grounds but from a philosophic viewpoint. Patient preferences, the morbidity of ICD shocks, and end-of-life decisions should be communicated openly between doctor and patient before implantation.

IMPLANTABLE CARDIOVERTER-DEFIBRILLATOR SHOCKS: INAPPROPRIATE, APPROPRIATE, AND NECESSARY

In the ideal setting, ICD therapy should only treat events that are imminently and inevitably fatal. However, clinical trial experience has revealed that up to 25% of patients receive inappropriate ICD shocks.[25] These shocks are commonly due to double counting, oversensing, ectopy, and supraventricular tachycardias, ranging from sinus tachycardia to atrial fibrillation (**Fig. 1**). ICD shocks have consistently been demonstrated to reduce overall quality of life and increase the incidence of depression and anxiety, while obligating strict driving restrictions. Aside from morbidity, these shocks may have attendant lethal risks, as patients receiving inappropriate shocks in SCD-HeFT were at higher risk for death (HR 1.57, 95% CI 0.99–2.50).[26]

An examination of randomized trials for primary and secondary prevention has shown that the number of appropriate shocks consistently exceeds the sudden death and overall mortality rate in the control group (**Fig. 2**).[25] Kadish and colleagues reported twice as many events in the ICD arm of DEFINITE when compared with controls (32 shocks/1 death, ICD vs 15 arrhythmic deaths, control).[27] Two plausible explanations have been proposed to explain this phenomenon. First, ICD therapies may not be a surrogate for sudden cardiac death, as many episodes may have been nonsustained, nonfatal events. This finding suggests that a distinction needs to be made between shocks that are appropriate and shocks that are necessary. Alternatively, implantation of the device may be directly or indirectly proarrhythmic. There are numerous speculated mechanisms by which an ICD may promote arrhythmogenesis including device malfunction, induction of arrhythmias from inappropriate shocks, pacemaker facilitated triggers, reversal of activation wavefronts from epicardial resynchronization, and increasing dispersion of refractoriness (see **Figs. 1** and **2**).[28–30] In addition, local

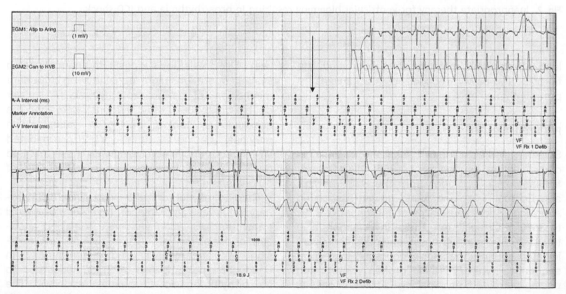

Fig. 1. Double proarrhythmia: (1) paced long-short initiation of ventricular tachycardia followed by a committed shock, which resulted in (2) nonsustained ventricular tachycardia.

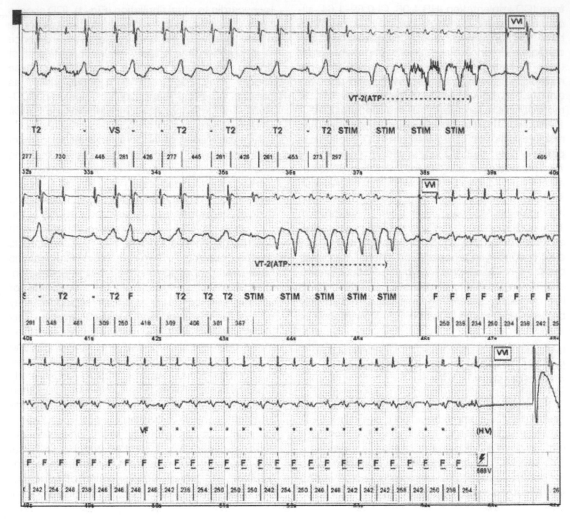

Fig. 2. Inappropriate therapy for ventricular bigeminy resulting in proarrhythmia and ICD shock.

lead effects with mechanical irritation and late fibrosis are newly recognized mechanisms of proarrhythmia.[31,32]

PACING HAZARDS

Sweeney and colleagues[33] analyzed the intracardiac initiation sequence of 1356 VT/ventricular fibrillation (VF) episodes from the PainFree RxII and EnTrust Trial, and found pacing-associated short-long-short sequences at the onset of 21% to 35% of all episodes. These investigators also found 29.8% sudden-onset episodes that were initiated during pacing. The short-long-short sequences were further broken down into pacing-permitted and pacing-facilitated onsets, with a higher rate of the former in managed ventricular pacing and VVI modes when compared

with DDD. This study suggests that normal pacing system operation might constitute an important mechanism of device proarrhythmia. A smaller double-crossover study demonstrated that the cessation of backup pacing in patients with previous pacing-facilitated VT-VF eliminated VT-VF recurrences compared with those that had backup pacing increased to a lower rate of 60 beats/min.[34]

Cardiac resynchronization with epicardial coronary sinus lead implantation reverses the typical transmural activation sequence, delaying endocardial depolarization and repolarization. Dispersion of refractoriness and heterogeneity in conduction patterns has been demonstrated to be arrhythmogenic in animal models.[35] The precipitation of ventricular arrhythmias immediately after cardiac resynchronization therapy has been reported. Extreme examples of VT storm that are only alleviated immediately after the discontinuation of left ventricular pacing have also been reported.[36,37]

HARDWARE MALFUNCTION

Despite advances in ICD system design and manufacturing, devices remain imperfect. Structural failure of an implanted device has tremendous adverse effects on patient morbidity, both medically and psychologically. Inappropriate sensing due to conductor or insulation fracture, sensing lead adapter failure, loose-set screws, or frank dislodgment can lead to oversensing of electrical noise with resultant inappropriate shocks. Kleeman and colleagues[38] reported on the suboptimal reliability of more than 20 lead models over a 13-year period. Overall, 148 (15%) of 990 ICD leads failed during follow-up, with estimated survival rates of 85% and 60% at 5 and 8 years after implant, respectively.

In 2001, Maisel and colleagues[39] reported a recall rate of 16.4 per 100 person-years, with 54% for hardware malfunctions and 41% for programming malfunctions. In 2005, all 3 of the major ICD manufacturing companies (St Jude Photon/Atlas, Guidant Ventak Prizm/Contak Renewal, Medtronic Marquis) issued advisories on the potential for ICD malfunction. Not unexpectedly, the public scrutiny of defibrillator recalls from 2005 brought the rampant implantation rate of ICD to a screeching halt. Yet in the aftermath of this, the highly publicized recall of the Sprint Fidelis lead was issued in October 2007.[40] The higher rates of lead fracture (2.3%–6.7% at 30 months) led to more media-provoked mass hysteria, as about 268,000 patients worldwide were at risk. Patients experiencing a lead complication are at risk for inappropriate shocks and ICD storm due to sensing of electrical noise. Five deaths linked to lead fracture induced proarrhythmia were reported in the initial advisory (**Fig. 3**).

Whereas the impact of recalls on patients is multiple and overt, the burden on physicians must not be overlooked as there is little guidance on how to manage the "at-risk" population. Routine explantation is not advised for patients who are not device-dependent, and individual cases are left up to the physician's discretion by the device companies. Several experienced centers reported a high rate of major complications (1.2%–7.3%) from replacement of devices under advisory, ranging from reoperation to pocket infections, hematomas, and even death.[41–44] From these data, the morbidity and mortality of device replacement must not be underestimated.

COST-INEFFECTIVENESS ANALYSES AND NATURAL HISTORY OF SHOCK RECIPIENTS

The multivariable calculus of cost-effectiveness analysis is critically dependent on event rates, start-up cost estimates, projected follow-up care, and a fundamental assumption of persistent treatment effect. Reynolds and colleagues[45] reported a 10.8% early complication rate in Medicare patients undergoing ICD implantation, associated with a mean cost $42,184 and mean length of stay of 4.7 days. This insight from a real-world registry demonstrates the potential for underestimating unforeseen costs with projected estimates.

Based on the previously mentioned overestimation of ICD efficacy and the underestimation of real-world complication rates, which leads to increased costs, the published time-extrapolated cost-effectiveness analyses are hypothetical "best-case scenario" estimates. A cost-effectiveness analysis based on the actual MADIT II study population within the study time frame supports this assertion. ICD therapy was associated with a threefold higher rate of hospitalizations, and the average survival gain was 2 months. Because of this modest benefit, the incremental cost-effectiveness ratio was an astounding $235,000 per year of life saved, unadjusted for quality of life. The cost-effectiveness approached the accepted range of $50,000 to $100,000 only when the data were extrapolated to 12 years.[46]

An analysis of SCD-HeFT found significant interaction between NYHA class and ICD therapy, and no incremental benefit despite higher costs in patients with NYHA III heart failure (**Fig. 4**). Furthermore, the incremental cost-effectiveness ratio was under $100,000 only after a sensitivity analysis extrapolated the time 3 years beyond the trial follow-up ($127,503 per life-years saved [LYS] at 5 years and $88,657 per LYS at 8 years).[47]

Sanders and colleagues[48] estimated the cost-effectiveness of ICD for primary prevention based on 8 randomized controlled trials. At a cost between $34,000 and $70,200 per quality-adjusted life-year (QALY), the investigators performed a sensitivity analysis that showed a cost-effectiveness ratio below 100,000, assuming that the benefit of ICD persisted after 7 years, to defray the costs. The projected life extension was 1.0 to 2.99 QALY based on the 6 trials that demonstrated ICD benefit.

The assumption that ICD therapy has a persistent effect on late survival has not been supported by data, and extrapolating ICD benefit beyond the timeframe of clinical trial boundaries is unfounded.

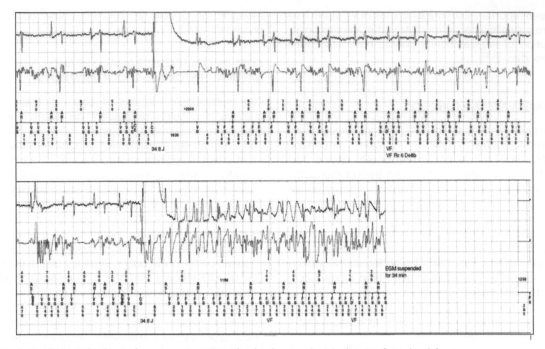

Fig. 3. Fatal proarrhythmia from inappropriate shocks due to electrical noise from lead fracture.

Patients who receive appropriate ICD shocks seem to have a declining prognosis. In SCD-HeFT, patients receiving appropriate shocks had a three-fold increase in risk for death. Eleven percent of patients in SCD-HeFT died within 24 hours after an appropriate shock, and the median life expectancy after one or more appropriate therapy was less than 1 year (168 days).[26] In MADIT II, the mortality rate of patients receiving therapy for VF was more than 50% at 2 years.[49] From these data, it seems that the natural history of patients receiving shocks (about 10%) is limited to 1 to 2 years, and it is implausible to believe that ICDs can save lives without delivering therapy.

A recent follow-up of MADIT II up to 6 years suggested that the extrapolation of constant risk is reasonable in this population, with a mortality rate of 8.5% per year in survivors.[50] There are 2 inherent limitations to this analysis. First, the control population was not followed and therefore, comparison is lacking to demonstrate the true impact of ICD mortality benefit.

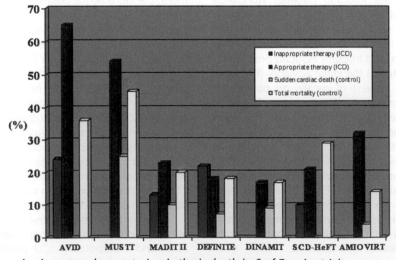

Fig. 4. Appropriate shocks outnumber control arrhythmic death in 6 of 7 major trials.

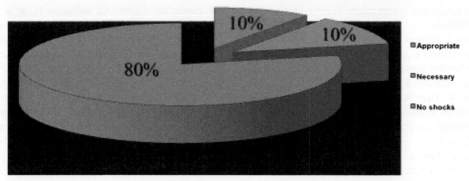

Fig. 5. In primary prevention, only 10% of patients receiving ICD implantation require life-saving therapy. Insurance comes with the following risks: 10% implant complication rate[45], 15% in appropriate shocks/2-3 years[1–4], 15% lead failure rate/5 years[38], 16 recalls/100 person-years[39], and 5% replacement complication.[42]

Second, data on device and pharmacologic therapies beyond the study-specific MADIT II follow-up are lacking. Therefore, the impact of ICD therapy on long-term mortality remains unknown.

Whereas many analyses attempt to adjust cost-effectiveness for quality of life, there are many intangible impacts on psychological well-being that cannot be made mathematically. Although many patients are comforted by having a "safety net," ICD-specific fears including fear of death, shock, and public embarrassment are commonly experienced by recipients. In one study, symptoms of anxiety and depression persisted in 40% to 63% of defibrillator recipients at 1 year.[51] Psychiatric studies have found that the aversive classical conditioning and dysfunctional cognition that occurs in defibrillator shock recipients makes them a prototypical model for anxiety development.[52,53] The adverse psychological effects of increasing shock frequency has been clearly demonstrated in the quality of life analysis from AVID, CIDS (Canadian Implantable Defibrillator Study), and DEFINITE.[54–56]

SUMMARY

As current guidelines have been broadened to include lower-risk groups with lower event rates, the cost-effectiveness of ICD therapy has become even less favorable. In the case of primary prevention in SCD-HeFT and MADIT II, a 20% appropriate shock rate approximates a 10% necessary life-saving therapy rate.[2,4] Therefore, 90% of patients who do not experience life-saving shocks are still exposed to the costs and risks of device-related complications (**Fig. 5**). A distinction between therapeutic efficacy and efficiency must be recognized.

In summary, the reasons why ICD therapy cannot be recommended to all patients meeting the current indications for primary prevention of sudden cardiac death include:

1. ICD therapy benefit has been amplified by imbalances in trial methodology.
2. ICD therapy has inherent risks that are under-appreciated and undercommunicated to patients.
3. The combination of amplified benefit, underestimated risks, underestimated incurred costs, and unsupported extrapolation of ICD benefit results in an overestimation of cost-effectiveness.
4. The discordance between trial inclusion criteria and real-world patients with multiple comorbidities may diminish real-world ICD efficacy.
5. The low incidence of events in the primary prevention setting leaves many more patients at risk from the device than those who will benefit from it.

Further studies are necessary for identifying the most appropriately "at-risk" population for primary prevention ICD therapies. An appreciation for the inherent limitations of ICD outlined will hopefully enable clinicians to more appropriately select those patients who are at highest risk for arrhythmic death, with the lowest risk for harm from ICD therapy and competing causes for overall mortality.

REFERENCES

1. Moss AJ, Hall WJ, Cannom DS, et al. Improved survival with an implanted defibrillator in patients with coronary disease at high risk for ventricular arrhythmia. Multicenter Automatic Defibrillator

Implantation Trial Investigators. N Engl J Med 1996; 335:1933–40.

2. Moss AJ, Zareba W, Hall WJ, et al. Prophylactic implantation of a defibrillator in patients with myocardial infarction and reduced ejection fraction. N Engl J Med 2002;346:877–83.

3. Kadish A, Dyer A, Daubert JP, et al. Prophylactic defibrillator implantation in patients with nonischemic dilated cardiomyopathy. N Engl J Med 2004; 350:2151–8.

4. Bardy GH, Lee KL, Mark DB, et al. Amiodarone or an implantable cardioverter-defibrillator for congestive heart failure. N Engl J Med 2005;352:225–37.

5. Epstein AE, DiMarco JP, Ellenbogen KA, et al. ACC/AHA/HRS 2008 guidelines for device-based therapy of cardiac rhythm abnormalities: a report of the American College of Cardiology/American Heart Association Task Force on Practice Guidelines (Writing Committee to Revise the ACC/AHA/NASPE 2002 Guideline Update for Implantation of Cardiac Pacemakers and Antiarrhythmia Devices) developed in collaboration with the American Association for Thoracic Surgery and Society of Thoracic Surgeons. J Am Coll Cardiol 2008;51:e1–62.

6. Goldenberg I, Vyas AK, Hall WJ, et al. Risk stratification for primary implantation of a cardioverter-defibrillator in patients with ischemic left ventricular dysfunction. J Am Coll Cardiol 2008;51: 288–96.

7. Hohnloser SH, Kuck KH, Dorian P, et al. Prophylactic use of an implantable cardioverter-defibrillator after acute myocardial infarction. N Engl J Med 2004; 351:2481–8.

8. Solomon SD, Zelenkofske S, McMurray JJ, et al. Sudden death in patients with myocardial infarction and left ventricular dysfunction, heart failure, or both. N Engl J Med 2005;352:2581–8.

9. Wilber DJ, Zareba W, Hall WJ, et al. Time dependence of mortality risk and defibrillator benefit after myocardial infarction. Circulation 2004;109: 1082–4.

10. Bansch D, Antz M, Boczor S, et al. Primary prevention of sudden cardiac death in idiopathic dilated cardiomyopathy: the Cardiomyopathy Trial (CAT). Circulation 2002;105:1453–8.

11. Strickberger SA, Hummel JD, Bartlett TG, et al. Amiodarone versus implantable cardioverter-defibrillator: randomized trial in patients with nonischemic dilated cardiomyopathy and asymptomatic nonsustained ventricular tachycardia— AMIOVIRT. J Am Coll Cardiol 2003;41:1707–12.

12. Echt DS, Liebson PR, Mitchell LB, et al. Mortality and morbidity in patients receiving encainide, flecainide, or placebo. The Cardiac Arrhythmia Suppression Trial. N Engl J Med 1991;324:781–8.

13. Waldo AL, Camm AJ, deRuyter H, et al. Effect of d-sotalol on mortality in patients with left ventricular dysfunction after recent and remote myocardial infarction. The SWORD Investigators. Survival with Oral D-Sotalol. Lancet 1996;348:7–12.

14. Kuck KH, Cappato R, Siebels J, et al. Randomized comparison of antiarrhythmic drug therapy with implantable defibrillators in patients resuscitated from cardiac arrest: the Cardiac Arrest Study Hamburg (CASH). Circulation 2000;102:748–54.

15. Myerburg RJ. Implantable cardioverter-defibrillators after myocardial infarction. N Engl J Med 2008;359: 2245–53.

16. Hreybe H, Razak E, Saba S. Effect of end-stage renal failure and hemodialysis on mortality rates in implantable cardioverter-defibrillator recipients. Pacing Clin Electrophysiol 2007;30:1091–5.

17. Lee DS, Tu JV, Austin PC, et al. Effect of cardiac and noncardiac conditions on survival after defibrillator implantation. J Am Coll Cardiol 2007;49: 2408–15.

18. Cuculich PS, Sanchez JM, Kerzner R, et al. Poor prognosis for patients with chronic kidney disease despite ICD therapy for the primary prevention of sudden death. Pacing Clin Electrophysiol 2007;30: 207–13.

19. Bruch C, Sindermann J, Breithardt G, et al. Prevalence and prognostic impact of comorbidities in heart failure patients with implantable cardioverter defibrillator. Europace 2007;9:681–6.

20. Zheng ZJ, Croft JB, Giles WH, et al. State-specific mortality from sudden cardiac death-United States, 1999. MMWR Morb Mortal Wkly Rep 2002;51:123–6.

21. Healey JS, Hallstrom AP, Kuck KH, et al. Role of the implantable defibrillator among elderly patients with a history of life-threatening ventricular arrhythmias. Eur Heart J 2007;28:1746–9.

22. Pellegrini CN, Lee K, Olgin JE, et al. Impact of advanced age on survival in patients with implantable cardioverter defibrillators. Europace 2008;10: 1296–301.

23. Panotopoulos PT, Axtell K, Anderson AJ, et al. Efficacy of the implantable cardioverter-defibrillator in the elderly. J Am Coll Cardiol 1997;29: 556–60.

24. Epstein AE, Kay GN, Plumb VJ, et al. Implantable cardioverter-defibrillator prescription in the elderly. Heart Rhythm 2009;6:1136–43.

25. Germano JJ, Reynolds M, Essebag V, et al. Frequency and causes of implantable cardioverter-defibrillator therapies: is device therapy proarrhythmic? Am J Cardiol 2006;97:1255–61.

26. Poole JE, Johnson GW, Hellkamp AS, et al. Prognostic importance of defibrillator shocks in patients with heart failure. N Engl J Med 2008;359:1009–17.

27. Ellenbogen KA, Levine JH, Berger RD, et al. Are implantable cardioverter defibrillator shocks a surrogate for sudden cardiac death in patients with non-ischemic cardiomyopathy? Circulation 2006;113: 776–82.

28. Healy E, Goyal S, Browning C, et al. Inappropriate ICD therapy due to proarrhythmic ICD shocks and hyperpolarization. Pacing Clin Electrophysiol 2004; 27:415–6.

29. Pinski SL, Fahy GJ. The proarrhythmic potential of implantable cardioverter-defibrillators. Circulation 1995;92:1651–64.

30. Basu Ray I, Fendelander L, Singh JP. Cardiac re-synchronization therapy and its potential proarrhythmic effect. Clin Cardiol 2007;30:498–502.

31. Tung R, Zimetbaum P, Josephson ME. A critical appraisal of implantable cardioverter-defibrillator therapy for the prevention of sudden cardiac death. J Am Coll Cardiol 2008;52:1111–21.

32. Lee JC, Epstein LM, Huffer LL, et al. ICD lead proarrhythmia cured by lead extraction. Heart Rhythm 2009;6.613–8.

33. Sweeney MO, Ruetz LL, Belk P, et al. Bradycardia pacing-induced short-long-short sequences at the onset of ventricular tachyarrhythmias: a possible mechanism of proarrhythmia? J Am Coll Cardiol 2007;50:614–22.

34. Himmrich E, Przibille O, Zellerhoff C, et al. Proarrhythmic effect of pacemaker stimulation in patients with implanted cardioverter-defibrillators. Circulation 2003;108:192–7.

35. Medina-Ravell VA, Lankipalli RS, Yan GX, et al. Effect of epicardial or biventricular pacing to prolong QT interval and increase transmural dispersion of repolarization: does resynchronization therapy pose a risk for patients predisposed to long QT or torsade de pointes? Circulation 2003;107:740–6.

36. Kantharia BK, Patel JA, Nagra BS, et al. Electrical storm of monomorphic ventricular tachycardia after a cardiac-resynchronization-therapy-defibrillator upgrade. Europace 2006;8:625–8.

37. Nayak HM, Verdino RJ, Russo AM, et al. Ventricular tachycardia storm after initiation of biventricular pacing: incidence, clinical characteristics, management, and outcome. J Cardiovasc Electrophysiol 2008;19:708–15.

38. Kleemann T, Becker T, Doenges K, et al. Annual rate of transvenous defibrillation lead defects in implantable cardioverter-defibrillators over a period of >10 years. Circulation 2007;115:2474–80.

39. Maisel WH, Sweeney MO, Stevenson WG, et al. Recalls and safety alerts involving pacemakers and implantable cardioverter-defibrillator generators. JAMA 2001;286:793–9.

40. Food and Drug Administration. Statement on Medtronic's voluntary market suspension of their Sprint Fidelis defibrillator leads. October 2007. Available at: http://www.fda.gov/NewsEvents/Newsroom/Press Announcements/2007/ucm109007.htm. Accessed August 1, 2009.

41. Gould PA, Krahn AD. Complications associated with implantable cardioverter-defibrillator replacement in response to device advisories. JAMA 2006;295: 1907–11.

42. Costea A, Rardon DP, Padanilam BJ, et al. Complications associated with generator replacement in response to device advisories. J Cardiovasc Electrophysiol 2008;19:266–9.

43. Kapa S, Hyberger L, Rea RF, et al. Complication risk with pulse generator change: implications when reacting to a device advisory or recall. Pacing Clin Electrophysiol 2007;30:730–3.

44. Byrd CL, Wilkoff BL, Love CJ, et al. Intravascular extraction of problematic or infected permanent pacemaker leads: 1994–1996. U.S. Extraction Database, MED Institute. Pacing Clin Electrophysiol 1999;22:1348–57.

45. Reynolds MR, Cohen DJ, Kugelmass AD, et al. The frequency and incremental cost of major complications among Medicare beneficiaries receiving implantable cardioverter-defibrillators. J Am Coll Cardiol 2006;47:2493–7.

46. Zwanziger J, Hall WJ, Dick AW, et al. The cost effectiveness of implantable cardioverter-defibrillators: results from the Multicenter Automatic Defibrillator Implantation Trial (MADIT)-II. J Am Coll Cardiol 2006;47:2310–8.

47. Mark DB, Nelson CL, Anstrom KJ, et al. Cost-effectiveness of defibrillator therapy or amiodarone in chronic stable heart failure: results from the Sudden Cardiac Death in Heart Failure Trial (SCD-HeFT). Circulation 2006;114: 135–42.

48. Sanders GD, Hlatky MA, Owens DK. Cost-effectiveness of implantable cardioverter-defibrillators. N Engl J Med 2005;353:1471–80.

49. Moss AJ, Greenberg H, Case RB, et al. Long-term clinical course of patients after termination of ventricular tachyarrhythmia by an implanted defibrillator. Circulation 2004;110:3760–5.

50. Cygankiewicz I, Gillespie J, Zareba W, et al. Predictors of long-term mortality in Multicenter Automatic Defibrillator Implantation Trial II (MADIT II) patients with implantable cardioverter-defibrillators. Heart Rhythm 2009;6:468–73.

51. Sears SF Jr, Todaro JF, Lewis TS, et al. Examining the psychosocial impact of implantable cardioverter defibrillators: a literature review. Clin Cardiol 1999; 22:481–9.

52. Godemann F, Ahrens B, Behrens S, et al. Classic conditioning and dysfunctional cognitions in patients with panic disorder and agoraphobia treated with an implantable cardioverter/defibrillator. Psychosom Med 2001;63:231–8.

53. Godemann F, Butter C, Lampe F, et al. Panic disorders and agoraphobia: side effects of treatment with an implantable cardioverter/defibrillator. Clin Cardiol 2004;27:321–6.

54. Schron EB, Exner DV, Yao Q, et al. Quality of life in the Antiarrhythmics Versus Implantable Defibrillators trial: impact of therapy and influence of adverse symptoms and defibrillator shocks. Circulation 2002;105:589–94.

55. Irvine J, Dorian P, Baker B, et al. Quality of life in the Canadian Implantable Defibrillator Study (CIDS). Am Heart J 2002;144:282–9.

56. Passman R, Subacius H, Ruo B, et al. Implantable cardioverter defibrillators and quality of life: results from the Defibrillators in Nonischemic Cardiomyopathy treatment evaluation study. Arch Intern Med 2007;167:2226–32.

Development and Industrialization of the Implantable Cardioverter-Defibrillator: A Personal and Historical Perspective

Robert G. Hauser, MD, FACC, FHRS

KEYWORDS

- Implantable cardioverter-defibrillator
- Lead • ICD • Battery • Medical device

It's not that it can't be done; [we] haven't found a way to do it. It's a question of mind, not facts.

Michel Mirowski, while developing the implantable defibrillator.

The implantable cardioverter-defibrillator (ICD) is the standard of care for preventing sudden cardiac death. Each year about 140,000 high-risk patients undergo initial ICD implantation and a further 30,000 to 40,000 patients receive an ICD pulse generator replacement. Qualified physicians can perform the surgical procedure safely in hundreds of hospitals worldwide. Contemporary ICDs are capable of providing a variety of therapeutic functions, including high-energy defibrillation, antitachycardia pacing, and sensor-based dual-chamber and resynchronization pacing. The ICD can automatically gather and store diagnostic data that offer valuable clinical and technical information to guide both device and drug therapy and alert caregivers of impending battery depletion or lead problems. Moreover, much of the diagnostic data can be monitored remotely, so that many patients can be evaluated in their homes.

The ICDs we have today are the result of a long journey (**Table 1**). I have had the privilege of traveling much of that road, which began with the first rudimentary automatic implantable defibrillator (AID) of the early 1980s. The ICD is the culmination of Michel Mirowski's remarkable vision, and the efforts of a small group of physicians, scientists, engineers, and businessmen who made that vision a reality. Most electrophysiologists do not know how difficult it was to gather the resources required to develop and commercialize the ICD. The $4-billion ICD market that exists today was inconceivable in 1970, when Mirowski and Mower[1] published their first manuscript. The information in this article is based as much on my personal recollections as it is on the published literature. I had the good fortune of being both an original AICD-B/BR investigator and a chief executive officer of Cardiac Pacemakers, Inc, which was the first company to commercialize ICDs.

EARLY DAYS

The ICD story has roots in the 1950s and 1960s when pioneering men and women thought they could stimulate the heart with a totally implantable, battery-powered electronic pacemaker connected to the heart by conductive wires and operating continuously for the life of the patient. My

Minneapolis Heart Institute Foundation, 920 E 28th Street, Suite 300, Minneapolis, MN 55407, USA
E-mail address: rhauser747@aol.com

Card Electrophysiol Clin 1 (2009) 117–127
doi:10.1016/j.ccep.2009.08.010
1877-9182/09/$ – see front matter © 2009 Published by Elsevier Inc.

Table 1
Key events in the development and industrialization of the implantable defibrillator

Event	Year
Michel Mirowski and Morton Mower defibrillate dog's heart with transvenous catheter and subcutaneous electrode.	1969
Prototype long-term implantable defibrillator successfully implanted in dogs. Intec is formed to produce rudimentary automatic implantable defibrillator for clinical trial.	1978
First rudimentary automatic implantable defibrillator implanted in humans at Johns Hopkins.	1980
Cardiac Pacemakers Inc/Eli Lilly acquires Intec. Food and Drug Administration approves the AICD for marketing in the United States.	1985
First human hybrid circuit ICD implanted.	1988
First human transvenous nonthoracotomy ICD lead implanted.	1988
Cardiac Arrhythmia Suppression Trial reports hazards associated with arrhythmic drug therapy.	1989
First human tiered-therapy ICD implanted.	1989
Researchers develop first ICD suitable for routine pectoral implant	1995
Researchers develop first ICD pulse generator under 50 cm³ in volume.	1997

introduction to these early pacemakers occurred late one summer night in 1968 when I was an intern at Presbyterian-St Luke's Hospital in Chicago (later Rush Medical Center). I assisted one of our cardiac surgeons as he repaired a fractured myocardial pacing lead in an elderly patient who had complete heart block. The hospital's biomedical department had developed and fabricated its own pacemaker and the woven pacing wires were fragile. So I spent many nights during that internship year crimping leads and replacing pulse generators whose mercury-zinc batteries depleted after months, not years, of fixed-rate pacing.

In 1968, while I was struggling with the vicissitudes of cardiac pacemakers, Michel Mirowski and Morton Mower were constructing the first prototype implantable defibrillator in the basement of Mt Sinai Hospital in Baltimore. Then in 1971, an editorial appeared in *Circulation* by Dr Bernard Lown,[2] a preeminent authority on sudden cardiac death, who wrote that the implantable defibrillator had no practical application in man. Subsequently Mirowski and Mower lost much of their financial support. But the following year, Dr Stephen Heilman, who owned Medrad, a small angiographic injector company in Pittsburgh, began working with Mirowski and Mower. In 1979, they formed Intec, the company that manufactured the first AID for human use. One technical challenge Intec had to solve was how to package 20 to 30 J of energy in an implantable device. Special batteries had to be built. It took Honeywell several years to come up with the first prototypes. Meanwhile, a large effort was devoted to optimizing the output

waveform and developing the fundamental ventricular fibrillation–recognition algorithm.

PACING'S MIDLIFE CRISIS

Pacing in the 1970s was replete with device problems and complications. Battery longevity was short, leads were displacing and breaking, and surgical pocket complications were common because of bulky pulse generators, which were necessarily thick to accommodate mercury-zinc batteries. Poor performance and the lack of communication and transparency by pacemaker manufacturers prompted Dr Michael Bilitch to start a multicenter registry, which was initially funded by the Food and Drug Administration (FDA) and would continue until 1993.[3] In 1976, Congress passed the Medical Device Amendments to empower the FDA to regulate medical devices, and the Good Manufacturing Practices regulations were established.

During the mid-1970s, manufacturers began to employ hybrid integrated electronic circuits in pacemakers, which had formerly used discrete electronic components mounted on miniature circuit boards and encapsulated or "potted" in epoxy (**Fig. 1**A, B). The hybrid integrated circuits offered many advantages. For example, such circuits enabled thousands of transistors to be contained in small, lightweight packages, making it possible for pacemakers to perform sophisticated functions while using less battery capacity. Unfortunately, the manufacturers failed to protect the hybrid integrated circuits from body fluids

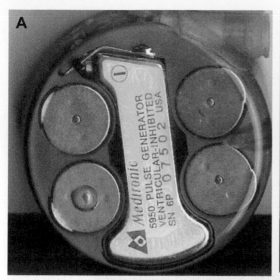

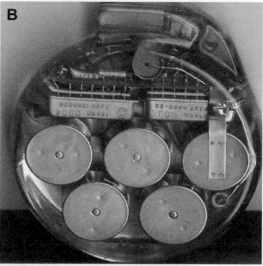

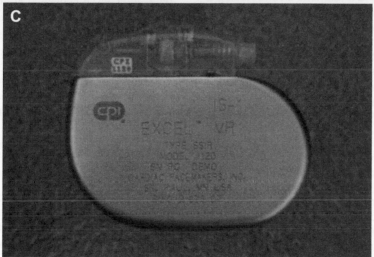

Fig. 1. Pacemaker pulse generators that used hybrid integrated electronic circuits, a technology that was key to the commercialization of the ICD. The Xytron (*A*) and the Omnicor (*B*) were prone to abrupt failure because they did not prevent moisture intrusion into the electronics' enclosures. Electronic reliability was achieved by hermetically sealing the electronics and battery in a single housing (*C*).

and the consequences were catastrophic for many patients. I vividly recall the sudden death of a pacemaker-dependent 42-year-old patient who was found by his wife on the doorstep of their home in Chicago. His Cordis hybrid integrated circuit pacemaker (see **Fig. 1**B) failed abruptly because of a short circuit caused by moisture on the hybrid, which was not detected by the manufacturer's faulty hermeticity tests.

Subsequently, many thousands of Medtronic Xytron pacemakers (see **Fig. 1**A) failed suddenly when moisture penetrated the hybrid-integrated circuit can, which was not hermetically sealed. To many of us, it appeared that hybrid integrated electronic circuits were unsafe. However, in

1977, Drs. Michael Bilitch, Victor Parsonnet, and Seymour Furman reported that hybrid integrated circuit pacemakers could perform reliably if all electronics, including the hybrid circuit and the lithium battery, were hermetically sealed inside a single metal housing (**Fig. 1**C). This study was the first of many contributions made by the Bilitch Registry that enhanced our understanding of rhythm management devices. Its findings were encouraging, and they set the technological stage for rapid advances in cardiac pacing and ultimately ICD therapy. These advances ushered in a vast array of functions and programmable features. Furthermore, in 1977, the lithium battery was proving to be the reliable energy source we needed to enable the development of sophisticated and long-lasting pacemakers. Thus, the modern pacemaker was born, and many of its technologies were transferred to the implantable defibrillator.

About this time the AID was undergoing chronic animal testing in preparation for the first human implants. (AID and AICD became trademarks for Intec's implantable defibrillator. *Implantable cardioverter-defibrillator* and *ICD* evolved later as generic terms.)

AUTOMATIC DEFIBRILLATION

At the 1979 World Symposium on Cardiac Pacing in Montreal, I viewed the remarkable film Mirowski and Mower had made of a conscious dog being resuscitated by a prototype implantable defibrillator. The demonstration was even more striking because it included a real-time electrocardiogram showing first sinus rhythm, followed by the induction of ventricular fibrillation, and then successful automatic defibrillation. Afterward I went to the small Intec booth in the exhibit hall and indicated my desire to be an investigator for the first human clinical trials. However, it would be 4 years before I could implant my first AICD.

Mirowski and colleagues[4] reported on the original human AID implant and the initial series of patients in 1980. Subsequently, a number of modifications were made to the device, including the addition of cardioversion capability, which required a synchronizing circuit. The original AID recognized ventricular fibrillation using a proprietary probability density function, which measured the time a rhythm spent near the isoelectric line. However, the probability density function could be confounded by electrode polarization potentials not seen during animal tests. Thus a rate-detection algorithm was added so that a shock was delivered if the rhythm satisfied both the probability density function and the rate criterion. An AICD that used the rate-detection algorithm alone was also developed and it became the standard for tachycardia recognition in future models.[5]

The automatic ICD (model AICD-B [**Fig. 2**]) we implanted in a 62 year-old survivor of multiple cardiac arrests at Rush Medical Center in 1983 weighed 292 g, occupied a volume of 112 cm^3, and delivered 25- to 30-J shocks via patch electrodes sewn onto the right and left ventricles through a midline sternotomy and tunneled to an abdominal pocket.[6] Ventricular fibrillation was induced using a common battery charger and the AICD required 40 seconds to recognize and terminate ventricular fibrillation. During those 40 seconds, there was no indication that the device was functioning until we heard the capacitors charging.

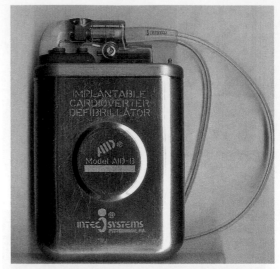

Fig. 2. Intec AID-B implanted at Rush Medical Center in 1983.

The clinical and technical problems associated with early ICDs have been told and retold. But the challenges of manufacturing ICDs, creating a viable business model, and evolving the therapy have received little attention. Intec was a small company described as a garage-type operation, without the capital to expand. Like most start-up companies, it had to either attract investors, partner with another company, or find a buyer. In retrospect, the ICD was one of the great medical device investments in history. But in 1984, the ICD was a therapy of last resort for patients who had suffered two or more cardiac arrests, and the device had yet to receive FDA approval. This was the era of electrophysiology studies, arrhythmia surgery, and multiple antiarrhythmic drug trials, and the sobering results of the Cardiac Arrhythmia Suppression Trial (CAST) were years away. Many thought leaders in pacing and electrophysiology were skeptical and vocal in their opposition to the ICD. Accordingly, major investors had serious reservations that the ICD would ever become a mainstream therapy and a viable product. Indeed, Medtronic had jettisoned its collaboration with Mirowski 10 years previously because it did not believe that the ICD could be a successful business in the twentieth century.

CARDIAC PACEMAKERS, INC

In 1983, Cardiac Pacemakers, Inc (CPI) was owned by the pharmaceutical manufacturer Eli Lilly and Company. CPI had flourished in the 1970s because it was the first company to commercialize the lithium battery pacemaker. Lilly wanted to enter the medical device business and it purchased CPI in 1978, when CPI's sales were peaking. CPI was a competent medical device manufacturer, but the company had lost its product development edge, and its market share eroded rapidly as Intermedics and Pacesetter developed user-friendly multiprogrammable pacemakers and as Medtronic introduced the first sensor-based activity pacemaker. Eventually, Lilly replaced CPI's management and Richard Strain, a Lilly pharmaceutical manager with no medical device experience, was named its chief executive officer.

CPR for CPI

CPI needed new products and a strategic direction. Its scientific advisory board, of which I was a member, recommended in 1983 that CPI/Lilly explore developing the ICD technology. The following year, Lilly made an offer to purchase Intec, but Michel Mirowski demurred: he was understandably concerned that CPI did not have the skills or resolve to develop and manufacture the ICD. I had a memorable conversation with Mirowski at a medical conference in Marseille where I expressed my belief that Lilly was in the business for the long term; besides, I said, Lilly had a lot of cash.

The Lilly-Intec transaction closed in June 1985 and the AICD received FDA approval later that year. CPI and the Intec team that had moved from Pittsburgh to St Paul were immediately confronted with the most complex technological challenge in medical device history: industrializing the ICD. They were ill prepared, and Lilly's management had underestimated the degree of difficulty and hence the time and money it would take to build a successful business. Mirowski's concerns proved prescient.

In 1985, Ronald Matricaria assumed the reins at CPI. Matricaria had been a Lilly pharmaceutical salesman and he was a very talented and focused manager who was concerned that CPI was losing a million dollars a month. Once a quarter Matricaria had to travel to Lilly headquarters in Indianapolis and report CPI's poor financial results to Lilly's senior management. It was a trying time for a young and ambitious executive. While a team of CPI and Intec engineers was transferring the AICD technology from Pittsburgh to St Paul, Matricaria was instituting a number of expense controls.

Late that year, I participated in a critical meeting at CPI that included Mirowski and Mower as well as Dr Philip Reid, who had joined Lilly from Johns Hopkins, where he had been a key participant in the first AID implants. The purpose of the meeting was to discuss future ICD products. All agreed that the next AICDs had to be programmable and that a transvenous lead should be developed. But the group could not reach a consensus for the design of the next-generation AICD pulse generators. There was great interest then in low-energy cardioversion because many patients were receiving painful high-voltage shocks for hemodynamically stable Ventricular tachycardia (VT). In addition, some patients needed back-up bradycardia pacing. The engineers thought they could develop a low-energy cardioversion model based on the first-generation hybrid circuit Ventak AICD, which was in the design phase. However, a tiered-therapy pulse generator (high- and low-energy shock, antitachycardia pacing, bradycardia pacing) would require a new electronic platform.

CPI made a fateful decision: It would develop both a high/low-cardioversion model, subsequently named the Ventak P, and a tiered-therapy device, which became the Ventak PRx. This product plan was an ambitious one for any company, but for years CPI had struggled to build a basic multiprogrammable pacemaker and it was not prepared for the leap into the high-tech world of ICDs. Moreover, CPI was trying to develop a rate-responsive pacemaker based on a complicated impedance stroke volume algorithm, while pushing the evolution of its other pacemaker product lines. It was too much for a company with limited technical and engineering resources and an owner, Lilly, that wanted profitability.

Technology Development

In 1985 and 1986, CPI began the laborious task of documenting Intec's circuits and component sources to meet the requirements of Good Manufacturing Practices.[7] Meanwhile Intec continued to manufacture the discrete component AID-B/BR. Each AID-B/BR was hand-built using outmoded manufacturing techniques and, as a result, many units failed the final qualification tests and had to be scrapped. This not only increased the costs of manufacturing (indeed CPI lost money on every AID-B/BR it sold), but it also created a backlog of patients who were hospitalized for weeks awaiting an ICD. Fabricating these discrete component devices was even more complicated because each AID-B/BR had to be painstakingly tuned on the manufacturing line to provide the tachycardia rate criterion and high-voltage output energy physicians desired for individual patients.

CPI had to develop a hybrid circuit ICD or it would not be able to manufacture reliable and affordable devices in volume and with the sophistication required of tiered-therapy models. The hybrid circuit presented a number of technical hurdles that took many months to overcome and even more time elapsed before the circuits could be produced in quantity. This was the first hybrid circuit ever used in a medical device that developed 800 V in the confined space of an implantable pulse generator. There were no predicate devices to show CPI the way. Prototype hybrids literally exploded on the bench.

A major problem was cracking of the hybrid ceramic substrate. CPI worked with Teledyne Technologies, a California electronics supplier, to solve the cracking problem and to manufacture the circuits. Teledyne's project manager was Don Washington, and he and his engineers solved the cracking problem by subjecting the ceramic substrate to high temperatures. Many of the electronic components on the hybrid were operating at the extremes of their rated tolerances. To further complicate the manufacturing process, CPI had to develop, build, and qualify the tools required for testing the various components on the hybrid before they could be hermetically sealed in the pulse generator.

Bob Larson and his manufacturing team changed how CPI built the first Ventak hybrid circuit AICD at CPI's facility in Minnesota. First they introduced just-in-time (JIT) manufacturing, which focuses on making multiple quality checks and eliminating the bottlenecks that stall products on the manufacturing line. Before JIT, there were just 11 inspections, and it took 400 hours to build one AID-B/BR. After JIT there were 33 quality control checks and the build time for a Ventak AICD was reduced to 17 hours. Furthermore, fewer ICD pulse generators were rejected at final inspection. Another Larson innovation was the introduction of pilot line manufacturing, whereby engineers refined the methods they would use to mass-produce pulse generators and leads.

I joined CPI in January 1987 after saying farewell to my colleagues and friends at Rush Medical Center. Dr Joseph Messer, the director of cardiology, had been my chief, mentor, and friend, and I regretted leaving his department. But the opportunity to participate in the growth and development of the ICD was irresistible, and I moved my family to Minnesota and entered the business world with a strong sense of purpose.

Indeed, although CPI did not then appreciate the full impact of our work, we and others would soon change the management of patients at risk for lethal ventricular tachyarrhythmias. During 1987, I was in charge of various medical services

at CPI and interacted with some very talented people, including Larson, whom Matricaria had recruited to run manufacturing, and Julie Overbeck, who directed the financial operations. Toward the end of 1987, Matricaria was promoted to run a new division at Lilly in Indianapolis, and I became CPI's president and chief executive officer.

Big Wave

CPI was confronted with a number of challenges in 1988. First, we were struggling with new product development and the company was feeling the strain of staying on plan and on budget. We needed to invest in our sales organization, information technology, supply chain, and financial systems, and the product development group had to have more engineering resources, instrumentation, and space. But CPI was barely profitable in 1987 and our 1988 financial goals precluded major investments in new technologies. Second, CPI/Lilly and Medtronic were going to trial in federal court in Philadelphia. At issue were the Mirowski ICD patents that Lilly had acquired in 1985 and Medtronic had infringed by developing an ICD without a license. If Medtronic prevailed, it could freely and at no cost gain access to the fledgling ICD market. We had a fiduciary responsibility to defend Lilly's intellectual property on behalf of its shareholders. The jury decided in favor of CPI/Lilly and the judge ordered Medtronic to cease all of its ICD development activities in the United States. This was a major legal victory, but the verdict and its aftermath unleashed a torrent of bombast directed at CPI by physicians who believed that Medtronic's ICD products should be available to patients. Medtronic appealed the decision on a technicality and eventually the parties settled the lawsuit. However, the patent litigation wars were only beginning.

In 1988, ICD therapy remained a distant second to antiarrhythmic agents as the treatment of choice for preventing sudden cardiac death. CPI was averaging 6 to 8 ICD pulse generator sales a day (the industry average in 2008 was about 600 per day). The introduction of a rate-programmable model based on the Ventak P platform boosted the number of implants but revenue growth was painfully slow. Fortunately, the addition of ICDs to CPI's product line helped its pacemaker sales, even though the models were notably undistinguished.

In the first quarter of 1988, an event occurred that has been overlooked for its significance. This was an internal CPI strategic analysis of what the ICD market could be if certain product developments occurred and if a substantial primary prophylactic indication for ICD implantation could be demonstrated. The principal products that needed to be developed were (1) a transvenous lead that could provide satisfactory defibrillation thresholds in 80% to 90% of patients and (2) a pulse generator small enough to permit pectoral implantation. The primary prevention indication was the large population of patients who had impaired left ventricular function after myocardial infarction.

The results of the analysis, for which Seah Nissam, Julie Overbeck, and Morton Mower deserve much credit, was designated the "Big Wave" because it clearly demonstrated that the ICD could be a billion-dollar market. We presented the study's results to the Lilly board of directors in the summer of 1988. The outcome was an increase in our budget for product development and manufacturing. The Big Wave was an important business milestone in the evolution of the ICD because this forecast justified the financial risks Lilly and others would willingly take to reap future profits.

Surprisingly, Lilly's chief financial officer shared the Big Wave study with the investment community. Soon interest in the ICD blossomed and the pace of investment accelerated. The money needed to supercharge ICD development began to flow everywhere. It catalyzed the evolution of ICD therapy by attracting key suppliers, accelerating technology development, and justifying the funding of such primary prevention trials as the Multicenter Automatic Defibrillator Implantation Trial (MADIT) under the direction of Dr Arthur Moss.

Transvenous Defibrillation

The single most critical factor for growing ICD therapy was the development of successful transvenous, nonthoracotomy defibrillation. Here CPI stumbled, and ultimately it cost Lilly shareholders at least $100 million in lost market share and product development costs. Initially Mirowski and Mower had conceived the ICD as a transvenous system, and Intec had built a prototype transvenous lead. However, the engineers at CPI rejected Intec's design and constructed the first Endotak ICD lead much like a pacemaker lead. After celebrating the first successful Endotak implant in 1988, I was deeply disappointed when Dr. Sanjeev Saksena, one of the clinical investigators, called me with the news that an Endotak had fractured in one of his patients and had caused multiple inappropriate shocks.[8] Subsequently, we convened a meeting of the Endotak trial investigators and I remember Dr Ralph Vicari of Johns Hopkins stating what I already knew: The Endotak

transvenous defibrillation trial had to stop until we had a lead that did not break. It was a major setback for the therapy, for CPI, and, most of all, for patients. It would take 18 months to fix the Endotak. The experience was a harbinger of the ICD lead problems that continue today.

A by-product of the first Endotak trial was the "hot can" concept, which came about by serendipity. Dr Saksena had agreed to perform a transvenous Endotak implant and broadcast it live to an audience at the Heart House in Bethesda, Maryland. I was sitting in the front row watching him place the subcutaneous patch, which was one of the three electrodes used in the lead system (the other two were on the dual-coil transvenous lead). Instead of placing the patch in the low left chest per protocol, Saksena moved it up to the prepectoral region, and commented that he was achieving lower defibrillation thresholds in that location. The implication was that the housing of a pectoral ICD pulse generator could serve as the third electrode. At that time, pulse generators were still large and were being implanted in the abdomen. But smaller models were under development, and CPI patented and eventually developed the "hot can" application for pectoral implants.

We assessed every technology that would enable transvenous defibrillation and reduce pulse generator size. One such technology was the biphasic waveform, which could decrease defibrillation thresholds and permit transvenous defibrillation in the vast majority of patients. However, CPI did not have a biphasic waveform and the intellectual property and technical knowledge belonged to a California start-up company, Ventritex, Inc. Ventritex was the brainchild of a group that included Michael Sweeney, who had started the pacemaker clinic with me at Rush Medical Center in 1974. Sweeney had gone onto Intermedics where he worked with many of the world's best electrophysiologists. Sweeney and others realized that antitachycardia pacing for VT without defibrillation backup was hazardous. He and an electrical engineer, Ben Pless, left Intermedics for Ventritex in the mid-1980s to develop a tiered-therapy biphasic ICD. CPI's objective in 1989 was to acquire Ventritex. Although CPI initially invested in Ventritex, Lilly's legal brain trust subsequently vetoed the acquisition because they feared it would invite a federal antitrust lawsuit.

Cardiac Arrhythmia Suppression Trial and Primary Prevention

The preliminary CAST results were published in 1989.[9] There was an excess of deaths in post–myocardial infarction patients with ventricular arrhythmias treated with encainide or flecainide; subsequently, CAST-II was terminated because moricizine-treated patients also had excess mortality. I heard the news from Dr Morton Mower, who had joined CPI as vice-president of medical services. Both of us had long believed that antiarrhythmic drugs were ineffective in high-risk patients, and CAST further validated our confidence in the ICD as the treatment of choice for preventing sudden cardiac death. Dr Tom Bigger, the principal investigator of CAST, approached CPI to help fund a National Institutes of Health prospective randomized primary prevention trial comparing surgical coronary artery revascularization plus prophylactic ICD implantation to coronary artery revascularization alone for the prevention of sudden cardiac death in patients who had impaired left ventricular function. The Coronary Artery Bypass Graft–Patch (CABG-Patch) trial, which was completed in 1997, did not favor prophylactic ICD implantation. But CPI had already funded the first MADIT trial in 1990 and that study would change everything. All that we did scientifically during that critical period of 1987 to 1992 was insignificant compared with CPI's decision to sponsor MADIT. Today the vast majority of ICD implants are for primary prevention and most of those flow from the MADIT trials.[10]

By 1990, the implantable defibrillator was beginning to share the clinical stage with antiarrhythmic therapy at the major scientific meetings. Now it is difficult for physicians to conceive that the ICD was ever an orphan therapy. But the ICD remained a second-line treatment until cardiologists recognized that electrophysiology testing and multiple drug trials were ineffective. The Arrhythmia Versus Implantable Defibrillation Trial (AVID) was in the planning stage but CPI declined to participate. Mower and I believed the trial was not needed: CAST had settled the drug issue. But in retrospect, we were mistaken, because the medical community, for a variety of good reasons, needed to conduct a prospective randomized study to prove that the ICD was superior to drugs.

Suppliers

All cardiac rhythm management companies depend on key suppliers, such as Wilson Greatbatch, Inc (WGL), which manufactures batteries and components for ICDs and pacemakers, and Lake Region, which provides wires for leads and other medical devices. WGL and Lake Region were (and are) high-quality suppliers and we valued their products and collaboration. The development and industrialization of the ICD

would have been impossible without these companies. Some suppliers did not meet the high-quality standards CPI required and we shed them rapidly. There were a few suppliers who were unfortunately indispensible but who were reluctant to provide components for medical devices because of perceived liability risks. CPI shielded its suppliers from most medical liability claims, but one microprocessor manufacturer demanded that it be indemnified against its own negligence. We had worked with that manufacturer's engineers for a year or more to develop the microprocessor's specifications, and for us to walk away over the indemnification issue was not a viable option. So we agreed and then designed this supplier's electronic components out of subsequent products.

Endotak II and Pacing for Heart Failure

The clinical trial of the Endotak transvenous lead resumed in 1990 after extensive revisions and bench testing (**Fig. 3**). We replaced the high-voltage conductors and made several changes to the electrodes. It closely resembled the lead Intec had sold Lilly in 1985. The quality-test engineers devised a bench fixture to flex and monitor the lead during many thousands of cycles; such testing is routine today but it was novel in 1990. We were not going to evaluate another lead that fractured in patients, and the company's future depended on it. The new Endotak functioned well and was reasonably durable. However, lead fractures continue to plague ICD therapy, and no bench test yet devised has been shown to predict a lead's clinical reliability.

While we were in the midst of developing the second-generation Endotak and a host of other products, Dr Morton Mower came to my office and said he had something of great importance to discuss. I remember sitting in the southwest corner of my office; it was late morning or early afternoon. Mower said we had to figure out a way to pace the left ventricle and that he and Mirowski were convinced that pacing for heart failure was going to be important. I was skeptical. Up to that point, a number of hemodynamic studies had appeared in the literature, but I was not aware of any positive results beyond sequential atrioventricular and rate-responsive pacing. Besides, I observed, we were sinking many millions of dollars into research and development while building a new manufacturing facility in Puerto Rico. "We need funding to get started," Mower said. I replied that I did not know where we were going to get the money. At this point, he uncharacteristically pounded the table and repeated the

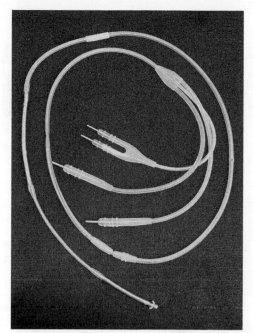

Fig. 3. Endotak II transvenous ICD lead. This lead was the redesign of the original Endotak lead that fractured during its clinical trial in 1988.

request and challenged me to find the money. I relented; after all, Mower and Mirowski had shown how far they could see beyond the horizon, and concepts related to pacing for heart failure deserved to be investigated. The money was found, and that was the start of cardiac resynchronization therapy at CPI.

End of the Beginning

Today, a subcutaneous electrode or thoracotomy approach is rarely needed to achieve satisfactory defibrillation thresholds. Transvenous defibrillation is 99% successful in most patient populations, and a single right ventricular coil to "hot can" pathway is commonly used. In 1990, no one thought that transvenous defibrillation would be successful in such a high percentage of patients. For me, the pivotal trial was performed in Germany, with the results presented at a CPI-sponsored conference in Brussels in 1991. I recall standing in the rear of the conference hall while Dr Michael Becker described a high success rate with the Endotak and other nonthoracotomy lead systems. This was an important milestone. The Endotak transvenous lead had been my number-one priority when I became the chief executive officer at CPI. It was clear that transvenous defibrillation was going to succeed and that this accomplishment would enable the ICD to be used in hundreds of thousands of patients who

otherwise would have remained at risk for sudden cardiac death. My work at CPI was done.

THE NEXT DECADE

The ICD market became very competitive during the 1990s and it remains so today. CPI grew rapidly and became the centerpiece for the medical device company Guidant, which Lilly spun off in 1994. Guidant's principal competitor was Medtronic, whose major strength was and is a powerful presence in virtually all important world markets. There was a flurry of acquisitions as St Jude under Matricaria, who had left Lilly, entered the cardiac rhythm management business when, in 1994, it acquired Pacesetter from Siemens for $500 million and Ventritex for $505 million. Then, in 1998, Guidant bought Intermedics for a reported $800 million, and the Big 3 was born, leaving Biotronik and ELA to operate principally outside the United States. There were many sideshows, including lawsuits among the Big 3 over patent infringement and unethical recruiting. Companies competed for every business advantage, including key physician opinion leaders to serve on their medical advisory boards.

ICD technology improved rapidly as each of the Big 3 ramped up its product development programs. AVID and MADIT demonstrated the value of ICD therapy in secondary and primary prevention trials. The ICD became a multibillion-dollar market that would continue to grow at a double-digit pace for years. What could go wrong? As it turned out many things could and did go wrong, but the therapy was so compelling that the industrialization of the ICD continued to evolve as the Big 3 companies began to integrate their manufacturing processes by building key components in-house and relying less on suppliers. Creative electrical and mechanical engineers and key suppliers found ways to shrink pulse generators (**Fig. 4**). Microprocessor power enabled the addition of more features and diagnostic tools. Programmers enabled physicians to interact with ICD diagnostics so that proper function could be verified and malfunctions recognized before they became clinically important.

To succeed, any company or business sector has to perform well at all levels, but it also needs to be lucky. As the number of ICD implants for the primary and secondary prevention of sudden cardiac death began to peak in 2000, the advent of cardiac resynchronization therapy opened up the huge heart-failure market. It was not simply luck, because CPI had launched its heart-failure research program in the pre-Guidant days, and Medtronic had also seen the opportunity early.

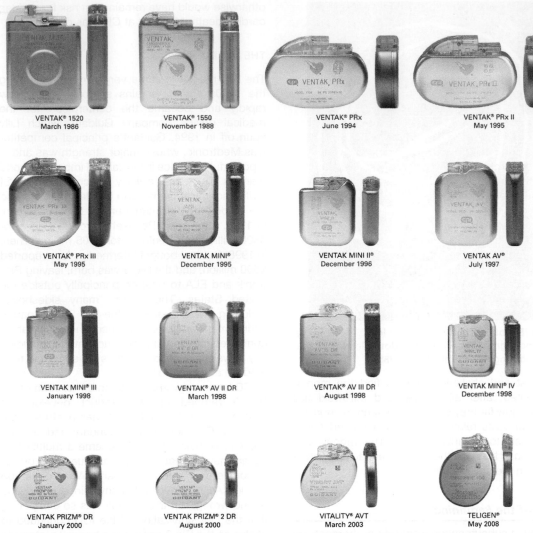

VENTAK® 1520
March 1986

VENTAK® 1550
November 1988

VENTAK® PRx
June 1994

VENTAK® PRx II
May 1995

VENTAK® PRx III
May 1995

VENTAK MINI®
December 1995

VENTAK MINI II®
December 1996

VENTAK AV®
July 1997

VENTAK MINI® III
January 1998

VENTAK® AV II DR
March 1998

VENTAK® AV III DR
August 1998

VENTAK MINI® IV
December 1998

VENTAK PRIZM® DR
January 2000

VENTAK PRIZM® 2 DR
August 2000

VITALITY® AVT
March 2003

TELIGEN®
May 2008

Fig. 4. Evolution of the ICD from the first nonprogrammable hybrid circuit single-chamber model (*upper left*) to a contemporary tiered-therapy cardiac resynchronization device (*lower right*). Significant reductions in volume and thickness began in 1995, even though the number of functions and features expanded rapidly with dual-chamber and cardiac-resynchronization pacing.

But the timing could not have been better, and the financial modeling showed that physicians would willingly implant a very expensive and relatively short-lived cardiac resynchronization therapy ICD in a large segment of the SCD population if the therapy improved cardiac function and enhanced quality of life. Today, more than a third of ICD unit sales and half of company ICD revenues can be attributed to cardiac resynchronization therapy–based devices.

2000 TO PRESENT

ICD product development cycles continued to shorten as companies focused on leap-frogging each other to grab market share when a market-share point was worth millions of dollars in after-tax profits and executive bonuses. Big 3 reliability engineers quietly complained that they were not being allowed to conduct adequate new-product testing because it would take too much time. Key suppliers were similarly pressured to stay on schedule. Rather than carefully introduce new ICD products to the market, companies launched them rapidly, often without any clinical testing. Hence large patient populations were exposed to a new lead or novel pulse generator without substantial in vitro life testing or any human safety data. The result was predictable: multiple ICD device problems that culminated in the product advisories of 2005 to 2007, from which the therapy and industry have yet to recover. During this turmoil, Boston Scientific acquired Guidant for $27.2 billion in 2006 after a bidding war with Johnson & Johnson.

The ICD industry continues to repeat the missteps of the 1970s, when pacemaker product issues affected thousands of patients. An occasional product problem is unavoidable because new technologies are inevitably accompanied by unforeseen failure modes. However, most ICD device problems are the result of poor engineering, inadequate testing, and senior management's desire to introduce new products before the competition. Furthermore, like Medtronic and Cordis before the lithium battery, ICD manufacturers are profiting from frequent ICD pulse generator replacements. The morbidity of replacing a pulse generator has been shown by studies of complications associated with the prophylactic replacement of recalled ICDs. Furthermore, the costs of replacing units for battery depletion are unsustainable in a struggling health economy. Eventually the patients and payers will insist that ICD manufacturers provide a battery that can last the lifetime of the average patient.

Modern ICD therapy is the result of vision, innovation, and good science and engineering. But the ICD would have remained an orphan without industry's vast technical and manufacturing resources. These resources became available only when the business opportunity emerged and investors embraced it. Similarly, MADIT and other primary prevention trials would have languished had industry looked elsewhere for growth. Industrializing the ICD has been a long journey, and it required the skills and expertise of thousands of dedicated people. Looking back, though, one has to marvel at Intec's amazing accomplishment. This was a small company existing on a shoestring and struggling for its next breath. Yet it managed to achieve the medical device equivalent of a lunar landing. As Michel Mirowski was fond of saying: It has been a road with a lot of bumps, but it was the right road, and here we are.

REFERENCES

1. Mirowski M, Mower MM, Staewen WS, et al. Standby automatic defibrillator. An approach to prevention of sudden coronary death. Arch Intern Med 1970;26:158–61.
2. Lown B, Axelrod P. Implanted standby defibrillators. Circulation 1972;46:637–9.
3. Furman S, Parsonnet V, Song S. The Bilitch Registry. Pacing Clin Electrophysiol 1993;10:1357–61.
4. Mirowski M, Reid PR, Mower MM, et al. Termination of malignant ventricular arrhythmias with an implanted automatic defibrillator in human beings. N Engl J Med 1980;303:322–4.
5. Winkle RA, Bach SM, Echt DS, et al. The automatic implantable defibrillator: local bipolar sensing to detect ventricular tachycardia and fibrillation. Am J Cardiol 1983;52:265–70.
6. Mirowski M. The Automatic implantable cardioverter defibrillator: an overview. J Am Coll Cardiol 1985;6:461–6.
7. Hauser RG, Heilman MS. The industrialization of the AICD. Pacing Clin Electrophysiol 1991;14:905–9.
8. Saksena S, Tullo NG, Krol RB, et al. Initial clinical experience with endocardial defibrillation using an implantable cardioverter/defibrillator with triple electrode system. Arch Intern Med 1989;149:2333–6.
9. The Cardiac Arrhythmia Suppression Trial (CAST) Investigators. Preliminary report: Effect of encainide and flecainide on mortality in a randomized trial of arrhythmia suppression after myocardial infarction. N Engl J Med 1989;321:406–12.
10. Moss AJ, Hall WJ, Cannom DS, et al. Improved survival with an implanted defibrillator in patients with coronary disease at high risk for ventricular arrhythmia. N Engl J Med 1996;335:1933–40.

The Wearable Cardioverter Defibrillator—Bridge to the Implantable Defibrillator

Helmut U. Klein, MD[a],*, Iwona Cygankiewicz, MD[a],
Christian Jons, MD[a], Frank Buhtz, RN[b], Steven Szymkiewicz, MD[c]

KEYWORDS
- Wearable cardioverter defibrillator
- Implantable cardioverter defibrillator
- Sudden cardiac death • Risk stratification
- External defibrillator

About 30 years ago, Mirowski introduced the implantable defibrillator (ICD),[1] causing a dramatic change in the treatment of life-threatening ventricular tachyarrhythmias to occur. For the first time, an effective weapon against sudden cardiac death was available. Initially, the ICD was used for secondary prevention to protect patients who had survived a cardiac arrest or had demonstrated ventricular tachycardia (VT) or ventricular fibrillation (VF).[2,3] With better ICD technology and convincing results of large randomized trials,[4–7] today, the implantable defibrillator is used more frequently for primary prevention of sudden death (ie, in patients who are considered of being at high risk, but have not experienced ventricular tachyarrhythmias so far). Both groups, however, have one thing in common. They have an arrhythmogenic substrate, often combined with reduced ventricular function and structural heart disease. Additionally, they suffer from heart failure or have genetically determined channelopathies, such as the long QT or Brugada syndromes.

Early defibrillation in cases of cardiac arrest caused by VF will decide upon survival. Every minute of delayed defibrillation will reduce the rate of survival by 7% to 10%. The automated external defibrillator (AED) has been demonstrated to be very effective at providing immediate defibrillation when used by trained lay responders, and public access defibrillation (PAD) programs will help to further improve survival of victims of cardiac arrest.[8] When defibrillation was provided within 3 minutes after onset of VF, 74% of cardiac arrest victims survived,[9] and lay AED defibrillation resulted in a threefold increase in survival after witnessed cardiac arrest compared with resuscitation procedures after arrival of the emergency medical service.[10] Similar beneficial results were achieved with the PAD study.[11]

Seventy percent to 80% of all cardiac arrest events occur at home, however, often unwitnessed or even during sleep. Although immediate defibrillation will improve survival, the problem of lack of bystanders to use the AED at home

Dr Klein received a research grant from Boston Scientific and lecture honoraria from Boston Scientific and ZOLL Lifecor.

[a] Heart Research Follow up Program, University of Rochester Medical Center, Box 653, 601 Elmwood Avenue, Rochester, NY 14642, USA
[b] CORIZON Gmbh, Heinrich-Hertz-Strasse 6, 50170 Kerpen, Germany
[c] ZOLL Lifecor Corporation, 121 Freeport Road, Pittsburgh, PA 15238-3495, USA
* Corresponding author.
E-mail address: helmut.klein@heart.rochester.edu (H.U. Klein).

Card Electrophysiol Clin 1 (2009) 129–146
doi:10.1016/j.ccep.2009.08.007
1877-9182/09/$ – see front matter © 2009 Published by Elsevier Inc.

remains unsolved. Even within a hospital setting, delayed defibrillation of 6 minutes or longer after cardiac arrest occurred in 22% of all cases, and resulted in survival to hospital discharge in only 10% to 15% of cases.[12]

Risk stratification for primary prevention of sudden death is quite challenging, because the various noninvasive risk parameters have a low positive predictive accuracy; the development of an arrhythmogenic substrate over time is unpredictable, and even invasive procedures such as programmed electrical stimulation are unreliable.

The indications for ICD implantation have been published,[13] and will be updated regularly according to new study results. The need for ICD intervention in primary prevention patients is relative low (ie, not more than 30% within the first 2 years after ICD implantation).

The arrhythmogenic risk, however, may be increased only temporarily as long as the proarrhythmic conditions persist. Improvement of left ventricular ejection fraction (LVEF) is often difficult to predict, and removal of correctable causes of an arrhythmic event may take time. Therefore, it is important to avoid unnecessary ICD implantation in cases of only temporary risk, but also protect these patients from sudden death during this period of uncertainty.

The wearable cardioverter defibrillator (WCD) is an alternative approach to protect patients with a temporary high risk and to prevent sudden arrhythmic death until either ICD implantation is indicated or the arrhythmic risk is considered significantly lower or even absent. The WCD was introduced into clinical practice 8 years ago,[14] and indications for its use are expanding. The intention of this article is to describe the technical characteristics of the WCD, to discuss its indications, and to report on the currently available experience with the WCD.

TECHNICAL CHARACTERISTICS OF THE WCD

The WCD is designed to detect and treat automatically ventricular tachyarrhythmias without the need of professional or bystander intervention. The WCD 3100 (LifeVest, ZOLL Lifecor Corporation (ZLC), Pittsburgh, PA) (**Fig. 1**) consists of a chest garment that holds two large posterior and one anterior self-gelling defibrillator electrodes and three (43 × 10 mm) nonadhesive capacitive dry tantalum oxide electrodes for long-term electrocardiogram (ECG) monitoring; the electrodes are mounted on an elastic belt of the chest garment. The ECG sensing electrodes provide two nonstandard leads, front–back (FB) and left–right (SS) bipolar ECG signals, for

continuous electrocardiographic analysis. The three defibrillation electrodes contain 10 gel capsules each, delivering electrode gel between the defibrillation electrode and the skin in order to lower the electrode–skin interface impedance for biphasic defibrillation, and to prevent skin irritation after shock delivery. Incorporated into the garment is a vibration plate to generate vibration as the first of a sequence of alarms once VT or VF is detected. The defibrillation electrodes are inserted into pockets of the garment, and they are exchangeable when the garment needs to be cleaned or replaced. The garment is connected with a cable to the defibrillator and monitor unit (815 g), which contains the battery, the biphasic defibrillation module with the capacitor and high-voltage converter, the monitor with the digital signal processor (DSP) circuit, a display unit, and the patient response buttons, offering the possibility to withhold defibrillator discharge as long as consciousness prevails. Integrated into the monitor unit are the alarm and voice system. The defibrillator unit is carried in a hip holster or with a shoulder strap (**Fig. 2**). As part of the LifeVest system, there is a battery charger (with less than 2 hours charging time), two batteries (each lasting 24 hours), and a telephone modem the patient uses to transmit ECG signals and the alarm and event history to a ZLC Web server.

Because the sensing ECG electrodes of the LifeVest system pick up more noise from skin movement than intraventricular lead recordings of the ICD, a sophisticated signal/noise detection algorithm is implemented in order to avoid unnecessary alarms or inappropriate defibrillator discharges.

After analog/digital conversion of the ECG electrode signal, a DSP evaluates the electrode skin contact for the presence of high frequency noise with 800 Hz clipping. Multiple input signals are analyzed from each of the two bipolar leads separately using a QRS complex detection system for rate and rate stability, a fast Fourier transformation (FFT) spectrum analyzer, and an analyzer that uses template matching from a vectorcardiographic ECG analysis. The processor also analyzes electrode fall off and has automatic gain control capacity.

Once the decision logic finds the programmed detection parameters fulfilled, a sequence of alarms is initiated, starting with vibration of the defibrillation electrodes, followed by two low- and high-volume alarm tones and a voice, warning that a shock may be delivered (**Fig. 3**). The patient is trained to press the response buttons within 20 seconds to withhold the capacitor discharge as long as consciousness prevails. If the response

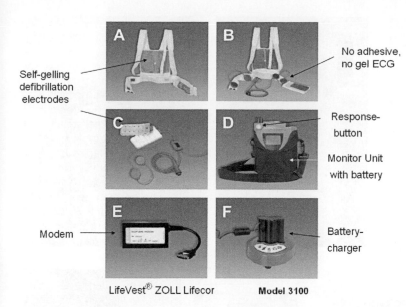

Fig. 1. The Wearable Cardioverter Defibrillator (LifeVest 3100, ZOLL Lifecor Corporation (ZLC), Pittsburgh, PA). Chest garment with back and front defibrillation electrodes (*A*). Elastic belt with electrocardiogram (ECG) monitoring electrodes (*B*). Self-gelling defibrillation electrode (*C*). Monitor unit with battery, capacitor, defibrillation module, digital signal processor and response buttons (*D*). Modem for ECG signal transmission via telephone (*E*). Battery charger (*F*). *Courtesy of* Zoll Lifecor Corporation, Pittsburgh, PA; with permission.

buttons are released or not used because of immediate unconsciousness caused by rapid VT or immediate VF, an impedance-adapted biphasic truncated exponential impulse is delivered through the defibrillation electrodes preceded by gel release from the gel capsules within the defibrillation electrodes. A predischarge test pulse measures transthoracic impedance. With a transthoracic impedance of 30 to 50 Ω, the two shock phases have the same pulse duration (2 to 4.5 milliseconds). With a higher impedance (between 50 and 100 Ω), the first phase of the shock impulse may vary, but the second impulse phase has a fixed duration of 4.5 milliseconds. Higher impedance will result in a lower amount of delivered shock energy. The LifeVest is able to deliver up to five shocks in case the arrhythmia is analyzed as not being terminated after the first shock.

Fulfilling the programmed VT/VF detection criteria lasts between 5 and 10 seconds; tachycardia confirmation lasts another 10 seconds, and the arrhythmia alarm runs for 25 seconds. Together with the necessary capacitor charging time and the attempt to synchronize the shock to the R-wave signal, the time elapsing between onset of the tachycardia and shock delivery is about 45 to 50 seconds, but generally not longer than 1 minute if the shock is not inhibited by holding the response buttons.

The tachycardia recognition cut-off rate is programmable for ventricular fibrillation between 120 and 250 bpm (default 200 bpm), and for stable VT, the rate is between 120 bpm and the VF setting (VT default 150 bpm). If R-wave synchronization is impossible (less than 3 seconds), an unsynchronized shock will be delivered. VF shock delay

can be programmed from 25 to 55 seconds, VT shock delay from 60 to 180 seconds. Further VT shock delay may be programmed for up to 30 seconds for an individually programmable nighttime (10PM to 7AM). The stored energy level of the defibrillator is programmable between 75 and 150 J (**Box 1**).

The LifeVest has a flash memory system integrated into the monitor unit that allows to store and to retrieve the ECG signal 30 seconds prior to the start of the arrhythmia alarms, and 15 seconds after the alarms stop. The current device has an overall event storage capacity of 70 minutes. All stored ECG event data are retrievable by the treating physician from the ZLC Web server once the data are transmitted by the patient via a modem, provided the treating physician has received access to the ZLC Web server for the particular patient. This data-transferring system also provides information about the patient's wearing compliance, ECG signal quality, alarm history, and noise occurrence (**Fig. 4**).

The WCD is not contraindicated in patients with implanted pacemakers. The pacing stimulus artifact, however, has to be smaller than the potential VF-ECG signal in order to avoid tracking of the pacing spike as a regular rhythm during VF. Patients who have a unipolar pacing mode with a stimulus artifact greater than 0.25 mV are at risk of having the pacing artifact during fine VF.[15] Baseline ECG recording to create a vector cardiographic template should be performed during nonpaced rhythms whenever possible. VT cut-off rate must be programmed high enough to avoid faster paced rhythms from being detected as a VT.

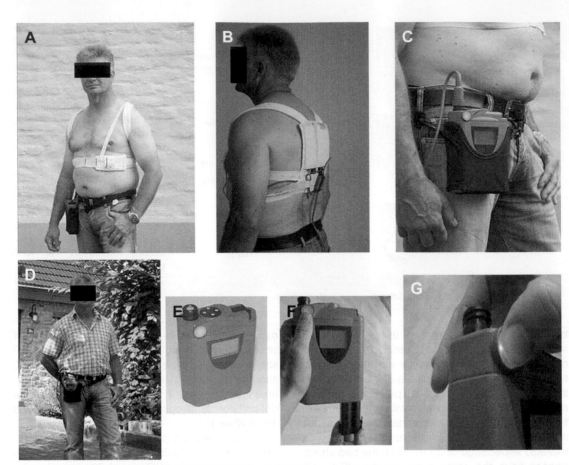

Fig. 2. Wearable cardioverter defibrillator (LifeVest 3100). Front defibrillation electrode and hip holster with monitor unit (*A*). Back defibrillation electrode (*B*). Hip holster with monitor unit (*C*). Hip holster with monitor unit (*D*). Monitor unit with electrocardiogram display and response button (*E*). Insertion of battery into monitor unit (*F*). Response buttons (*G*).

Because the LifeVest is a therapeutic approach that needs patient cooperation, careful explanation and training of the patient are mandatory to guarantee appropriate device use and assembling (**Fig. 5**). This most often is done by specialized nursing staff. The WCD (LifeVest) can be programmed to a training mode in order to allow the patient

> To become familiar with the difference between noise alarms and true arrhythmia alarms
> To assemble the garment with the electrodes
> To charge and exchange the battery every day
> To use the modem correctly for signal transmission over the telephone

A weekly transmission of the wearing data is requested, and a monthly visit at the physician's office is recommended. After each shock delivery, the garment has to be replaced immediately in order to have new self-gelling defibrillation electrodes available in case there will be further events. The LifeVest system also can deliver a bradycardia alarm, and starts ECG recording with severe bradycardia (less than 20 bpm), but the current device does not have pacing capability. Future generations of the WCD will have a lower weight of the monitor unit, a larger signal storage capacity, and an easier automatic data transmission system that will allow permanent ECG signal control by the treating physician, transforming the WCD system into a real long-term Holter recording system.

In 1998, for the first time the successful clinical testing of the WCD in 10 patients was reported.[16] Induced VT/VF was terminated in 9 of 10 patients in the catheterization laboratory, with the first automatically delivered monophasic shock of 230 J with a mean transthoracic impedance of 53 Ω after a mean of 32 seconds. In one patient, erroneously disconnected sensing electrodes prevented

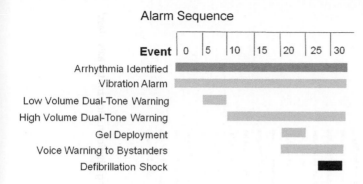

Alarm Sequence

Fig. 3. Sequence of alarms after identification of the tachycardia. Time 0 to 30 seconds. Vibration alarm continues over the whole alarm time. While the patient uses the response buttons, the shock will not be delivered. If the response buttons are released, the alarms sequence starts again prior to shock delivery.

adequate VT detection. In 2003, a new WCD generation was introduced using impedance-compensating biphasic truncated exponential waveforms. Under electrophysiology laboratory conditions it was able to demonstrate a 100% first shock termination success of 22 VT/VF episodes in 12 patients, using 70 J of stored energy in 12, and 100 J in 10 shocks respectively. Transthoracic impedance varied between 47 to 79 Ω.[17]

The clinical benefit of the WCD to detect and treat life-threatening ventricular arrhythmias effectively first was demonstrated with the wearable defibrillator investigative trial and bridge to ICD in patients at risk of arrhythmic death studies.[14] In 289 patients with LVEF less than or equal to 30% and either severe heart failure, acute myocardial infarction (MI) or recent coronary artery bypass graft surgery (CABG), the WCD was worn for up to 4 months. When the prespecified safety and efficacy boundaries of the sequential study design were met, six out of eight successful defibrillations of spontaneous VT/VF episodes had occurred. Two defibrillation attempts were unsuccessful because of incorrectly placed defibrillation electrodes. In 901 months of WCD use, six unnecessary shocks occurred in six patients (0.67% inappropriate shocks per month of use). It was concluded from this combined study that in ambulatory patients with a high risk of sudden death, who have a time-limited need of protection from life-threatening arrhythmias but who are not candidates for immediate ICD implant, the WCD is able to effectively bridge this time period.

WHEN SHOULD THE WEARABLE CARDIOVERTER DEFIBRILLATOR BE USED?

The WCD is an important tool for patients considered at high risk for sudden arrhythmic events. It should be used as long as there is uncertainty of how long such a risk will persist, for periods of longer-lasting risk stratification after syncope of unknown origin, interrupted protection from an already implanted ICD, temporary inability to implant an ICD, and in some cases with refusal of an indicated ICD by the patient.

EARLY PHASE AFTER MYOCARDIAL INFARCTION

The current approach to the acute coronary syndrome has reduced the overall mortality of an acute MI significantly. The relative percentage of sudden cardiac death (SCD) in the early phase of infarction, however, remained intolerably high, with the highest sudden death mortality of 1.4% per month for the first 3 months after an acute MI, particularly those with LVEF less than or equal to 35%.[18–20]

It has been demonstrated that implantable defibrillators significantly reduce sudden arrhythmic death in the remote phase of infarction.[4–7] Overall mortality, however, was not reduced when the ICD

Box 1
Programming parameters of the wearable cardioverter defibrillator

Rate programming

Ventricular tachycardia (VT) (default 150 bpm)

Programmable from 120 bpm to ventricular fibrillation (VF) setting

VT shock delay from 60 to 180 seconds (default 60 seconds)

Additional shock delay at night programmable between 0 and 30 seconds

Ventricular fibrillation

Programmable from 120 to 250 bpm (default 200 bpm)

VF shock delay from 25 to 55 seconds (default 25 seconds)

No additional VF shock delay at night

Shock energy

75 to 150 J

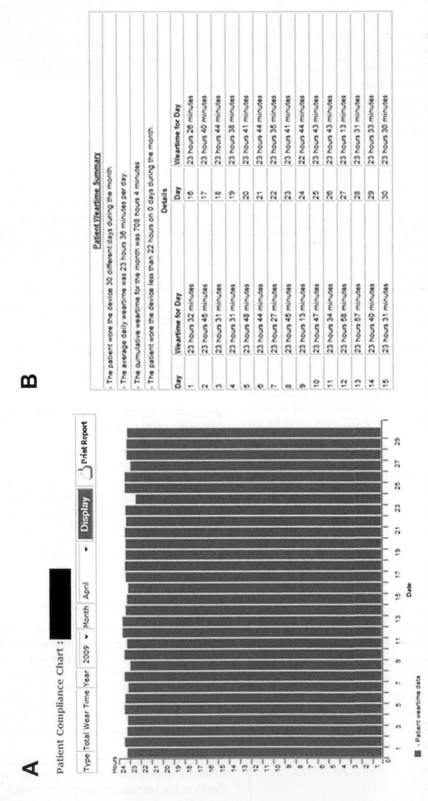

Fig. 4. Wearable cardioverter defibrillator (WCD) wearing compliance report of a patient sent via modem and telephone to treating physician. Horizontal axis: days/month of wearing. Vertical axis: hours per day; each bar represents WCD wearing time per day (A). List of wearing time (B).

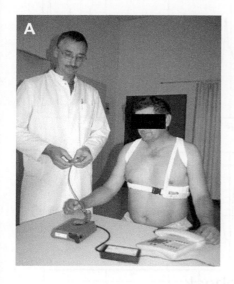
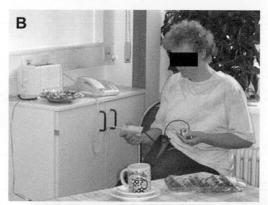
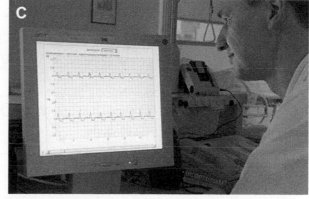

Fig. 5. Training to use the wearable cardioverter defibrillator (*A*). Patient transmits electrocardiogram (ECG) via modem and telephone to ZLC Web server (*B*). Treating physician analyzes transmitted ECG (*C*).

was implanted within the first 40 days of infarction.[21] Therefore, current guidelines do not recommend ICD implantation early after infarction in patients with an LVEF less than or equal to 35%.[13] The recently launched VEST prevention of early sudden death trial and prediction of ICD therapies study will show if the WCD is a valid approach to close the defibrillator in acute myocardial infarction trial gap.[22]

The WCD should be used in patients with an acute MI who demonstrate poor left ventricular (LV) function (LVEF less than or equal to 35%) within the first few days after the onset of infarction, particularly if the initial phase is accompanied by symptoms of heart failure or early episodes of VT/VF or cardiac arrest. The WCD will protect the patient during the first 2 to 3 months after infarction until LVEF has improved (LVEF greater than 35%) and lowered the risk of sudden arrhythmic events, or the criteria for an ICD are fulfilled, if low LVEF persists. About 30% of the initial patient cohort with an acute MI will continue to demonstrate a low LVEF of less than or equal to 35%, or will develop further remodeling of ventricular function.[19] The WCD bridges the time until final decision to implant an ICD is possible, and in

case of improved LV function, will help to avoid unnecessary ICD implantation (**Fig. 6**).

AFTER HEART SURGERY WITH POOR VENTRICULAR FUNCTION

Patients who undergo open heart surgery, in particular coronary bypass graft surgery, and have reduced LV function prior to the surgical procedure, have a high postoperative 30- day mortality of 4.3% to 5.1%.[23] About 50% of the patients who die within the early postoperative phase, either while still in the hospital or during surgical rehabilitation, will die from sudden arrhythmic death.[24] These patients have an LVEF less than or equal to 30%, may suffer from intra- or early postoperative MI, and may have needed a ventricular assist device, intra-aortic balloon pumping, or had ventricular tachyarrhythmias early after surgery. Because it is unclear if their ventricular function will improve later on, the WCD represents a bridging tool against sudden death during the first few months after surgery. The decision for an ICD can be safely postponed until the permanent risk for SCD becomes more obvious.

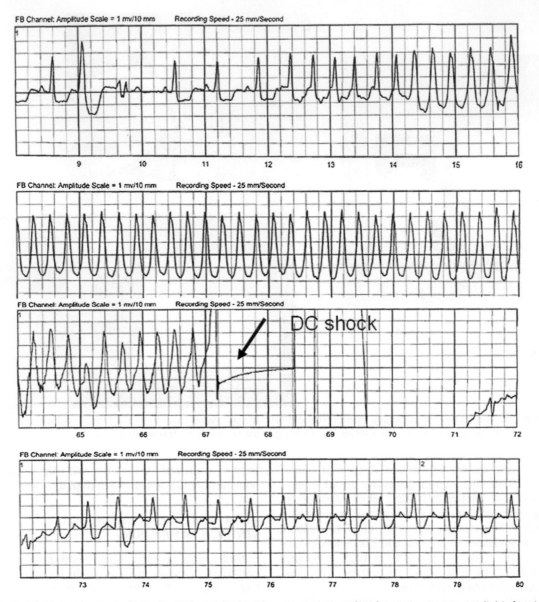

Fig. 6. Rapid ventricular tachycardia (VT) spontaneously occurring 5 weeks after an acute myocardial infarction (left ventricular ejection fraction 24%) in a 58 year-old man. VT terminated by wearable cardioverter defibrillator shock of 150 J 55 seconds after onset of VT (numbers under electrocardiogram strips: seconds after beginning of recording).

ACUTE HEART FAILURE AND BRIDGING UNTIL HEART TRANSPLANTATION

Sudden death is a frequent event among patients with acute congestive heart failure or when waiting for heart transplantation, because heart failure is a strong risk factor for lethal arrhythmic events.[25] Overall mortality was 25% in patients waiting for heart transplantation, and 66% of them died of sudden death.[26] Therefore, ICD implantation was recommended for these patients even without prior tachyarrhythmic episodes.[27] Besides the issue of cost, ICD implantation in patients waiting for heart transplant is not without risk, considering the need for ICD testing during implant, and a tendency towards a higher device infection rate. Without doubt, even after heart transplantation, when immunosuppression is needed during severe rejection, the risk of life-threatening arrhythmias is high, particularly if this is combined with an acute remodeling of the donor heart.

The WCD can be considered as an alternative approach to ICD implantation for 6 to 9 months, particularly once the patient is listed as candidate for heart transplantation. Even after a successfully terminated VT/VF episode, the WCD continues to be a lifesaving tool until transplantation is performed. Patients with organ rejection should be protected with the WCD as long as there is poor ventricular function.

SYNCOPE OF UNKNOWN ORIGIN

The underlying mechanism of syncope with or without cardiac arrest is often difficult to assess. Although there is a tendency towards immediate ICD implantation, ICD implantation is debatable in many of these patients, particularly when VT/VF is the assumed cause of syncope, but has not been documented. It often remains uncertain if the risk of VT/VF recurrence persists, and about 20% of all cardiac syncopes or arrests have no shockable rhythm at the time of arrest. The cause of such an event may be bradycardia, asystole, or even electromechanical dissociation. Unfortunately, current risk stratification techniques are inconclusive, time-consuming, and have a low positive predictive accuracy.

In cases of acute myocarditis with an arrhythmic event as the first symptom of the disease, the stability of the arrhythmic substrate, and the potential progress into a dilated cardiomyopathy with poor ventricular function, is often totally unpredictable.[28,29] Similar problems may be encountered in rare cases of a Takotsubo cardiomyopathy that can be accompanied by VT or VF episodes.[30] An unclear collapse in young athletes without detectable structural abnormalities or electrocardiographic signs of genetic abnormalities may be caused by VT/VF. Syncope or aborted cardiac arrest in patients with hypertrophic cardiomyopathy with or without obstruction needs careful consideration for an implantable defibrillator,[31] because not all such events are caused by ventricular tachyarrhythmias. Current guidelines do not recommend ICD implantation when correctable or reversible causes of the arrhythmic event may be present or cannot be excluded.[13] The WCD system allows a safe bridging during the period of risk assessment for a few months until a persistent arrhythmic risk can be confirmed or has reliably disappeared (**Figs. 7** and **8**).

PATIENTS WITH INHERITED ARRHYTHMOGENIC DISORDERS

The prevalence of inherited cardiac arrhythmias such as the long QT syndrome, Brugada-syndrome,

short-QT syndrome or catecholaminergic polymorphic VT is not high; however, the risk, the clinical course, and the electrocardiographic appearance are variable owing to incomplete genetic penetration. Careful risk stratification is necessary to select the appropriate candidates for ICD implantation. Assessment of the typical ECG changes after syncope or a tachycardia episode is often difficult and inconclusive. Electrophysiologic testing in patients with assumed arrhythmogenic disorders is still a matter of debate; the beneficial effect of drugs such as beta-blockers or specific antiarrhythmic agents is difficult to assess, and genetic testing is not always available and is time-consuming.

Although ICD implantation in some individuals with inherited cardiac arrhythmias, and an established high risk for SCD, is recommended,[13] ICD therapy in these often young patients is not without problems, particularly when accompanied with serious psychological distress or frequent inappropriate ICD firing. The WCD is able to bridge the time of risk stratification and decision making for the right therapeutic direction, which may last weeks or even months (**Fig. 9**).

ICD INFECTION OR TEMPORARY LOSS OF ICD PROTECTION

ICD system infection is a complication that occurs even in experienced centers. Chronic device infection requires device removal and prolonged antibiotic treatment.[32] Removal of the ICD system deprives the patient of the protection against potential life-threatening VTs, particularly if ICD implantation was performed for secondary prevention of SCD. Close monitoring of these patients is mandatory until infection is cured completely and a new ICD device can be implanted (**Fig. 10**).

There are clinical settings when ICD implantation is indicated, but the clinical condition of the patient may not allow immediate ICD implant. This can occur with signs of a general infectious disease, a dangerous metabolic disturbance, amiodarone-induced hyperthyroidism, or with a severe electrolyte disorder, particularly in patients with renal failure or after intense diuretic therapy. In these clinical situations that go along with a temporary loss of ICD protection or a need to postpone indicated ICD implantation, the use of the WCD is mandatory in order to avoid long-lasting and cost-intensive hospitalizations on a monitor unit.

For various reasons, patients occasionally refuse to have an ICD although their risk for SCD is high, they need time to agree to ICD

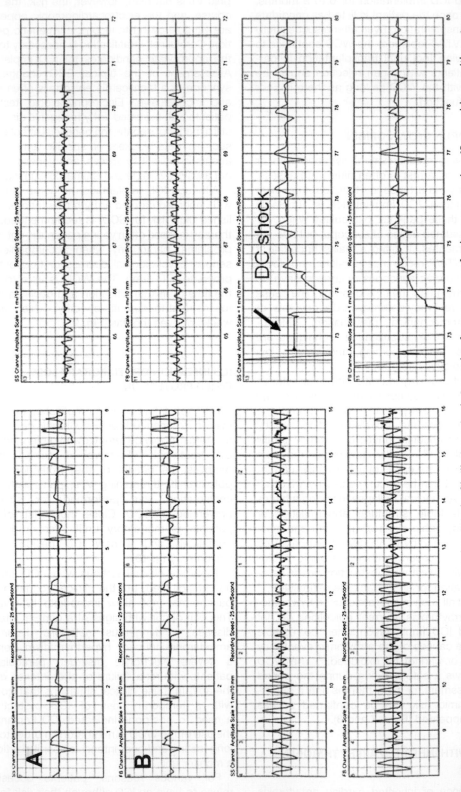

Fig. 7. Wearable cardioverter defibrillator terminated ventricular fibrillation episode 2 months after a syncope of unknown cause in a 43 year-old man with acute myocarditis; recorded are both electrocardiogram leads (*A* = site-site [SS] and *B* = front–back [FB]).

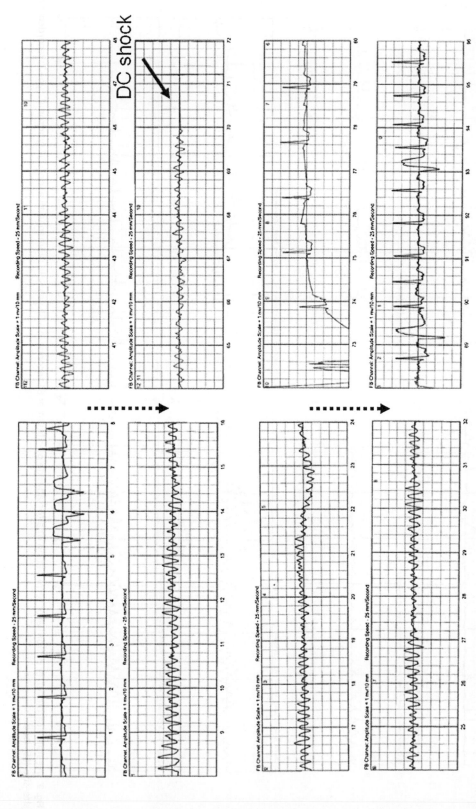

Fig. 8. Termination of a spontaneous ventricular tachycardia episode in a 61 year-old woman with no structural heart disease 5 weeks after a cardiac arrest of unknown cause. Discontinuously recorded front–back (FB) electrocardiogram lead.

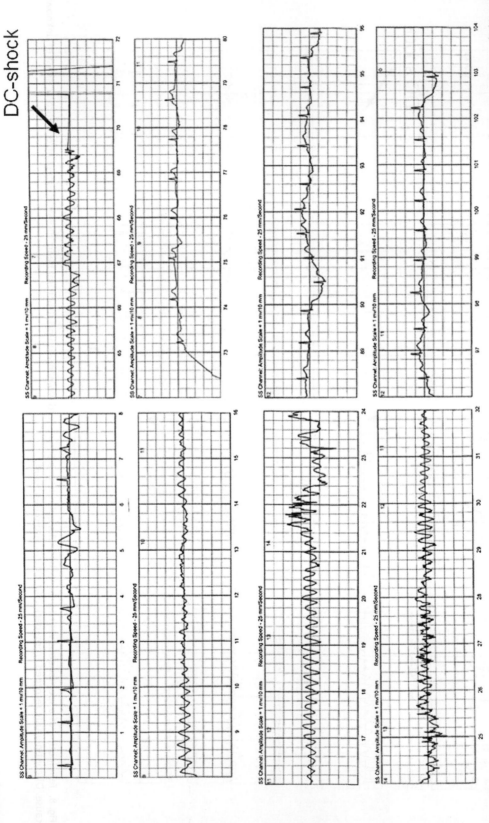

Fig. 9. Wearable cardioverter defibrillator termination of a torsades de pointes after 61 seconds in a 38 year-old woman with a long QT syndrome, type 2; recorded is only site–site (SS) lead.

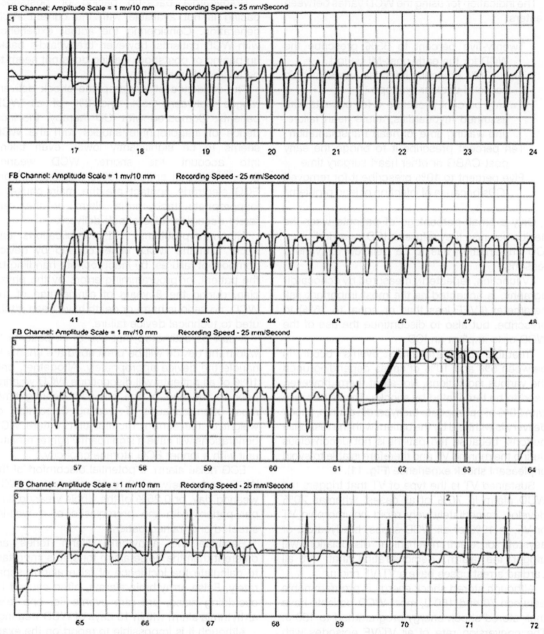

Fig. 10. Wearable cardioverter defibrillator termination of a spontaneous ventricular tachycardia in a 73 year-old man 17 days after removal of an infected implantable defibrillator; recorded is the front–back (FB) lead.

implantation, or the clinical conditions with an uncertain life expectancy do not favor ICD therapy. The WCD may be another option or can help to postpone the definitive therapeutic approach.

CLINICAL ASPECTS OF THE WCD

Approximately 18000 patients have used the WCD during the 8 years since its introduction for clinical use in the United States and in a few countries in Europe. The wearing time per patient varies between 2 and 3 months depending upon the indication for its use. Some patients had the WCD for 1 or 2 weeks only, whereas few patients continued to wear the device for more than a year; the longest time now is almost 8 years. The wearing compliance is astonishingly high, with about 90% of all patients using the WCD for 22 to 24 hours per day, interrupting the protection only to have a shower or bath, or when they replace the garment.

The indication for using the WCD varies between centers:

Twenty-five percent to 35% prescribe the WCD for the early post-MI period

About 30% prescribe it for risk assessment in cases of unclear syncope

Twenty percent prescribe it for patients with assumed myocarditis, acute heart failure, and waiting time for heart transplantation

Ten percent prescribe it to bridge the early post-CABG or other heart surgery time

Five percent to 10% prescribe it for removed ICDs because of infection or lead problems

Only a small percentage of patients wear the device because they refuse an ICD, or an indicated ICD implantation has to be delayed for various reasons.

LV function, repeatedly measured by echocardiography, is accepted as the most important risk parameter (LVEF less than or equal to 35%) to prescribe, but also to discontinue the use of the WCD or to implant an ICD.

Treatable tachyarrhythmia events occur in between 5% and 10% of cases depending upon the various indications. Not all of them, however, need to be terminated by shocks. This is because with 20% of appropriate tachycardia alarms, shock delivery is withheld by the patient with the response buttons, because the patient is not unconscious during the running VT and therefore is able to avoid unpleasant shock experience (**Fig. 11**).

Sustained VT is the type of VT that triggers the WCD alarm in 70% of all cases, whereas 20% develop immediately very rapid polymorphic VT or VF. In 10% of all WCD cases, bradycardia or asystole or electromechanical dissociation will trigger the alarm, demonstrating that not all cardiac arrest cases have a VT/VF origin.

Although stored shock energy is programmable between 70 and 150 J, most WCD patients have their stored shock energy programmed to 150 J. The conversion rate of all VT/VF episodes with the first delivered shock is 95% to 98%. Only very few episodes need a second shock to terminate VT/VF. All VT/VF episodes are terminated within 60 seconds except when shock delivery is withheld by the patient, or additional VT/VF response delay is programmed. Withholding of shock occurs in 20% of tachycardia alarms.

Survival of shock-treated tachycardia events ranges between 90% and 95%. Patients with documented bradycardia or asystole events have a significantly lower survival, particularly those with asystole as a sign of a dying heart or after electromechanical dissociation (**Fig. 12**).

Bradycardia back-up pacing or postshock pacing is not available with the current WCD generation. Considering the actual experience with WCD patients, however, bradycardia back-up pacing or postshock pacing does not seem to be absolutely mandatory.

The incidence of inappropriate shock delivery ranges between 1.5% and 2% of all WCD patients. Compared with ICD therapy, the incidence of inappropriate shocks with the WCD seems to be significantly lower, even taking into account the shorter WCD wearing time.[33,34] Signal artifacts (60%) caused by poor ECG electrode contact are the main cause of inappropriate tachycardia alarm or the very rarely occurring false shock delivery.

Although problems and complications can occur with the WCD, either caused by device component failures, by inappropriate handling by the patient, or programming errors by the physician, during the 8 years of clinical use of the WCD, no serious harm or death have been attributed to technical device failure.

It can be estimated that 5% of all patients to whom the device will be prescribed are unable to handle the device appropriately. Altogether, only 10% of all patients will discontinue WCD wearing prior to the end of the planned wearing time, most often because of wearing discomfort or weight of the current monitor unit. Future WCD generations will have a significantly lighter monitor unit with a longer ECG storage capacity.

ECG noise alarm, a potential discomfort of the WCD, varies between 2 to 15 minutes per WCD wearing day, or 0.25% of the whole wearing time per patient with the prerequisite of a well-instructed and trained patient.

Because the arrhythmia alarm tones are different than the noise alarm tone, it is important to calculate the incidence of false alarms separately. False arrhythmia alarms, often caused by overriding noise, are rare events (ie, one false arrhythmia alarm within 13 days of WCD wearing).

Although it is impossible to report on the exact mode of therapy after the patients had finished WCD wearing without having experienced WCD shocks, data retrieved from a small cohort of WCD patients in Germany show that only half of the WCD patients received ICDs after they had the WCD. This is interesting, because most of these patients initially would have been potential ICD candidates (unpublished data from Klein H, 2009).

ROLE OF THE WCD BETWEEN ICD AND AED

Current experience demonstrates that the WCD is an effective tool to protect patients identified as

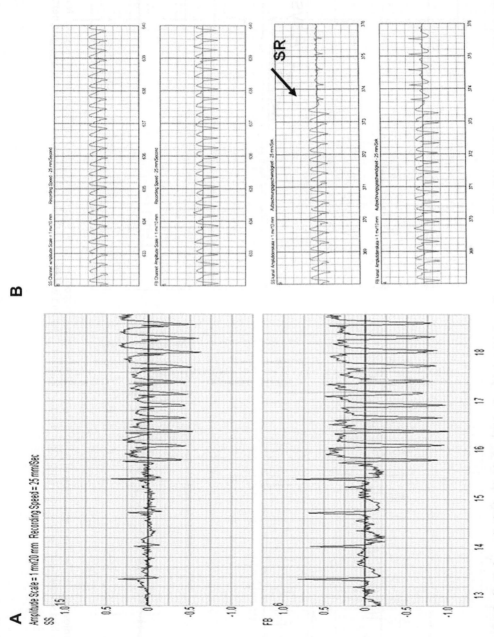

Fig. 11. Spontaneous ventricular tachycardia (VT) episode in a 64-years-old man 71 days after acute myocardial infarction (left ventricular ejection fraction 19%); pushing the response buttons (time not indicated) withholds wearable cardioverter defibrillator shock until self-termination of VT after 373 seconds (A) Onset of VT. (B) Self-termination of VT into sinus rhythm (SR).

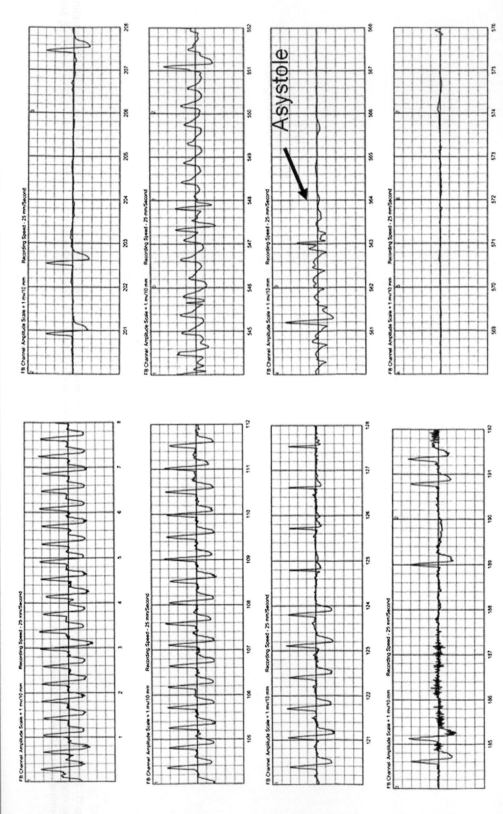

Fig. 12. Wearable cardioverter defibrillator recording of a rapid rhythm that terminates spontaneously into bradycardia and finally lethal asystole. No therapy delivered. The 61 year-old man had severe heart failure (left ventricular ejection fraction 12%) and was listed for heart transplant; he was found dead the next morning at home.

being at high risk of SCD. The main purpose for using the WCD is to bridge a temporary risk period prior to deciding whether ICD implantation is mandatory or not necessary. Life-threatening VTs are terminated reliably within less than 1 minute, and device complications are tolerably low. Additionally, patient compliance is excellent, and WCD therapy acceptance by the patient is astonishingly high, allowing about 70% of patients to continue their daily life activities without major restrictions.

The WCD can help to prevent unnecessary ICD implantation, and thereby contribute to the improvement of quality of life and reduce healthcare costs. The WCD has characteristics of an ICD, but does not need to be implanted. It detects and terminates VT/VF almost as fast as the ICD, offering the possibility of withholding painful defibrillation as long as consciousness persists. The WCD has a lower incidence of inappropriate shocks compared with ICD therapy without reducing the safety of arrhythmia termination.

Because it is of great importance to analyze the long-term arrhythmia profile of patients at high risk of SCD, the WCD provides uninterrupted long-term information on all arrhythmia events over months, with an event storage capacity of more than 1 hour with quick ECG event retrieval via the ZLC website. This tool gives the WCD characteristics of a real long-term Holter monitoring unit in addition to SCD protection.

The WCD has similarities with an AED, but it does not need bystander help to apply the lifesaving defibrillation shock when needed. The home use of automated external defibrillators for sudden cardiac arrest (HAT) trial[35] aimed to determine whether the AED in the home of patients at risk of SCD can improve survival when placed in the home of patients who were not ICD candidates but considered at risk after anterior MI. Use and efficacy of the AED were compared to emergency medical service (EMS) intervention. After somewhat more than 3 years of follow-up, it was demonstrated that the AED at home yields no better overall survival than immediate arrival of EMS personnel. The request of the authors from the HAT trial that "some form of a home automated alert system might be of value"[35] will be satisfied only by the WCD. Even if the defibrillation electrodes of the AED are applied by home bystanders, the time to terminate VT/VF is simply too long. This can be seen by the fact that AED recordings of the arrhythmia events exclusively demonstrated VF, whereas WCD recordings show VT in most cases, allowing the conclusion that even when witnessed, the time for the AED to be able to deliver life-saving therapy is too long to achieve a higher survival rate.

The WCD does not compete with the ICD or with the AED. The ICD has its undeniable role in the long-term prevention of SCD, and the concept of the AED in all public places together with improved knowledge of lay providers of basic life support is very promising to further reduce SCD.

SUMMARY

The WCD is an effective tool to provide immediate life-saving defibrillation for patients at risk for sudden arrhythmic death. It is a reliable and safe approach for patients in whom indications for an ICD remain undecided, when ICD therapy needs more time for risk stratification, or when already existing ICD protection mandates temporary interruption. The value of the WCD lies in its contribution to better selection of patients for ICD therapy, and wearing the WCD diminishes the risk of patients to die suddenly when bystanders for the AED shock delivery are not available within the shortest possible time.

REFERENCES

1. Mirowski M, Mower MM, Reid PR. The automatic implantable defibrillator. Am Heart J 1980;100: 1089–92.
2. The Antiarrhythmics Versus Implantable Defibrillators (AVID) Investigators. A comparison of antiarrhythmic drug therapy with implantable defibrillators in patients resuscitated from near-fatal ventricular arrhythmias. N Engl J Med 1997; 337(22):1576–83.
3. Kuck K, Cappato R, Siebels J, et al. Randomized comparison of antiarrhythmic drug therapy with implantable defibrillators in patients resuscitated from cardiac arrest: the Cardiac Arrest Study Hamburg (CASH). Circulation 2000;102(7):748–54.
4. Moss AJ, Hall WJ, Cannom DS, et al. Improved survival with an implanted defibrillator in patients with coronary disease at high risk for ventricular arrhythmia. Multicenter Automatic Defibrillator Implantation Trial Investigators. N Engl J Med 1996;335(26):1933–40.
5. Moss AJ, Zareba W, Hall WJ, et al. Prophylactic implantation of a defibrillator in patients with myocardial infarction and reduced ejection fraction. N Engl J Med 2002;346(12):877–83.
6. Buxton AE, Lee KL, Fisher JD, et al. A randomized study of the prevention of sudden death in patients with coronary artery disease. Multicenter Unsustained Tachycardia Trial Investigators. N Engl J Med 1999;341(25):1882–90.
7. Bardy GH, Lee KL, Mark DB, et al. Amiodarone or an implantable cardioverter–defibrillator for congestive heart failure. N Engl J Med 2005;352(3):225–37.

8. Rho RW, Page RL. The automated external defibrillator. J Cardiovasc Electrophysiol 2007;18(8):896–9.

9. Valenzuela TD, Roe DJ, Nichol G, et al. Outcome of rapid defibrillation by security officers after cardiac arrest in casinos. N Engl J Med 2000;343(17):1206–9.

10. Capucci A, Aschieri D, Piepoli MF, et al. Tripling survival from sudden cardiac arrest via early defibrillation without traditional education in cardiopulmonary resuscitation. Circulation 2002;106(9):1065–70.

11. Hallstrom AP, Ornato JO, Weisfeldt M, et al. Public-access defibrillation and survival after out of hospital cardiac arrest. N Engl J Med 2004;351(7):637–46.

12. Chan PS, Krumholz HM, Nichol G, et al. Delayed time to defibrillation after in-hospital cardiac arrest. N Engl J Med 2008;358(1):9–17.

13. Zipes DP, Camm AJ, Borggrefe M, et al. ACC/AHA/ESC 2006 guidelines for management of patients with ventricular arrhythmias and the prevention of sudden death: a report of the American College of Cardiology/American Heart Association Task Force and the European Society of Cardiology Committee for practice guidelines. J Am Coll Cardiol 2006; 48(5):e247–346.

14. Feldman A, Klein H, Tchou P, et al. Use of a wearable defibrillator in terminating tachyarrhythmias in patients at high risk for sudden death: results of WEARIT/BIROAD. Pacing Clin Electrophysiol 2004;27(1):4–9.

15. Lapage MJ, Canter CE, Rhee EK. A fatal device-device interaction between a wearable automated defibrillator and a unipolar ventricular pacemaker. Pacing Clin Electrophysiol 2008;31(7):912–5.

16. Auricchio A, Klein H, Geller CJ, et al. Clinical efficacy of the wearable cardioverter defibrillator in acutely terminating episodes of ventricular fibrillation. Am J Cardiol 1998;81(10):1253–6.

17. Reek S, Geller JC, Meltendorf U, et al. Clinical efficacy of a wearable defibrillator in acutely terminating episodes of ventricular fibrillation using biphasic shocks. Pacing Clin Electrophysiol 2003; 26(10):2016–22.

18. Huikuri HV, Tapanainen JM, Lindgren K, et al. Prediction of sudden cardiac death after myocardial infarction in the beta-blocking era. J Am Coll Cardiol 2003;42(4):652–8.

19. Solomon SD, Zelenkofske S, McMurray JJ, et al. Sudden death with myocardial infarction and left ventricular dysfunction, heart failure, or both. N Engl J Med 2005;352(25):2581–8.

20. Adabag AS, Therneau TM, Gersh BJ, et al. Sudden death after myocardial infarction. JAMA 2008; 300(17):2022–9.

21. Hohnloser SH, Kuck KH, Dorian P, et al. Prophylactic use of an implantable cardioverter defibrillator after acute myocardial infarction. N Engl J Med 2004; 351(24):2481–8.

22. Olgin J, Evaluating the effectiveness of the LifeVest defibrillator and improving methods for determining the use of implantable cardioverter defibrillators (The VEST/PREDICTS Study). Available at: http://www.clinicaltrials.gov; NCT:00628966.

23. Vaughan-Sarrazin MS, Hannan EL, Gormley CJ, et al. Mortality in Medicare beneficiaries following coronary artery bypass graft surgery in states with and without certificate of need regulation. JAMA 2002;288(15):1859–66.

24. Toda K, Mackenzie K, Mehra MR, et al. Revascularization in severe ventricular dysfunction (15% ≤LVEF ≤30%): a comparison of bypass grafting and percutaneous intervention. Ann Thorac Surg 2002;74(6):2082–7.

25. Goldenberg I, Moss AJ, Hall WJ, et al. Causes and consequences of heart failure after prophylactic implantation of a defibrillator in the multicenter automatic defibrillator implantation trial II. Circulation 2006;113(24):2810–7.

26. Sandner SE, Wieselthaler G, Zuckermann A, et al. Survival benefit of the implantable cardioverter-defibrillator in patients on the waiting list for cardiac transplantation. Circulation 2001;104:171–6.

27. Da Rosa MR, Sapp JL, Howlett JG, et al. Implantable cardioverter defibrillator as a bridge to cardiac transplantation. J Heart Lung Transplant 2007; 26(12):1336–9.

28. Kawai C. From myocarditis to cardiomyopathy: mechanisms of inflammation and cell death. Learning from the past for the future. Circulation 1999;99(8):1091–100.

29. De Cobelli F, Pieroni M, Esposito A, et al. Delayed gadolinium-enhanced cardiac magnetic resonance in patients with chronic myocarditis presenting with heart failure or recurrent arrhythmias. J Am Coll Cardiol 2006;47(8):1649–54.

30. Matsuoka K, Okubo S, Fujii E, et al. Evaluation of the arrhythmogenecity of stress-induced Takotsubo cardiomyopathy from the time course of the 12-lead surface electrocardiogram. Am J Cardiol 2003;92(2):230–3.

31. Maron BJ, Shen WK, Link MS, et al. Efficacy of implantable cardioverter defibrillators for the prevention of sudden death in patients with hypertrophic cardiomyopathy. N Engl J Med 2000;342(6):365–73.

32. Chua JD, Wilkoff BL, Lee I, et al. Diagnosis and management of infections involving implantable electrophysiologic cardiac devices. Ann Intern Med 2000;133(8):604–8.

33. Daubert JP, Zareba W, Cannom DS, et al. Inappropriate implantable cardioverter defibrillator shocks in MADIT II. J Am Coll Cardiol 2008;51(14):1357–65.

34. Poole JE, Johnson GW, Hellkamp AS, et al. Prognostic importance of defibrillator shocks in patients with heart failure. N Engl J Med 2008;359(8):1009–17.

35. Bardy GH, Lee KL, Mark DB, et al. Home use of automated external defibrillators for sudden cardiac arrest. N Engl J Med 2008;358(17):1793–804.

Subcutaneous Implantable Cardioverter-Defibrillator Technology

Anurag Gupta, MD, Amin Al-Ahmad, MD, FACC*,
Paul J. Wang, MD, FACC

KEYWORDS

- Subcutaneous ICD • Implantable cardioverter-defibrillator
- Defibrillation • Sudden death • Tachyarrhythmias

The first human implant of the implantable cardioverter-defibrillator (ICD) in 1980 ushered in an era of improved recognition and therapy for sudden cardiac death (SCD).[1] Initial epicardial ICD lead systems required a thoracotomy for placement of epicardial defibrillation patches and epicardial rate-sensing leads. Advances in ICD technology over the last 3 decades have led to decreased device size and the design of effective transvenous defibrillation leads. In addition, there have been significant improvements in ICD detection and discrimination algorithms and improved shock waveforms. This had led to the current paradigm of endocardial ICD lead systems in which endocardial leads (including pace-sense components and shocking coils) are placed transvenously, thus obviating the need for thoracotomy.

Indications for ICD therapy have also changed over the years based upon the results of well-conducted large-scale clinical trials. Whereas, initially, the ICD was only indicated after aborted SCD, current ICD indications have expanded to include prophylactic implantation in individuals who have a high risk of SCD, greatly increasing the pool of potentially eligible candidates.[2–5]

Despite these advancements, there continues to be significant barriers in offering this therapy to appropriately indicated patients. ICD delivery can be technically challenging and expensive. Furthermore, current ICD systems have associated risk, including but not limited to procedural

risks, inappropriate device therapy, and long-term device-related complications that prominently include lead failure.

Recently, subcutaneous or so-called leadless ICD systems have been developed that offer a potential new paradigm for facilitating ICD implantation. Though heterogeneous in design, these systems typically share a common theme of using electrodes that are placed subcutaneously without requirement for leads in or on the heart. Although not clinically approved, this article will examine studies investigating the subcutaneous ICD and discuss its possible advantages and disadvantages as compared with current transvenous ICD systems.

EXPERIMENTAL EVIDENCE FOR THE SUBCUTANEOUS ICD
Initial Studies

Defibrillation with implantable devices using noncardiac electrodes is not a new concept. In 1970, Schuder and colleagues[6] demonstrated the efficacy of a completely automatic implantable defibrillator that weighed approximately 1037 g and that used extrathoracic electrodes in three canines. Energy delivery across the chest wall ranged between approximately 23 to 37 J, and the time between induction of ventricular fibrillation to shock delivery ranged between 14 seconds to 40 seconds with later inductions. The first shock

Department of Internal Medicine, Division of Cardiovascular Medicine, Cardiac Arrhythmia Service, Stanford University School of Medicine, 300 Pasteur Drive, Room H2146, Stanford, CA 94305-5233, USA
* Corresponding author.
E-mail address: aalahmad@cvmed.stanford.edu (A. Al-Ahmad).

Card Electrophysiol Clin 1 (2009) 147–154
doi:10.1016/j.ccep.2009.08.012
1877-9182/09/$ – see front matter © 2009 Published by Elsevier Inc.

was successful in terminating ventricular fibrillation in 67 of 73 induced episodes, and no animal required external defibrillation.

Subcutaneous Defibrillation in Children

Subcutaneous defibrillation has only been more recently reported in humans. Clinicians wishing to avoid or unable to place fully transvenous or epicardial ICD systems in pediatric patients with complex cardiac disease have reported cases of effective defibrillation using a subcutaneous array as the high-voltage lead.[7–12] For example, Gradaus and colleagues[7] reported successful subcutaneous defibrillation in two patients aged 12- and 14-years-old with a single-chamber ICD with a transvenous and epicardial bipolar pace-sense lead, respectively. Using an active abdominal can and a single subcutaneous array placed dorsolaterally in the left thorax, they reported successful conversion of ventricular fibrillation with defibrillation threshold (DFT) less than or equal to 20 J. Likewise, Berul and colleagues[8] reported successful defibrillation with threshold less than or equal to 14 J using an active abdominal can and a single subcutaneous array in a 2-year-old girl with a single chamber ICD using an epicardial bipolar rate-sensing lead.

Stephenson and colleagues[13] reported a larger, multicenter retrospective review of subcutaneous defibrillation (that is, not using transvenous high-voltage coils or epicardial patches) in children with mean age of 8.9 years and complex cardiac disease. Of 22 patients examined, 14 had a subcutaneous coil system while the remaining 8 had the coil placed on the epicardium; all patients had an epicardial or transvenous bipolar ventricular pace-sense lead and used an active can configuration. While a true DFT was not obtained in all patients, subcutaneous lead placement was associated with a higher DFT than the epicardial system (19 ± 7 vs 13 ± 4 J, $P = .03$). Though 7 of the 22 patients required system revisions, this study again demonstrated the feasibility of subcutaneous defibrillation in children.

Experimental Models of Subcutaneous Defibrillation in Adults

There have also been studies examining a subcutaneous lead system in adults indicated for and receiving transvenous ICDs. Grace and colleagues[14] examined the DFT for subcutaneous ICD systems using various dual electrode configurations between the ICD can and subcutaneous electrode. In one study, 41 patients were enrolled in a multicenter, prospective study comparing

DFT between a standard transvenous ICD system and a subcutaneous system. For the subcutaneous system, the active can was placed in the anterolateral axillary line at the sixth intercostal space and the subcutaneous electrode was placed 3 cm left of the sternum with the coil centered at the fifth intercostal space. The DFT for the subcutaneous system was 39 J. As expected, this was higher than the 12 J DFT of the transvenous system but still within a technically feasible range.

Optimal electrode configurations were further examined by Grace and colleagues[15] in a study of 10 patients undergoing standard transvenous ICD implantation. Four electrode configurations were tested: (1) 60 cc lateral can and 8 cm parasternal coil, (2) 60 cc lateral can with a 5 cm squared parasternal disk electrode, (3) 60 cc pectoral can with a 4 cm paraxiphoid coil, and (4) 60 cc pectoral can with a 8 cm inframammary coil electrode. In this study, though the optimal configuration appeared to require a lateral can position, all groups were thought to be in a technically feasible range of defibrillation with mean DFT for the four groups ranging between 27 to 39 J.

Similarly, Lieberman and colleagues[16] examined the efficacy of a nontransvenous defibrillation, this time using an anteroposterior shock pathway. Specifically, 33 patients undergoing standard transvenous ICD implantation had an anterior low pectorally-placed active can emulator and a 25 cm coil tunneled subcutaneously around the back of the left thorax between the 6th and 10th intercostal space. A standard electrophysiology catheter was placed for sensing and for ventricular fibrillation induction. Biphasic shocks with a 50%-50% tilt and total waveform time of 16 ms were delivered and defibrillation testing was performed using a stepwise protocol. Eighty one percent of patients had successful defibrillation using less than or equal to 35 J.

Likewise, Burke and colleagues[17] estimated the subcutaneous defibrillation energy requirement in 20 adults indicated for an ICD, this time using anterior-anterior vector. In their experimental model, a cutaneous electrode patch, acting as a surrogate for a subcutaneous electrode, was first placed at the inferior border and apex of the left heart. Next, a standard transvenous ICD was implanted and DFT testing was performed. The DFT using the standard transvenous system was 10.4 ± 6.5 J. The device was then removed (replaced at the end of study) and an emulator was placed in the device position. Defibrillation was retested for the investigational, nontransvenous configuration using an external defibrillator that delivered a shock between the pectoral subcutaneous emulator and the apical cutaneous electrode patch, 10 seconds after induction of ventricular fibrillation. Using the nontransvenous system, successful defibrillation at 50 J was achieved in 17 of 20 (85%) patients including 7 of 9 (78%) patients with successful defibrillation tested at 30 J. Only two patients required more than 70 J for successful defibrillation.

A follow-up study by Burke and colleagues,[18] again using cutaneous electrode patches as surrogates for subcutaneous electrodes, suggested that subcutaneous signals could distinguish ventricular fibrillation from sinus rhythm when using sensing and detection algorithms typical for ICDs. Gold and colleagues[19] also showed reliable arrhythmia detection in an experimental model using subcutaneous equivalent cutaneous electrode configurations that were compared with detection from single-chamber transvenous ICD systems. Based upon the recorded signals from 43 induced ventricular arrhythmias and 45 induced atrial arrhythmias with rate greater than or equal to 170 beats per minute, the subcutaneous system showed significantly improved specificity and not different, excellent sensitivity greater than 98% for the detection of ventricular arrhythmias. Unlike prior studies and case reports that demonstrated the feasibility of subcutaneous defibrillation, these experiments suggested that a subcutaneous ICD system could further be used to reliably detect ventricular arrhythmias. Studies such as these paved the way for investigations in humans using totally subcutaneous ICD systems.

Totally Subcutaneous ICD Systems in Adults

Recently, early experience with a total-purpose, totally subcutaneous ICD system has been reported by Crozier and colleagues.[20] This device, manufactured by Cameron Health, Inc (San Clemente, CA) is an approximately 69 cc, 145 g defibrillator that is able to discharge 80 J and provide limited postshock pacing. The system consists of a subcutaneously placed pulse generator and a subcutaneous lead that is placed along the left side of the sternum (**Fig. 1**). Sensing occurs via one of three electrode configurations: from the distal subcutaneous lead to the can, from the proximal subcutaneous lead to the can, or from the distal to proximal subcutaneous lead. The device has a projected longevity of 5 years.

The initial clinical experience regarding this device was recently reported.[20] In a multicenter study, 55 patients with an indication for a standard ICD underwent implantation of a subcutaneous ICD without the use of fluoroscopy. The patients had a mean age of 56 years and mean ejection fraction of 34 ± 13% and the majority of individuals had ischemic heart disease (67%). Implant time and testing was 74 ± 38 minutes. Specifically, the procedure involved subcutaneous implantation of the pulse generator over the sixth rib in the anterior axillary line and tunneling of the subcutaneous lead in a parasternal position, 1 to 2 cm left of midline and midway between the xiphoid and sternomanubrial junction. The primary study objective was to describe device detection and conversion efficacy for induced ventricular fibrillation.

The subcutaneous ICD was able to successfully detect ventricular fibrillation in all 137 episodes of induced ventricular fibrillation among the 53 patients able to complete the protocol (100% sensitivity). Moreover, the device had 98% (52 of 53 patients) conversion efficacy, defined as two consecutive successful conversions of ventricular fibrillation using a 65 J shock per maximum four inductions. Thus, the majority of patients had a 15 J safety margin, as the device is able to deliver 80 J. Of note, the charge time to deliver a shock was 14 ± 2.5 seconds. In addition, over a brief follow-up period, there was one case of appropriate detection and treatment and two cases of inappropriate oversensing due to noise from a loose setscrew and from T-wave oversensing. The lead was also found to have moved in four patients, requiring repositioning in two individuals. Despite some initial encouraging results, the clinical experience with totally subcutaneous ICD systems remains preliminary and limited.

LIMITATIONS WITH CURRENT ICD SYSTEMS

A primary drawback of epicardial ICD systems is that they require invasive procedures associated with higher periprocedural risk. The perioperative mortality associated with lead implantation via thoracotomy may be as high as 5%, acknowledging that heterogeneity exists between operators and patients (including for example need for concomitant cardiac surgery) within and between surgical series.[21,22] Epicardial systems may pose other unique challenges such as difficulty in removing fibrosed epicardial leads or patches, potential for triggering a restrictive pericardial process, possibility of complicating future cardiac surgery, or risk of hindering external cardioversion due to increased transthoracic impedance.[23]

Epicardial ICD systems have been largely supplanted by endocardial ICD systems using transvenous delivery of leads. Though the procedure is substantially safer, less expensive, and easier to perform, procedural risks remain. For

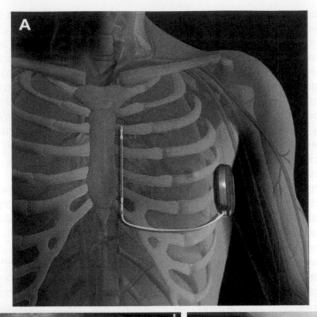

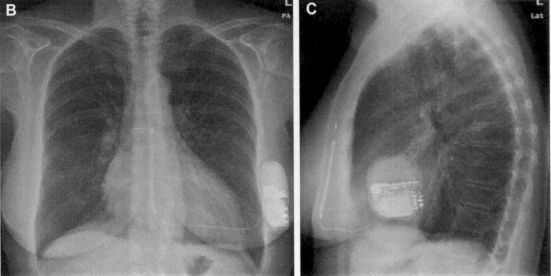

Fig. 1. (*A*) Schematic depiction. (*B*) Posterior to anterior chest radiograph. (*C*) Lateral chest radiograph of an individual implanted with a totally subcutaneous ICD system. The pulse generator is located approximately over the sixth rib in the anterior axillary line and is connected to a tunneled subcutaneous lead approximately 1 cm left of the sternum between the xiphoid and sternomanubrial junction. The subcutaneous electrode consists of a high-voltage, low-impedance, shocking coil electrode and low-voltage, high-impedance, sensing electrodes (*Courtesy of* Cameron Health, Inc, San Clemente, CA, USA; with permission.)

example, among a cohort of the ICD Registry of 111,293 initial ICD implantations reported between 2006 and June of 2007, Curtis and colleagues[24] reported that 1.5% of all patients experienced a major in-hospital procedural complication and 3.7% of all patients experienced any complication. In this study, complications stemming from transvenous lead delivery were prominent with reported complications specifically including hematoma (1.1%), lead dislodgement (1%), pneumothorax (0.5%), and cardiac arrest (0.3%) and a less than or equal to 0.1% rate of hemothorax, cardiac perforation, pericardial tamponade, stroke, conduction block, myocardial infarction, infection, phlebitis, transient ischemic attack, drug reaction, arteriovenous fistula, peripheral nerve injury, and cardiac valve injury.

Moreover, transvenous lead delivery can be technically challenging, potentially restricting dissemination of this technology to eligible patients. In the same study performed by Curtis and colleagues,[24] they reported that 70.9% of the 111,293 ICD implantations were performed by certified electrophysiologists. Interestingly, in comparison to electrophysiologists, the risk of complications in both unadjusted and adjusted analyses was higher when performed by nonelectrophysiologist cardiologists (who performed 21.9% of implants) or thoracic surgeons (who performed 1.7% of implants).

Beyond periprocedural risks of transvenous lead delivery, such leads pose long-term challenges. For example, late infection, vessel occlusion, lead dislodgment, and valvular dysfunction may be observed with endocardial leads.[25] Most notably, defibrillation lead failure is common, potentially leading to need for procedural revision, lead extraction with its attendant risks, accelerated battery depletion, failure to deliver appropriate therapy, or inappropriate shocks. For example, Kleemann and colleagues[26] examined 990 patients with first implantation of transvenous ICD between 1992 and May of 2005 from five manufacturers, excluding patients requiring device explant due to infection and patients with lead dislodgement. They estimated lead survival rates of 85% at 5 years and 60% at 8 years, and reported an annual incidence of lead failure up to 20% in 10-year-old leads. The majority of lead defects were due to insulation defects (56%). However, leads were implanted at a single center and approximately 95% of implantations were via the subclavian vein.

Eckstein and colleagues[27] reported a lower incidence of lead malfunction among a series of 1317 consecutive patients with transvenous ICDs implanted between 1993 and 2004 followed for a median 6.4 years. Specifically, they reported a cumulative incidence of lead failure requiring surgical revision of 2.5% at 5 years and 4.6% at 10 years. Though variable incidences of lead defects have been reported in smaller series, likely due to a combination of factors such as definitions of lead performance, ICD models examined, patient and physician characteristics, and tools used to detect lead failure, the rate of lead dysfunction remains clinically relevant.[28] Nonetheless, a vast clinical experience documenting the efficacy of transvenous lead technology along with continued technological advances have solidified its primary role in ICD therapy.

POTENTIAL ADVANTAGES AND DISADVANTAGES OF SUBCUTANEOUS ICD SYSTEMS
Advantages of Subcutaneous ICD Systems

Although clinical experience is required with subcutaneous ICD systems before meaningful comparisons can be derived with current transvenous ICD systems, they do offer multiple potential advantages and disadvantages. The primary potential strengths of subcutaneous ICD systems are that implantation and explantation may be easier and may be associated with fewer complications. In their pilot studies with a totally subcutaneous ICD system, Crozier and colleagues[20] reported implantation time including testing of 74 ± 38 minutes for the first three implants per operator, then 60 ± 22 minutes thereafter. Notably, fluoroscopy, intravascular access, and instrumentation in the heart are not required for implantation or explantation.

These features have significant implications in select populations for whom placing transvenous or epicardial leads is not possible or is especially unpalatable. This may include individuals in whom long-term device therapy is indicated and who are thus anticipated to have higher rates of lead-related complications or failure, leading to more potential device revisions or removals. This may include ICD-indicated pediatric patients with cardiac disease, younger patients with channelopathies (such as long or short QT, Brugada syndrome, or catecholaminergic polymorphic ventricular tachycardia), and younger patients with cardiomyopathies (such as hypertrophic cardiomyopathy, arrhythmogenic right ventricular cardiomyopathy, dilated cardiomyopathy, or acquired disease).[29] A subcutaneous ICD may also have a role in individuals at risk for ventricular arrhythmias though with potential for improvement, such as those individuals awaiting cardiac transplantation or high-risk individuals immediately postinfarction.[29]

Beyond potential indications in niche populations, subcutaneous ICD systems, by perhaps representing a simpler and safer method of implant, offers the potential for greatly expanding ICD therapy in the overall pool of potentially eligible patients. Though individual estimates of appropriate ICD use vary widely, with one analysis approximating the current prevalence of individuals in the United States eligible for, yet without, prophylactic ICD therapy to be 820,000,[29] all studies consistently demonstrate underutilization.[30,31] The reasons for low implantation are multifactorial and require further definition. However, challenges with transvenous implantation including its expense, requirement for access to technical expertise, and associated morbidity may all be contributory factors that may somewhat be ameliorated by use of subcutaneous ICD systems.

Disadvantages of Subcutaneous ICDs

Notwithstanding, subcutaneous ICD systems have limited clinical experience and have several significant potential limitations. First, current subcutaneous ICD systems can provide temporary, but not long-term, pacing support. At present, such devices would not be appropriate for the significant pool of ICD-indicated patients requiring pacing for cardiac resynchronization therapy or bradycardia. Moreover, many of the patients requiring bradycardia support cannot be identified at implant owing to the development of drug-induced, progressive, or acquired disease.[32] In addition, current subcutaneous ICDs cannot deliver pacing support for ventricular tachyarrhythmias (eg, antitachycardic pacing [ATP]), a cornerstone of ventricular tachycardia management. Multiple studies have demonstrated high efficacy of ATP in terminating slow and fast ventricular tachyarrhythmias.[33,34] For example, Wathen and colleagues[34] demonstrated that for fast ventricular tachyarrhythmias with rates between 188 and 250 beats per minute, a strategy of initial empiric ATP therapy was effective in terminating 72% of fast ventricular episodes and was overall equally safe as a strategy of shock-only therapy.

In addition, intracardiac leads potentially offer advantages over subcutaneous leads with respect to (1) lower DFTs; (2) decreased charge times; and (3) improved sensing of intracardiac ventricular and atrial activity, thus enhancing tachyarrhythmia detection and discrimination using established algorithms. Data to establish the performance, reliability, and stability of sensing and defibrillation in subcutaneous ICDs will be critical before such comparisons can be made and before subcutaneous ICD technology can be adopted.

Whereas subcutaneous ICDs avoid intravascular access and potentially offer a safer method of implantation and explantation, operator skill is still critical and the potential for significant device-related complications remain. Subcutaneous systems do not mitigate pocket-related complications such as skin erosion; hematoma and seroma; infection; dehiscence; and device migration. In fact, if larger pulse generators were required to deliver more energy, the rate of such complications may in theory increase. In addition, leadless ICD is a misnomer for most current subcutaneous ICD systems, which employ subcutaneous leads. These leads are likewise subject to mechanical stress, albeit different from transvenous leads, and are vulnerable to failure, erosion, infection, and migration and may cause irritation to the patient. The optimal subcutaneous electrode configuration, size, shape, and material all require definition. Current data prospectively examining subcutaneous lead performance is also required, though an older study prospectively examining the performance of 398 patients with transvenous ICDs employing subcutaneous high voltage electrodes reported a 93.7%, 5-year cumulative survival of these leads.[35]

SUMMARY

The advent of subcutaneous ICD systems represents a major paradigm shift for the detection and therapy of ventricular tachyarrhythmias. Despite critical advances in lead technology that have permitted widespread adoption of highly effective transvenous ICDs, problems remain including requirement for technical expertise; periprocedural complications during implantation and explantation; and long-term lead failure. Although subcutaneous ICD systems may mitigate some of these risks, they provide new shortcomings, such as inability to provide pacing therapy for bradyarrhythmias, ventricular tachyarrhythmias, and cardiac resynchronization. Moreover, despite promising initial experimental studies and clinical reports, the safety, efficacy, cost, reliability, and long-term performance of subcutaneous ICDs require thorough investigation before adoption into clinical practice. Though promising, ongoing clinical evaluation and development are required before the role of subcutaneous ICDs as an adjunctive or primary therapy can be defined.

REFERENCES

1. Mirowski M, Reid PR, Mower MM, et al. Termination of malignant ventricular arrhythmias with an implanted automatic defibrillator in human beings. N Engl J Med 1980;303:322–4.
2. Moss AJ, Hall WJ, Cannom DS, et al. Improved survival with an implanted defibrillator in patients with coronary disease at high risk for ventricular arrhythmia. Multicenter Automatic Defibrillator Implantation Trial Investigators. N Engl J Med 1996;335:1933–40.
3. Buxton AE, Lee KL, Fisher JD, et al. A randomized study of the prevention of sudden death in patients with coronary artery disease. Multicenter Unsustained Tachycardia Trial Investigators. N Engl J Med 1999;341:1882–90.

4. Moss AJ, Zareba W, Hall WJ, et al. Prophylactic implantation of a defibrillator in patients with myocardial infarction and reduced ejection fraction. N Engl J Med 2002;346:877–83.

5. Bardy GH, Lee KL, Mark DB, et al. Amiodarone or an implantable cardioverter-defibrillator for congestive heart failure. N Engl J Med 2005;352:225–37.

6. Schuder JC, Stoeckle H, Gold JH, et al. Experimental ventricular defibrillation with an automatic and completely implanted system. Trans Am Soc Artif Intern Organs 1970;16:207–12.

7. Gradaus R, Hammel D, Kotthoff S, et al. Nonthoracotomy implantable cardioverter defibrillator placement in children: use of subcutaneous array leads and abdominally placed implantable cardioverter defibrillators in children. J Cardiovasc Electrophysiol 2001;12:356–60.

8. Berul CI, Triedman JK, Forbess J, et al. Minimally invasive cardioverter defibrillator implantation for children: an animal model and pediatric case report. Pacing Clin Electrophysiol 2001;24:1789–94.

9. Thogersen AM, Helvind M, Jensen T, et al. Implantable cardioverter defibrillator in a 4-month-old infant with cardiac arrest associated with a vascular heart tumor. Pacing Clin Electrophysiol 2001;24:1699–700.

10. Madan N, Gayno JW, Tanel R, et al. Single-finger subcutaneous defibrillation lead and "active can": a novel minimally invasive defibrillation configuration for implantable cardioverter-defibrillator implantation in a young child. J Thorac Cardiovasc Surg 2003;126:1657–9.

11. Greene AE, Moak JP, Di Russo G, et al. Transcutaneous implantation of an external cardioverter-defibrillator in a small infant with recurrent myocardial ischemia and cardiac arrest simulating sudden infant death syndrome. Pacing Clin Electrophysiol 2004;27:112–6.

12. Luedemann M, Hund K, Stertmann W, et al. Implantable cardioverter defibrillator in a child using a single subcutaneous array lead and an abdominal active can. Pacing Clin Electrophysiol 2004;27:117–9.

13. Stephenson EA, Batra AS, Knilans TK, et al. A multicenter experience with novel implantable cardioverter defibrillator configurations in the pediatric and congenital heart disease population. J Cardiovasc Electrophysiol 2006;17:41–6.

14. Grace AA, Smith WM, Hood M, et al. A prospective, randomized comparison in humans of defibrillation efficacy of a standard transvenous ICD system with a totally subcutaneous ICD system (the S-ICD system) [abstract]. Heart Rhythm 2005;2:1036.

15. Grace AA, Hood M, Smith WM, et al. Evaluation of four distinct subcutaneous implantable defibrillator (S-ICD) lead systems in humans [abstract]. Heart Rhythm 2006;3:S128–9.

16. Lieberman R, Havel WJ, Rashba E, et al. Acute defibrillation performance of a novel, non-transvenous shock pathway in adult ICD indicated patients. Heart Rhythm 2008;5:28–34.

17. Burke MC, Coman JA, Cates AW, et al. Defibrillation energy requirements using a left anterior chest cutaneous to subcutaneous shocking vector: implications for a total subcutaneous implantable defibrillator. Heart Rhythm 2005;2:1332–8.

18. Burke MC, Haefner PA, Gilliam R, et al. Feasibility of left chest cutaneous electrode configurations to distinguish ventricular fibrillation from sinus rhythm. Heart Rhythm 2006;3(Suppl 1):S156.

19. Gold MR, Theuns DA, Knight BP, et al. Arrhythmia detection by a totally subcutaneous S-ICD® system compared to transvenous single-chamber ICD systems with morphology discrimination [abstract]. Heart Rhythm 2009;6:S34–5.

20. Crozier I, Melton I, Park RE, et al. Clinical evaluation of the subcutaneous implantable defibrillator (S-ICD) system [abstract]. Heart Rhythm 2009.

21. Gartman DM, Bardy GH, Allen MD, et al. Short-term morbidity and mortality of implantation of automatic implantable cardioverter-defibrillator. J Thorac Cardiovasc Surg 1990;100:353–9.

22. Saksena. Defibrillation threshold and perioperative mortality associated with either endocardial and epicardial defibrillation lead systems. The PCD investigators and participating institutions. Pacing Clin Electrophysiol 1993;16:202–7.

23. Russo AM, Marchlinski FE. Engineering and construction of pacemaker and implantable cardioverter-defibrillator leads. In: Ellenbogen KA, Kay GN, Lau CP, et al, editors. Clinical cardiac pacing, defibrillation, and resynchronization therapy. 3rd edition. Philadelphia: Saunders Elsevier; 2007. p. 161–200.

24. Curtis JP, Luebbert JJ, Wang Y, et al. Association of physician certification and outcomes among patients receiving an implantable cardioverter-defibrillator. JAMA 2009;310:1661–70.

25. Gold MR, Peters RW, Johnson JW, et al. Complications associated with pectoral implantation of cardioverter defibrillators. Pacing Clin Electrophysiol 1997;28:208–11.

26. Kleemann T, Becker T, Doenges K, et al. Annual rate of transvenous defibrillation lead defects in implantable cardioverter-defibrillators over a period of >10 years. Circulation 2007;115:2474–80.

27. Eckstein J, Koller MT, Zabel M, et al. Necessity for surgical revision of defibrillator leads implanted long-term: causes and management. Circulation 2008;117:2727–33.

28. Maisel WH, Kramer DB. Implantable cardioverter-defibrillator lead performance. Circulation 2008;117:2721–3.

29. Santini M, Cappato R, Andresen D, et al. Current state of knowledge and experts' perspective on the subcutaneous implantable cardioverter-defibrillator. J Interv Card Electrophysiol 2009;25:83–8.

30. Fonarow GC, Yancy CW, Albert NM, et al. Heart failure care in outpatient cardiology practice setting: findings from IMPROVE HF. Circ Heart Fail 2008;1:98–106.

31. Shah B, Hernandez AF, Liang L, et al. Hospital variation and characteristics of implantable cardioverter-defibrillator use in patients with heart failure: data from the GTWG-HF (Get With The Guidelines-Heart Failure) Registry. J Am Coll Cardiol 2009;53:416–22.

32. Saksena S. The leadless defibrillator or the return of the subcutaneous electrode: episode III in the ICD saga? J Interv Card Electrophysiol 2005;13:179–80.

33. Peinado R, Almendral J, Rius T, et al. Randomized, prospective comparison of four burst pacing algorithms for spontaneous ventricular tachycardia. Am J Cardiol 1998;82:1422–5.

34. Wathen MS, DeGroot PJ, Sweeney MO, et al. Prospective randomized trial of empirical antitachycardic pacing versus shocks for spontaneous rapid ventricular tachycardia in patients with implantable cardioverter defibrillators. Pacing Fast VT Reduces Shock Therapies (PainFREE Rx II) Trial Results. Circulation 2004;110:2592–6.

35. Pratt TR, Pulling CC, Stanton MS. Prospective post-market device studies versus returned product analysis as a predictor of system survival. Pacing Clin Electrophysiol 2000;23:1150–5.

Inappropriate Implantable Cardioverter-Defibrillator Therapy

Sivakumar Ardhanari, MD, Ashok J. Shah, MD, Nitesh Gadeela, MD, Ranjan K. Thakur, MD, MPH, FHRS*

KEYWORDS
- Inappropriate shock • Antitachycardia therapy
- Implantable cardioverter-defibrillator
- Ventricular arrhythmia • Atrial arrhythmia
- Sinus tachycardia • Supraventricular tachycardia discrimination • Proarrhythmia • Oversensing

Mortality benefit of the implantable cardioverter-defibrillator (ICD) in patients at risk of sudden cardiac death (SCD) is well established.[1–7] Since the first human implant of the ICD in 1980 and its subsequent approval by the US Food and Drug Administration (FDA) in 1985, the ICD has evolved rapidly and gained widespread patient acceptance.[8] Initially, the ICD was implanted exclusively for secondary prevention of SCD. Accumulating evidence of mortality benefit with ICD use for primary prevention has extended its use to patients who are at risk of SCD without any prior history of sustained ventricular arrhythmias or sudden death. Presently, primary prevention of SCD is the most common indication for ICD implantation worldwide. This has been driven by clinical trials demonstrating survival benefit in wider patient populations, significant technological advances, and patient acceptance. ICD implants have increased almost tenfold over a decade: 29,000 in 1997 to 260,000 in 2008.[9–11] Implants in the United States account for almost 70% of all ICD implants worldwide. Growing numbers of ICD implants combined with younger recipients and increasing life expectancy of these patients have led to an increasing prevalence of patients living with ICDs. This has brought new challenges in the management of ICD patients.

From its introduction as a bulky and primitive device, the ICD has evolved to a compact and complex multiprogrammable device capable of delivering tiered therapy (antitachycardia pacing (ATP), low- and high-energy shocks), back-up bradycardia pacing, and data storage. Although the ICD serves its purpose of preventing arrhythmic SCD caused by ventricular tachycardia (VT) or ventricular fibrillation (VF), a stage of perfection has not yet been reached, and this quest likely never will be attained. Inappropriate ICD therapy (IT) may be defined as an unintended ICD intervention (ATP or shock) for which the device was not designed or programmed. Inappropriate therapy remains a common occurrence and a significant detractor of this life-saving treatment. The most common causes of IT are atrial arrhythmias (**Figs. 1** and **2**).

ICD shocks reduce the quality of life (QoL), increase rehospitalization rates, and if frequent, may reduce the battery life of the ICD generator. Older-generation ICDs only had the ability to deliver a shock. Shocks are effective but painful, and among the ICD recipients, patients who receive shocks suffer more anxiety and depression and a (QoL) than ICD recipients who do not experience any shocks.[12] The mortality in patients with inappropriate ICD therapies, however, is

Arrhythmia Services, Thoracic and Cardiovascular Institute, Sparrow Health System, Michigan State University, Lansing, MI 48910, USA

* Corresponding author. Thoracic and Cardiovascular Institute, 405 West Greenlawn, Suite 400, Lansing, MI 48910.
E-mail address: thakur@msu.edu (R.K. Thakur).

Card Electrophysiol Clin 1 (2009) 155–171
doi:10.1016/j.ccep.2009.08.002
1877-9182/09/$ – see front matter © 2009 Published by Elsevier Inc.

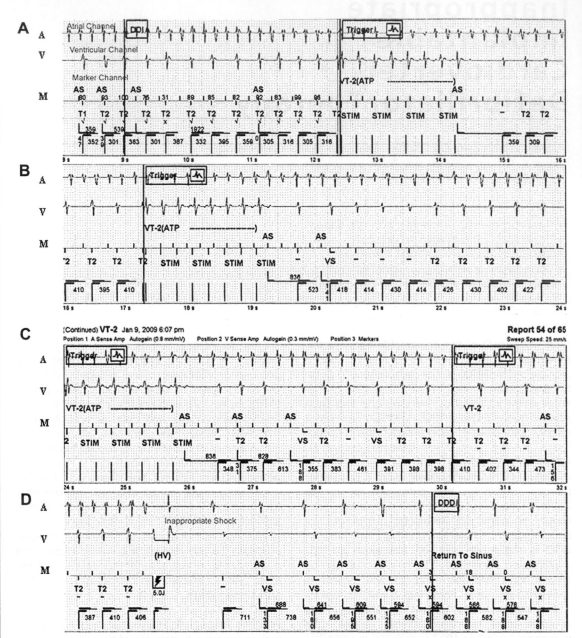

Fig. 1. Stored intracardiac electrograms during an episode of atrial arrhythmia with fast ventricular rates inappropriately diagnosed and treated as ventricular tachycardia (VT). Panels *A, B, C,* and *D* represent continuous electrograms. Panel *A* shows fast atrial rhythm leading to mode switch (DDI). Ventricular channel shows irregular V-V intervals at high rates binned in VT-2 zone leading to inappropriate diagnosis of VT. It ensues into inappropriate delivery of programmed therapy with adenosine triphosphate (ATP). Understandably, ATP was unsuccessful in terminating fast ventricular rates. Device continues to diagnose it as persistent VT in VT-2 zone and inappropriately delivers two more unsuccessful therapies with ATP followed by an inappropriate high voltage 5 J shock as shown in panels *B, C,* and *D.* Though inappropriate, shock therapy converts atrial arrhythmia to sinus rhythm, leading to restoration of DDD pacing mode after satisfying the exit count (*top channel*: bipolar atrial EGM; *middle channel*: bipolar ventricular EGM; *bottom channel*: marker channel with interval windows). *Abbreviations:* A, atrial channel; AS, atrial sensed event; ATP, antitachycardia pacing; DDD, atrioventricular synchronous pacing mode; DDI, nontracking mode; HV, high voltage shock delivery; M, marker channel; STIM, ventricular stimulation during antitachycardia pacing; T2, ventricular sensed event binned in VT-2 zone; V, ventricular channel; VERSUS, ventricular sensed event; VT-2, ventricular tachycardia zone 2; √, template match with %; X, template nonmatch with %. Numbers below the marker channels represent A-A, V-V, and A-V intervals.

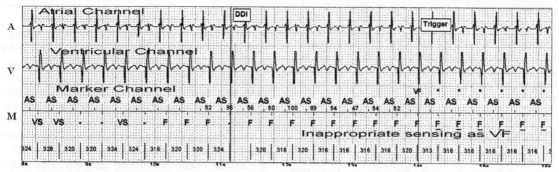

Fig. 2. Stored intracardiac electrograms during an episode of supraventricular tachycardia (SVT) at greater than or equal to 185 beats per minute with 1:1 atrioventricular (AV) conduction inappropriately diagnosed as ventricular fibrillation (VF). High atrial rates during SVT satisfy the entry count for atrial mode switch to DDI. Latter part of the figure shows therapy being triggered off and ongoing confirmation of the inappropriately diagnosed VF simultaneously with accumulation of charge (*) on the capacitors (*top channel*: bipolar atrial EGM; *middle channel*: bipolar ventricular EGM; *bottom channel*: marker channel with interval windows). *Abbreviations:* A, atrial channel; AS, atrial sensed event; DDI, nontracking mode; F, ventricular sensed event binned in the VF zone; F̲, ongoing confirmation of the diagnosed event as VF; M, marker channel; V, ventricular channel; R̲, ongoing confirmation of the diagnosed event as VF; VERSUS, ventricular sensed event; *, process of charge accumulating on the capacitors before high-voltage therapy; X, template nonmatch with %; numbers below the marker channels represent V-V intervals. Panels A and B show stored intracardiac electrograms during an episode of irregular fast supraventricular tachycardia (SVT) with 1:1 AV conduction inappropriately diagnosed as VF. Some of the fast and irregular ventricular sensed events occurred at sufficiently close intervals to be binned in the VF zone. As the entry criteria satisfied the programmed parameters for diagnosis of VF, the device triggered off the therapy and performed confirmation of the inappropriately diagnosed VF simultaneously with accumulation of charge (*) on the capacitors. Delivery of high-voltage therapy for inappropriate diagnosis of VF did not change the underlying rhythm, which is seen to persist in the latter half of panel B. SVT discriminators were disabled, because arrhythmia was detected in the VF zone. Process of charge accumulating on the capacitors before high-voltage therapy, √, template match with %. Numbers below the marker channels represent A-A, A-V & V-V intervals.

similar to that among patients without inappropriate therapies.[13] Evidence also suggests that the emotional stress and depression associated with ICD shocks can by itself trigger potential arrhythmias requiring ICD therapies, establishing a vicious cycle.[14–16] The secondary heightened sympathetic overactivity can trigger heart failure or ventricular arrhythmias that may complicate management issues further. This is especially true for ICD recipients for secondary prevention because of their greater likelihood of receiving ICD therapies compared with ICD recipients for primary prevention. In ICD recipients for primary prevention, the proportionately higher incidence of inappropriate-to-appropriate shocks may worsen the risk–benefit ratio.

There has been a continuous and constant effort to minimize ICD shocks. In 1970, Wellens recognized ATP as a painless means of terminating monomorphic VT.[17] In the late 1970s, ATP was used in pacemaker recipients with VT.[18] But the potential for the ATP to accelerate VT into VF made the treatment of VT by standalone antitachycardia pacemakers too risky. The later introduction of low-energy cardioversion also fell out of favor for the same reasons.[19] The introduction of high-energy

cardioversion has led to the inclusion of ATP in commercially available ICDs since 1993.[20] The introduction of ATP brought in a new concept of tiered ICD therapy aimed at reducing ICD shocks.

The pacing reduces shocks for fast ventricular tachycardia II (PainFREE Rx II) trial II showed the success rate of ATP in terminating a fast and slow VT to be 81% and greater than 90% respectively. There was also a substantial (70%) reduction in the number of shock episodes and a significant improvement in QoL as compared with the ICD recipients who received shocks.[13] Although appropriate ATP is effective in terminating VT and avoiding painful shocks, it can result in acceleration of well-tolerated VT into VF; this is more likely to occur in faster VT with more variable cycle length. Other studies also confirmed this result, with success rates of termination of spontaneous VT occurring in 63% to 94% of episodes with ATP. Acceleration to faster VT and degeneration into VF occurred in 17% and 21% of patients, respectively, in the ATP group. Neither the efficacy of ATP nor the acceleration of VT showed any statistical significance when compared with the low-energy cardioversion group.[21–23] Inappropriate ATP can be proarrhythmic, inducing ventricular arrhythmias that may require a shock.[24–26] Although rarely fatal, this is associated with significant morbidity.[27] The proarrhythmic potential of the ICD, however, can be minimized by optimizing the electrical therapy prescription, because suboptimal programming contributes to this complication as much as the technological limitations of the ICD.

ETIOLOGY OF INAPPROPRIATE THERAPY

Detection of a rapid ventricular rate (actual or apparent) is a prerequisite for delivery of any ICD therapy. IT results from inappropriate sensing of any stimulus other than a rapid ventricular arrhythmia. This can be a consequence of actual rapid ventricular rate conducted from a supraventricular rhythm or apparent sensing of rapid ventricular activity caused by overcounting of non-ventricular signals due to oversensing of T-waves, electromagnetic interference (EMI), myopotentials, or lead-related sensing problems (**Figs. 3–6**). **Box 1** offers a classification for the reasons for inappropriate therapies.

RISK FACTORS

History of prior atrial arrhythmias, AV nodal conduction, antiarryhthmic medications that influence AV nodal conduction or the occurrence of atrial arrhythmias, and device programming for therapy and detection of arrhythmia can influence the occurrence of IT. Risk factors include age greater than or equal to 70 years, ejection fraction (EF) less than or equal to 0.35, New York Heart Association (NYHA) class greater than 2, preoperatively documented AF, a maximum heart rate during exercise close to the detection interval, and a low detection rate.[2,28]

INCIDENCE

On review of the literature on IT, approximately 20 studies were published between 1986 and 2008, and the incidence of inappropriate ICD therapies varied between 11% and 66% (**Table 1**).[13,28–54] In 1989, Fogoros and colleagues published the first report of actuarial incidence of appropriate and inappropriate ICD therapies in 43% to 81% and 15% to 21% of patients, respectively, during

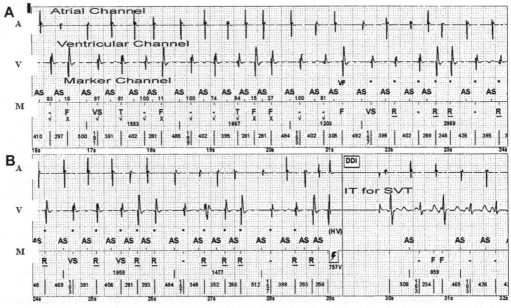

Fig. 3. Panels *A* and *B* show stored intracardiac electrograms during an episode of irregular fast supraventricular tachycardia (SVT) with 1:1 AV conduction inappropriately diagnosed as ventricular fibrillation (VF). Some of the fast and irregular ventricular sensed events occurred at sufficiently close intervals to be binned in the VF zone. As the entry criteria satisfied the programmed parameters for diagnosis of VF, the device triggered off the therapy and performed confirmation of the inappropriately diagnosed VF simultaneously with accumulation of charge (*) on the capacitors. Delivery of high-voltage therapy for inappropriate diagnosis of VF did not change the underlying rhythm, which is seen to persist in the latter half of panel *B*. SVT discriminators were disabled, because arrhythmia was detected in the VF zone (*top channel*: bipolar atrial EGM; *middle channel*: bipolar ventricular EGM; *bottom channel*: marker channel with interval windows). *Abbreviations:* A, atrial channel; AS, atrial sensed event; DDI, nontracking mode; F, ventricular sensed event binned in the VF zone; M, marker channel; R, ongoing confirmation of the diagnosed event as VF; V, ventricular channel; VERSUS, ventricular sensed event; X, template nonmatch with %; *, process of charge accumulating on the capacitors before high voltage therapy; √, template match with %. Numbers below the marker channels represent A-A, A-V & V-V intervals.

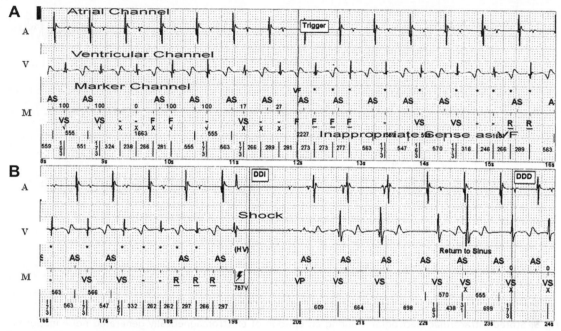

Fig. 4. Panels *A* and *B* show stored intracardiac electrograms during an episode of intermittent T-wave oversensing, which led to inappropriate diagnosis of ventricular fibrillation (VF). During 1:1 A-V rhythm, two ventricular events get sensed intermittently for one event on the atrial channel. This is caused by oversensing of T-waves, which bins such events into the VF zone. On meeting the entry criteria, therapy is triggered off, and confirmation of the inappropriately diagnosed VF simultaneously occurs with accumulation of charge (*) on the capacitors, leading to delivery of high-voltage therapy (panel B). SVT discriminators were disabled, because arrhythmia was detected in the VF zone (*top channel*: bipolar atrial EGM; *middle channel*: bipolar ventricular EGM; *bottom channel*: marker channel with interval windows). *Abbreviations:* A, atrial channel; AS, atrial sensed event; DDD, atrioventricular synchronous pacing mode; DDI, non tracking mode; F, ventricular sensed event binned in the VF zone; M, marker channel; R, ongoing confirmation of the diagnosed event as VF; V, ventricular channel; VERSUS, ventricular sensed event; X, template nonmatch with %. *, process of charge accumulating on the capacitors before high voltage therapy; √, template match with %. Numbers below the marker channels represent V-V intervals.

a follow-up of over 4 years.[32] In recent reports, incidence of appropriate defibrillator therapies was found to be 46% and 24% of patients included in antiarrhythmics versus implantable defibrillators (AVID) and multicenter automatic defibrillator implantation trial (MADIT) trials respectively. Irrespective of the indication for an ICD, approximately one third of the therapies were reported to be inappropriate in PainFREE Rx II trial.[13]

But the estimation of the incidence of IT and conclusions about its incidence based on these studies are not without limitations. First, the primary indication for the ICD implant in the earlier studies was secondary prevention of SCD, whereas presently, the most common indication for the ICD is primary prevention. Second, the earlier studies measured only the inappropriate shocks, whereas the studies done later analyzed both the shocks and ATPs. Third, the incidence of IT was reported as percentage of patients who suffered IT and a proportionate number of patients who suffer IT as compared with appropriate therapy. With

follow-up duration ranging from 1 year to 4 years among the studies, there is no standardization for the follow-up for comparison. Fourth, before introduction of third-generation ICDs with capabilities to store electrograms, the therapies were classified unreliably as inappropriate based on severity of the patient's symptoms and if available, surface electrocardiogram, telemetry, or Holter. However, symptoms do not correlate well with the arrhythmia diagnosis.[55] Finally, none of the studies reported so far was done prospectively, to reliably estimate the incidence of IT.

Patients with Brugada syndrome (BS) and hypertrophic cardiomyopathy (HCM) deserve special mention, because these patients are younger and may be exposed to the potential complications of ICD for decades.

BS is an inherited arrhythmic syndrome with potential high risk for SCD in some patients. An ICD is the recommended therapy in patients with high-risk clinical features. Investigators, however, have reported a high incidence of IT in BS patients

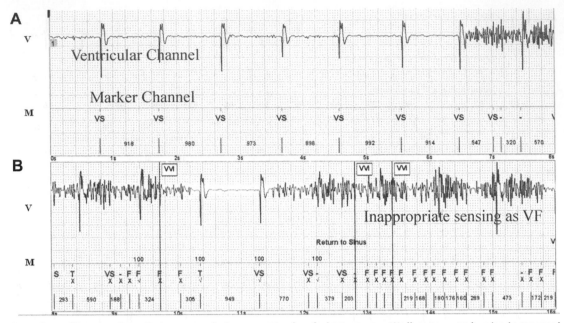

Fig. 5. Stored intracardiac electrograms during an episode of electromagnetically generated noise inappropriately diagnosed as ventricular fibrillation (VF) in a person with single chamber device while operating a weed whacker. High-frequency noise sensed as ventricular event in the fibrillation zone is evident on the ventricular channel in panel *B* (*top channel*: bipolar ventricular EGM; *bottom channel*: marker channel with interval windows). *Abbreviations:* F, ventricular sensed event binned in the VF zone; F̲, ongoing confirmation of the diagnosed event as VF; M, marker channel; T, ventricular sensed event binned in VT zone; V, ventricular channel; VERSUS, ventricular sensed event; VVI, ventricular inhibited pacing. *, process of charge accumulating on the capacitors before high-voltage therapy. Numbers below the marker channels represent V-V intervals.

with ICD.[37,38] This is because of the active younger population in this group who can have their sinus rates accelerated more than the cut-off rates for the detection of VT. Also, they are prone to atrial arrhythmias that are more common in patients with BS. The worsening pattern on sinus tachycardia (ST) elevation with beta-blockers has led to underusage of the drug in these patients, making ventricular rate control a difficult task. The only feasible way to reduce IT in these patients is to reprogram the device for a higher rate cutoff for delivery of therapy. In another study by Sachar and colleagues,[53] lead failure was the most common cause of IT, occurring in almost half of the patients with IT. A major finding from that study was that inappropriate shocks were 2.5 times more frequent than the appropriate ones. They also concluded that a history of SVT and T-wave oversensing were among the predictors of inappropriate shock.

Other special patients are those who receive ICD for HCM. Incidence of IT as reported in studies ranged between 20% and 33%.[54,56–58] IT rates are higher when compared with non-HCM patients. IT, however, occurs in 50% of non-HCM children and adolescents who receive ICDs, and this rate is comparable to the patients with HCM who receive ICD.[42] Determinants of IT in this group of patients include younger age at implantation and pre-existing AF.

PATHOPHYSIOLOGY OF IT

The detection of arrhythmia by an ICD, in general, requires the heart rate exceeding a programmed rate cutoff as the defining criteria. Other parameters, such as sustained heart rate duration, QRS duration or morphology, also may be available as additional discriminators. Any ventricular rate above this cutoff rate will be recognized as arrhythmia, and the ICD will deliver the therapy as programmed. Although the cutoff rates are programmed to avoid delivering therapies for conducted supraventricular rhythms, some episodes of ST, AF and atrial flutter exceed these cutoff rates and results in IT. Because of the tendency of the rates of the ventricular and the supraventricular rhythms to overlap, it is difficult to predict an ideal cutoff value, either generally or in an individual patient. In addition, inappropriate detection of high ventricular rates can occur with oversensing of T-waves, leading to double counting, lead-related problems, and EMI. Various strategies have evolved through pharmacologic approaches

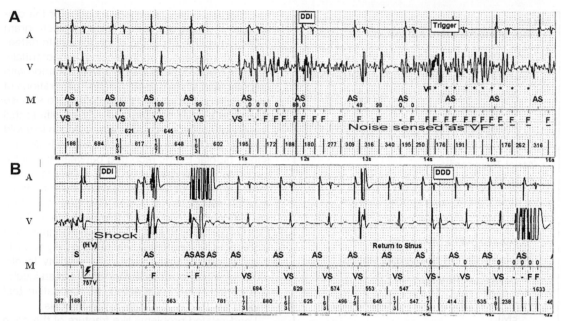

Fig. 6. Stored intracardiac electrograms during an episode of electromagnetically generated noise inappropriately diagnosed as ventricular fibrillation (VF). High-frequency noise sensed as ventricular event in the fibrillation zone is evident on the ventricular channel in panel A. As therapy is being triggered off, confirmation of the inappropriately diagnosed VF simultaneously occurs with accumulation of charge (*) on the capacitors, leading to delivery of high-voltage therapy (panel B). Because it was not fibrillation but noise, the latter continues to intermittently occur on both the channels after high-voltage therapy (*top channel*: bipolar atrial EGM; *middle channel*: bipolar ventricular EGM; *bottom channel*: marker channel with interval windows). *Abbreviations:* A, atrial channel; AS, atrial sensed event; DDD, atrioventricular synchronous pacing mode; DDI, nontracking mode; F, ventricular sensed event binned in the VF zone; F̲, ongoing confirmation of the diagnosed event as VF; M, marker channel; V, ventricular channel; VERSUS, ventricular sensed event. *, process of charge accumulating on the capacitors before high-voltage therapy. Numbers below the marker channels represent V-V intervals.

and technological advances in ICD to overcome these problems.

DETECTION OF RAPID VENTRICULAR RATE
AF and Other Supraventricular Arrhythmias

AF is common in ICD recipients and may result in increased incidence and triggering of ventricular arrhythmias.[59,60] Dual tachycardia is defined as occurrence of ventricular arrhythmia during or preceded by AF or atrial tachycardia, and it is estimated to occur in approximately 9% of dual-chamber ICD recipients and at least once in 20% of ventricular event episodes.[61] This may be a direct effect of tachycardia-induced changes in ventricular refractoriness or indirectly caused by hemodynamic alterations, ischemia, or neurohumoral activation. Elevated left atrial pressures in ICD recipients with heart failure (HF) are also risk factors for increased incidence of atrial arrhythmias. The inhomogeneous repolarization secondary to the irregular ventricular excitation in AF and proarrhythmic potential of short-long-short ventricular excitation sequence explains the association of AF in

patients with HF.[62] The incidence of AF in symptomatic HF patients is reported to be as high as 40%.[63] Also, 25% of patients with AF suffer HF. AF begets not only AF but also HF, perpetuating AF burden. Inherited arrhythmic syndromes like BS and long QT syndrome have been shown to be a common link between ventricular events and AF. The presence of AF in patients with HF predisposes them to increased hospitalization rates and mortality, but it does not seem to reduce the efficacy of ICD. AF with intact AV conduction, however, can result in faster ventricular rates that predispose the patient to IT, and it remains the most common reason for IT.

Oversensing of Ventricular Activity

T-wave oversensing, P-wave oversensing, EMI, myopotential oversensing, oversensing caused by sensing lead dysfunction, and double QRS detection result in overcounting of ventricular sensed events.[64,65] Ventricular oversensing occurs in up to 25% of patients with dual-chamber ICDs[66] and results in inappropriate shocks in 2.3% to 3.9% of the ICD population.[67,68]

Box 1
Etiology of inappropriate ICD therapy

Actual detection of rapid ventricular rate

    Re-entrant Supraventricular Tachycardia (SVT)

        Atrioventricular (AV) nodal re-entry tachycardia

        Accessory pathway-mediated tachycardias

    Atrial Fibrillation (AF) and Atrial Flutter

    Atrial Tachycardia

    Sinus Tachycardia

False detection of rapid ventricular rate

    Overdetection of Non-QRS Cardiac Signals

        T-wave oversensing

    Overdetection of Noncardiac Signals

        Device malfunction

        Lead fracture

        EMI

        Oversensing of myopotentials

Reconfirmation error due to premature ventricular complexes (PVC)

T-wave oversensing occurs when the amplitude of the T-wave exceeds the threshold for the detection of the R-wave (see **Fig. 5**). It may occur when the R-waves are small in amplitude (arrhythmogenic right ventricular (RV) dysplasia or sarcoidosis), when the T-waves are abnormally tall (electrolyte abnormalities, drugs, and short QT syndrome), or when there is a long distance between the R-wave and the T-wave (long QT syndrome).[69] When it occurs because of low R-wave amplitude, the low amplitude may be persistent or transient. If the R-wave amplitude is persistently low (below 5 mV), it requires lead revision, either revising the defibrillator lead, or implanting an additional sensing lead.[70] Automatic adjustment of the sensitivity threshold, a programmable time delay before the decay in ventricular sensitivity, and the possibility of customizing the initial value of ventricular sensitivity as a percentage of the R-wave amplitude may prevent T-wave oversensing and IT.

P-wave oversensing is a ventricular sensing problem affecting function of 11% of dual-chamber devices with integrated bipolar lead systems, and this type of lead is significantly more susceptible to T-wave and P-wave oversensing than dedicated bipolar leads. Patients with cardiomyopathies may be more prone to oversensing than patients with other heart diseases.[66]

Myopotentials are high-frequency, low-amplitude electrical signals generated by skeletal muscles, including intercostal muscles or the diaphragm.[71] These appear as noise on electrogram (EGM). Inhibition of pacing or inappropriate detection of VF may ensue upon sensing myopotentials. Sensing myopotentials was relatively common with unipolar lead system used in earlier generations of pacemakers. Pacemakers and defibrillators these days use bipolar sensing and rely on differential amplification and common mode rejection to avoid sensing pectoral myopotentials. Some ICDs use shock bipolar EGMs recorded between the pulse generator and a proximal or distal coil as a template to discriminate between supraventricular rhythms and VT. Myopotential noise generated in or near the ICD pocket can distort this template and has been reported to interfere with such discrimination algorithms. Myopotential oversensing may occur in case of programming maximal sensitivity levels, although in most cases it is indicative of an insulation defect. When suspected, a provocative test should be used to stimulate myopotentials.

Lead-related problems like fracture of the pace sense conductor and coil and the high-voltage conductor can manifest as inappropriate shocks caused by oversensing and high impedance. In a study by Daoud and colleagues,[72] defective leads were found in 1.7% of total implanted leads. In a head-to-head comparison between small- and large-diameter leads, small-diameter, high-voltage leads were 10 times more prone to early failure. These leads were associated with incidence of inappropriate therapies in 33% of patients.[73] Activation of available alert features triggered when the lead impedance value is out of a programmable range can avoid IT. Ventricular oversensing, however, may be an early sign of lead dysfunction, preceding lead fracture and a rise in impedance values. In these cases, IT is the first clue to lead malfunction, and its occurrence cannot be prevented by the activation of alert features.

EMI is an important cause of pacemaker or ICD malfunction that can falsely activate or inhibit the devices, leading to complications (see **Figs. 3** and **6**). In a study of 341 ICD recipients, an incidence of 0.75% per patient–year of follow-up was found, and the risk for receiving inappropriate shocks because of EMI was found to be less than 1% per patient–year.[74] Intermittent EMI can result in shock delivery even in noncommitted devices. Improvement of EMI detection algorithms and advances in lead technology may minimize this risk further. Newer-generation devices with hermetic shielding in metal cases, filtering, interference rejection circuits, and bipolar sensing leads have made the devices less susceptible to EMI.[75]

Double counting occurs in biventricular defibrillators because of simultaneous R-wave sensing in both the RV and left ventricular (LV) leads. Double counting can occur under the following circumstances: loss of tracking of ST above the upper rate (P waves buried in a relatively longer post ventricular atrial refractory period) and double counting caused by SVT and VT. If reprogramming does not help, repositioning of one of the ventricular leads, LV-only pacing, ablation of the AV junction, or other measures may be needed.[76,77]

PREVENTION OF RECURRENCES
Pharmacologic Approaches

Antiarrhythmic medications can reduce the frequency of ICD shock by reducing the tendency for sustained VT, by (**Box 2**) slowing of episodes of spontaneous VT, rendering it more amenable to ATP, and by suppressing atrial tachyarrhythmias that lead to IT or that can even trigger ventricular tachyarrhythmias.[61] Sotalol reduces the incidence of recurrent sustained ventricular tachyarrhythmias and lowers the risk of death or delivery of an ICD shock.[78] Azimilide has been found to reduce appropriate ICD therapies at all doses,[79,80] In the Optical Pharmacologic Therapy in Cardioverter Defibrillator Patients (OPTIC) study, amiodarone plus β-blocker was the most effective regimen at reducing ICD shocks when compared with β-blocker or sotalol alone.[81] Statins may have antiarrhythmic effects and may reduce the occurrence of ICD shocks.[82] Antiarrhythmic medications are associated with elevated defibrillation thresholds (DFTs), proarrhythmia, and noncardiac adverse effects. Perhaps the most important potential risk is the possibility of increasing the ventricular defibrillation threshold. Amiodarone can increase DFT, but this is unlikely in the cases of sotalol or azimilide, which have no effect or may even lower the DFT.[79,83,84] Proarrhythmia is particularly common with sotalol and is associated with a higher risk of torsades de pointes.[85] A reasonable approach would be to start with b-blockers in all patients with ICDs. In patients with recurrent ICD shocks, sotalol or amiodarone is a reasonable first option. Azimilide is not approved by the FDA. Drug therapy to prevent occurrence of atrial tachyarrhythmias in ICD recipients may be unsatisfactory because of its limited efficacy, ventricular proarrhythmia, drug–device interaction, and frequent inability to tolerate antiarrhythmic therapy because of adverse effects.[86–88]

Device Reprogramming

Newer-generation ICDs are capable of delivering tiered therapy with ATP, low- and high- energy shocks. This gives the physician the luxury to program the ICD to function optimally according to the patient's needs.

ATP and low-energy shocks are used in patients with ventricular arrhythmia of longer cycle lengths for the purpose of reducing painful shocks. This strategy, however, may misdirect the ICD to treat SVT. This occurs, because the lower rate cutoffs do not exclude SVTs based on heart rate alone. ATP may accelerate the ventricular rate, resulting in VT or VF, resulting in a painful shock.[24,25] With lower rate cutoff, the overlap of rates between longer cycle length VT and SVT reduces the effectiveness of rate criterion to reliably distinguish SVT from ventricular arrhythmia. Additional rhythm discriminators have been used to overcome this difficulty. These include sudden arrhythmia onset, rate stability or regularity, sustained rate duration, probability density function, atrial sensing, and sensing of electrogram configuration and vector timing correlation (VTC).

The cycle lengths of inappropriately detected SVTs may be different between primary and secondary prevention patients, possibly related to mechanisms of SVT.[50] Additionally, some studies have reported that the cycle lengths of appropriately detected VT may be longer in secondary than in primary prevention patients and that the difference in cycle lengths between appropriately detected VT and inappropriately detected SVT may be greater in primary prevention patients.[50,89] One possible interpretation of these data is that rate-based programming to achieve the optimal balance between VT detection and SVT rejection is different between primary and secondary prevention patients. ICD programming must find a balance between reducing the probability of inappropriate therapies by eliminating a slow-VT detection zone with the risk of failing to treat unanticipated VT.[90]

INTERVAL-BASED DISCRIMINATORS (SINGLE-CHAMBER ICDs)

Sudden onset refers to the degree of prematurity of the initial beat of the tachycardia with respect to the previous ones. This may help to distinguish ST from VT, because ST starts gradually, unlike VT, which starts suddenly. But this criterion may provoke some discrimination errors, including VTs induced by ST, gradual acceleration of VT and ST, premature ventricular beats simulating a sudden onset, and regular atrial tachycardia simulating a VT.[91]

Rate stability refers to the degree of regularity of the arrhythmia.[92] Stability window and stability duration are the two criteria used in the stability algorithms. The former is defined as the preprogrammed acceptable deviation (plus or minus milliseconds) from the mean cycle length of the

Table 1
Incidence of inappropriate therapy

Study	Type	Study Year	Published in	Journal	Ind	Total	Therapy	Num IT	Incidence	MC Reason	Inc AT	Mean Follow-up	F/U
Francis et al			1986	Ann Intern Med 1986;104:481–488	S	26	Shocks	4/6	66	AF/ST	N/A	13 ± 6 mo	Holter
Gabry et al		1982–1986	1987	JACC 1987;9:1349–56	S	22	Shocks	9	41	AF/ST	50	19.6 mo	
Kelly et al		1983–1987	1988	JACC 1988;11:1278–86	S	90	Shocks	17	19	AF	52	17 ± 10 mo	
Fogoros et al			1989	PACE 1989;12:1465–73	S	65	Shocks	25	21	AF	64	25 ± 21 mo	
Maloney et al		1984–1988	1991	PACE 1991 Vol. 14, Feb, Pt2	N/A	105	Shocks	12	13	SVT	44	13 ± 8 mo	
Fromer et al	CT	1989–1991	1992	CIRC 1992;86;363–374	S	102	B	10	9	AF	43	9.4 ± 5.8 mo	
Grimm et al		1983–1991	1992	PACE 1992;15:1667–73	S	241	Shocks	54	22	AF	N/A	24 ± 20 mo	
Schmitt et al			1994	PACE, Vol. 17, March 1994, Part I	S		B	14	16	AF		17 ± 9 mo	
Nunain et al			1995	CIRC 1995;91:2204–13	S	154	Shocks	32	26	AF/ST	55	15.3 ± 9.7 mo	
Weber et al			1996	Z CARDIOL 1996;85(11):809–19	N/A	462	Shocks	82	18	AF	N/A	15 ± 13 mo	
Rosenquist et al	P	1993–1994	1998	CIRC 1998;98:663–670	S	778	B	111	14	N/A	N/A	4 ± 4.6 mo	
Grimm et al		1992–1998	1999	PACE 1999;22:206–11	B[a]	144	Shocks	16	16	SVT	N/A	21 ± 15 mo	
Gradaus et al (EURID reg)		1998–2000	2003	PACE 2003;26:1511–18	S 68%; P 32%	3344	Both	23	16.2		40	12.4 ± 2 mo	
Klein et al (AVID trial)		1993–1997	2003	JCE 2003;14:940–48	S	449	Both	106	22	AF	64		
Wilkoff et al (MIRACLE ICD)	R	1999–2002	2004	JCE 2004;15:1002–1009	B	978	Both	289	30	AF/ST			

Study	Design	Years	Year	Reference	Type	n	Therapy	Num IT	Inc AT	Indication	IT	F/U
Rinaldi et al		1984–2001	2004	Heart 2004;90:330–331	Bᵃ	155	Both	22	14	AF/Afl	N/A	N/A
Korte et al		1990–1999	2004	PACE 2004;27:924–932	S	20	Both	10	50	SVT	75	51 ± 31 mo
Alter et al		1994–2004	2005	PACE 2005;28:926–32	S 66%; P 34%	440	Both	54	12	SVT	N/A	46 ± 37 mo
Sweeney et al (Painfree trial)	R		2005	CIRC 2005;111:2898–2905	B	582	Both	89	15	SVT	22	11 ± 3 mo
Chen et al	R	2000–2005	2006	CHINESE MED J 2006;119(7):557–563	S	50	Both	11	22	AF	N/A	N/A
Dwarakraj et al	R	N/A	2006	PACE 2006;29:810–815	B	386	Both	71	18	ST/AF	49	N/A
Sachar et al	R	1993–2005	2006	CIRC 2006;114:2317–2324	B (Brugada)	220	Shocks	45	20	Lead failure	8	38 ± 27 mo
Anselme et al	MA	1997–2003	2007	PACE 2007;30:S128–S133	Bᵃ	802	Both	117	15	ST	27	302 ± 113d
Stuber et al	O	1995–2002	2007	SWEDISH MED WKLY 2007;137:228–233	B	214	Both	58	27	AF/Afl	N/A	2.7 y
Sarkozy et al	R	1996–2004	2007	Eur HJ 2007;28,334–344	P (Brugada)	47	Shocks	17	36	ST	15	47.5 mo
Maron et al	R	1986–2003	2007	JAMA 2007;298(4):405–412	B (HOCM)	506	Shocks	136	27	N/A	20	3.7 y
Daubert et al (MADIT II)			2008	JACC 2008;51:1357–65		719	Shocks	83	11.5	AF	23	
Almendral et al (DATAS)	CT	2000–2003	2008	Europace 2008;10:528–535	B	334	Shocks	23	7	AF	7	16 mo

Few patients received ICDs for primary prevention.

ᵃ Small percentage of primary prevention patients.

Abbreviations: AF, atrial fibrillation; B, both primary and secondary prevention; CT, controlled trial; DATAS, Dual Chamber and Atrial Tachyarrhythmias Adverse Events Study; F/U, follow-up; ICD, implantable cardioverter-defibrillator; Inc AT, incidence (percentage) of appropriate therapy; Ind, indication; IT, inappropriate ICD therapy; MA, meta-analysis; N/A, not available; Num IT, number of IT; O, observational; P, primary prevention; R, retrospective; S, secondary prevention; ST, sinus tachycardia; SVT, supraventricular tachycardia.

Box 2
Strategies to prevent recurrences of inappropriate therapy

Pharmacologic therapy
Device-based
    Interval-Based
        Onset
        Stability
        Sustained rate duration
    Morphology-Based Discrimination
        Probability density function
        EGM width discriminator
        Vector timing and correlation
        Wavelet transform algorithm
    AV Association

last few intervals, and the latter is defined as the preprogrammed number of intervals the ICD will evaluate the stability of the arrhythmia.[93] Pseudoregularization of the ventricular rate in patients with AF with rapid response can satisfy these criteria and decrease the diagnostic accuracy of the algorithm.[94,95] There is also a possibility for underdetection of VT that may be irregular, as in polymorphic VT, ischemic VTs with dynamic changes in the re-entrant circuit, and also some cases of monomorphic VT that may be irregular.[96]

ST is gradual in onset and regular, contrary to AF, which is sudden and irregular. The capacity of the ICD to recognize sudden onset and regularity may improve detection specificity.[94,97] There may be a potential risk of underdetection of life-threatening VT, however, and this had led to the underuse of these parameters.[98] To address this concern, another criterion was established, the sustained rate duration, which is the amount of time the device would wait to eventually deliver the rate-criterion-based therapy even if the onset and stability criteria are not met. Use of these parameters has been shown to reduce the incidence of IT because of decreases in misidentification of AF as VT.[99]

Detection enhancements have to be prescribed cautiously and have to be individualized. The stability criterion is useful for discrimination of AF, the most common cause of IT. These enhancements should be avoided in patients with hemodynamically unstable VT, and short detection times should be used to ensure rapid therapy delivery. Reprogramming for IT because of supraventricular arrhythmia should include onset, stability, sustained rate duration, and medical treatment to control AV nodal conduction

time.[99] Because sensitivity is not 100% in detecting VTs, these detection criteria only can be programmed if a security backup mechanism such as sustained rate duration is available.[92] In an analysis of various algorithms, sudden onset greater than 9% and stability less than 40 milliseconds were found to have the greatest specificity and sensitivity, and application of sustained rate duration criteria increased the sensitivity to detect VT episodes to 100%.[100]

MORPHOLOGY-BASED DISCRIMINATORS

Probability density function and the EGM width algorithm were the early morphology discriminators used in the ICD.[101,102] The EGM width algorithm measures the time span of the ventricular depolarization in the intracardiac electrogram as the only feature to discriminate between atrial and ventricular tachyarrhythmias, achieving a sensitivity of 64%.[103] This algorithm has limited utility:

> In a patient with an intrinsic wide QRS complex
> If the patients develops a rate-dependent bundle branch block
> If there are changes in QRS duration caused by antiarrhythmic drug therapy or electrolyte disturbance

As a single parameter, this algorithm has an unacceptably low sensitivity.

Later, morphology-based algorithms used the changes in the ventricular electrogram during VT compared with supraventricular baseline rhythm. This algorithm constructs a quantitative representation of each ventricular complex determined by the peak amplitudes, polarities, number of peaks, and order of peaks. After alignment of the tachycardia and stored template complex, differences in surface areas are calculated. These differences are translated into a similarity score, which represents the percent template match score.[104] As a single function, morphology discrimination algorithm also is not sufficient for reliable discrimination of VT from a supraventricular rhythm.

Recently, more advanced morphology algorithms, based on more complex comparisons, have been implemented. The vector timing and correlation (VTC) algorithm uses two vectors of electrical activity: a bipolar signal from the right ventricular pace/sense lead and a far-field signal constructed between the defibrillation coils and pulse generator. Morphology discrimination with this algorithm is based on the measurement of voltage differences over time. In an initial study, the VTC algorithm demonstrated 99% sensitivity for induced VTs. In the same study, the combination of this algorithm with interval-based discriminators achieved a sensitivity of 100%.[105] In case of a dual-chamber ICD implantation, the VTC algorithm was incorporated into the atrial and ventricular rate comparison and its stability above AF threshold. VTC algorithm showed high sensitivity and specificity for discriminating between ventricular and supraventricular arrhythmias, with sensitivity of 100% in patients with dual-chamber ICDs.[106]

Another morphology-based algorithm, the wavelet transform algorithm, uses a far-field electrogram source constructed between the distal defibrillation coil and the pulse generator. Morphology discrimination with this algorithm is based on comparison of electrogram morphology, with the stored baseline electrogram template constructed by a Harr wavelet transform. The wavelet transform algorithm demonstrated a sensitivity of 100% for VT detection.[107]

Morphology discrimination alone resulted in a limited sensitivity for detecting VT. The loss in sensitivity is compensated by combinations with interval-based discriminators in single-chamber devices and by rate branch analysis in dual-chamber devices. With these combinations, morphology discrimination can be activated with nominal values to achieve high sensitivity and specificity for arrhythmia discrimination.

AV RELATIONSHIP (DUAL-CHAMBER ICDs)

A dual-chamber ICD has the advantage of atrial sensing capabilities that enable correlation of atrial and ventricular electrical activity. A tachycardia with AV dissociation and ventricular rate exceeding the atrial rate will properly distinguish most VTs from SVTs. This criterion, however, will fail when there is a 1:1 relationship between the atrial and ventricular rates or in the case of dual tachycardias, such as the case of VT with concomitant AF. In these situations, ICDs may use sophisticated algorithms analyzing the relationship between sensed atrial and ventricular activity to diagnose the tachycardia.[108–110] Several randomized, prospective studies comparing single-chamber versus dual-chamber ICDs have shown no benefit of dual-chamber ICDs in reducing inappropriate shocks.[111–113] A larger randomized crossover study of 400 patients comparing single-chamber with dual-chamber ICD detection algorithms demonstrated a nearly 50% reduction in the rate of inappropriate detection when using a dual-chamber algorithm.[114] In another study by Theuns and colleagues,[115] there was a reduction of number of inappropriately treated episodes with dual-chamber ICD, but there was no decrease in the number of patients who were treated inappropriately.

SUMMARY

Although ICD therapy has improved greatly, problems remain. Inappropriate delivery of therapy is a big problem that impacts the QoL0 of ICD recipients. While is now a clear understanding that atrial arrhythmias are the main cause, physicians have not been very successful in preventing inappropriate therapy. Although many discriminators have been shown to be helpful, it is not clear that there is a particular combination that is ideal for all patients. Until such an algorithm is developed (which may not be possible), a detailed knowledge and use of all available programming options, guided by special characteristics of each unique patient, are the only paths available. Finally, one must face the prospect that this problem cannot be vanquished, but only ameliorated.

REFERENCES

1. The AVID Investigators. A comparison of antiarrhythmic drug therapy with implantable defibrillators in patients resuscitated from near-fatal ventricular arrhythmias. The Antiarrhythmics Versus Implantable Defibrillators (AVID) investigators. N Engl J Med 1997;337(22):1576–83.
2. Connolly SJ, Gent M, Roberts RS, et al. Canadian implantable defibrillator study (CIDS): a randomized trial of the implantable cardioverter defibrillator against amiodarone. Circulation 2000;101(11):1297–302.
3. Moss AJ, Hall WJ, Cannom DS, et al. Improved survival with an implanted defibrillator in patients with coronary disease at high risk for ventricular arrhythmia. N Engl J Med 1996;335(26):1933–40.
4. Moss AJ, Zareba W, Hall WJ, et al. Prophylactic implantation of a defibrillator in patients with myocardial infarction and reduced ejection fraction. N Engl J Med 2002;346(12):877–83.
5. Kadish A, Dyer A, Daubert JP, et al. Prophylactic defibrillator implantation in patients with nonischemic dilated cardiomyopathy. N Engl J Med 2004; 350(21):2151–8.
6. Buxton AE, Lee KL, Fisher JD, et al. A randomized study of the prevention of sudden death in patients with coronary artery disease. Multicenter Unsustained Tachycardia Trial Investigators. N Engl J Med 1999;341(25):1882–90.
7. Bardy GH, Lee KL, Mark DB, et al. Amiodarone or an implantable cardioverter-defibrillator for congestive heart failure. N Engl J Med 2005;352(3):225–37.
8. Mirowski M, Reid PR, Mower MM, et al. Termination of malignant ventricular arrhythmias with an implanted automatic defibrillator in human beings. N Engl J Med 1980;303(6):322–4.
9. Bernstein AD, Parsonnet V. Survey of cardiac pacing and implanted defibrillator practice

patterns in the United States in 1997. Pacing Clin Electrophysiol 2001;24(5):842–55.

10. Zhan C, Baine WB, Sedrakyan A, et al. Cardiac device implantation in the United States from 1997 through 2004: a population-based analysis. J Gen Intern Med 2008;23(Suppl 1):13–9.

11. Josephson ME, Callans DJ, Buxton AE. The role of the implantable cardioverter-defibrillator for prevention of sudden cardiac death. Ann Intern Med 2000;133(11):901–10.

12. Sears SF, Lewis TS, Kuhl EA, et al. Predictors of quality of life in patients with implantable cardioverter defibrillators. Psychosomatics 2005;46(5):451–7.

13. Sweeney MO, Wathen MS, Volosin K, et al. Appropriate and inappropriate ventricular therapies, quality of life, and mortality among primary and secondary prevention implantable cardioverter defibrillator patients: results from the Pacing Fast VT REduces Shock ThErapies (PainFREE Rx II) trial. Circulation 2005;111(22):2898–905.

14. Lampert R, Joska T, Burg MM, et al. Emotional and physical precipitants of ventricular arrhythmia. Circulation 2002;106(14):1800–5.

15. Whang W, Albert CM, Sears SF Jr, et al. Depression as a predictor for appropriate shocks among patients with implantable cardioverter-defibrillators: results from the Triggers Of Ventricular Arrhythmias (TOVA) study. J Am Coll Cardiol 2005;45(7):1090–5.

16. Dunbar SB. Psychosocial issues of patients with implantable cardioverter defibrillators. Am J Crit Care 2005;14(4):294–303.

17. Wellens HJJ. Electrical stimulation of the heart in the study and treatment of tachycardias. Baltimore (MD): University Park Press; 1971.

18. Lister JW. A new technology: patient-triggered pacemakers. Ann Intern Med 1978;88(1):120–1.

19. Miles WM, Prystowsky EN, Heger JJ, et al. The implantable transvenous cardioverter: long-term efficacy and reproducible induction of ventricular tachycardia. Circulation 1986;74(3):518–24.

20. Wathen M. Implantable cardioverter defibrillator shock reduction using new antitachycardia pacing therapies. Am Heart J 2007;153(Suppl 4):44–52.

21. Nasir N Jr, Pacifico A, Doyle TK, et al. Spontaneous ventricular tachycardia treated by antitachycardia pacing. Cadence investigators. Am J Cardiol 1997;79(6):820–2.

22. Brady GH, Poole JE, Kudenchuk PJ, et al. A prospective randomized repeat-crossover comparison of antitachycardia pacing with low-energy cardioversion. Circulation 1993;87(6):1889–96.

23. Ip JH, Winters SL, Schweitzer P, et al. Determinants of pace-terminable ventricular tachycardia: implications for implantable antitachycardia devices. Pacing Clin Electrophysiol 1991;14:1777–81.

24. Johnson NJ, Marchlinski FE. Arrhythmias induced by device antitachycardia therapy due to diagnostic nonspecificity. J Am Coll Cardiol 1991; 18(5):1418–25.

25. Pinski SL, Fahy GJ. The proarrhythmic potential of implantable cardioverter-defibrillators. Circulation 1995;92(6):1651–64.

26. Gottlieb C, Rosenthal M, Marchlinski FE. Initiation of a sustained ventricular arrhythmia resulting from R wave-synchronous AICD discharge. Am Heart J 1988;115(4):915–7.

27. Messali A, Thomas O, Chauvin M, et al. Death due to an implantable cardioverter defibrillator. J Cardiovasc Electrophysiol 2004;15(8):953–6.

28. Rosenquist M, Beyer T, Block M, et al. Adverse events with transvenous implantable cardioverter-defibrillators: a prospective multicenter study. European 7219 Jewel ICD investigators. Circulation 1998;98(7):663–70.

29. Marchlinski FE, Flores BT, Buxton AE, et al. The automatic implantable cardioverter-defibrillator: efficacy, complications, and device failures. Ann Intern Med 1986;104(4):481–8.

30. Gabry MD, Brodman R, Johnston D, et al. Automatic implantable cardioverter-defibrillator: patient survival, battery longevity, and shock delivery analysis. J Am Coll Cardiol 1987;9(6):1349–56.

31. Kelly PA, Cannom DS, Garan H, et al. The automatic implantable cardioverter-defibrillator: efficacy, complications and survival in patients with malignant ventricular arrhythmias. J Am Coll Cardiol 1988;11(6):1278–86.

32. Fogoros RN, Elson JJ, Bonnet CC. Actuarial incidence and pattern of occurrence of shocks following implantation of the automatic implantable cardioverter defibrillator. Pacing Clin Electrophysiol 1989;12(9):1465–73.

33. Maloney J, Masterson M, Khoury D, et al. Clinical performance of the implantable cardioverter defibrillator: electrocardiographic documentation of 101 spontaneous discharges. Pacing Clin Electrophysiol 1991;14:280–5.

34. Grimm W, Flores BF, Marchlinski FE. Electrocardiographically documented unnecessary, spontaneous shocks in 241 patients with implantable cardioverter defibrillators. Pacing Clin Electrophysiol 1992;15:1667–73.

35. Schmitt C, Montero M, Melichercik J. Significance of supraventricular tachyarrhythmias in patients with implanted pacing cardioverter defibrillators. Pacing Clin Electrophysiol 1994;17:295–302.

36. Nunain SO, Roelke M, Trouton T, et al. Limitations and late complications of third-generation automatic cardioverter-defibrillators. Circulation 1995; 91(8):2204–13.

37. Weber M, Block M, Brunn J, et al. Inadequate therapies with implantable cardioverter-defibrillators-incidence, etiology, predictive factors and preventive strategies. Z Kardiol 1996;85(11):809–19.

38. Grimm W, Menz V, Hoffman J, et al. Complications of third-generation implantable cardioverter defibrillator therapy. Pacing Clin Electrophysiol 1999;22:206–11.

39. Gradaus R, Block M, Brachmann J, et al. Mortality, morbidity, and complications in 3344 patients with implantable cardioverter defibrillators: results from the German ICD Registry EURID. Pacing Clin Electrophysiol 2003;26:1511–8.

40. Klein RC, Raitt MH, Wilkoff BL, et al. Analysis of implantable cardioverter defibrillator therapy in the antiarrhythmics versus implantable defibrillators (AVID) trial. J Cardiovasc Electrophysiol 2003;14(9):940–8.

41. Rinaldi CA, Simon RD, Baszko A, et al. A 17-year experience of inappropriate shock therapy in patients with implantable cardioverter-defibrillators: are we getting any better? Heart 2004;90(3):330–1.

42. Korte T, Koditz H, Niehaus M, et al. High incidence of appropriate and inappropriate ICD therapies in children and adolescents with implantable cardioverter defibrillator. Pacing Clin Electrophysiol 2004;27(7):924–32.

43. Alter P, Waldhans S, Plachta E, et al. Complications of implantable cardioverter defibrillator therapy in 440 consecutive patients. Pacing Clin Electrophysiol 2005;28(9):926–32.

44. Chen RH, Chen KP, Wang FZ, et al. Incidence and causes of inappropriate detection and therapy by implantable defibrillators of cardioversion in patients with ventricular tachyarrhythmia. Chin Med J (Engl) 2006;119(7):557–63.

45. Soundarraj D, Thakur RK, Gardiner JC, et al. Inappropriate ICD therapy: does device configuration make a difference. Pacing Clin Electrophysiol 2006;29(8):810–5.

46. Anselme F, Mletzko R, Bowes R, et al. Prevention of inappropriate shocks in ICD recipients: a review of 10,000 tachycardia episodes. Pacing Clin Electrophysiol 2007;30(Suppl 1):S128–33.

47. Stuber T, Eigenmann C, Delacretaz E. Inappropriate interventions during the long-term follow-up of patients with an implantable defibrillator. Swiss Med Wkly 2007;137:228–33.

48. Daubert JP, Zareba W, Cannom DS, et al. Inappropriate implantable cardioverter-defibrillator shocks in MADIT II: frequency, mechanisms, predictors, and survival impact. J Am Coll Cardiol 2008; 51(14):1357–65.

49. Fromer M, Brachmann J, Block M, et al. Efficacy of automatic multimodal device therapy for ventricular tachyarrhythmias as delivered by a new implantable pacing cardioverter-defibrillator. Results of a European multicenter study of 102 implants. Circulation 1992;86(2):363–74.

50. Wilkoff BL, Hess M, Young J, et al. Differences in tachyarrhythmia detection and implantable cardioverter defibrillator therapy by primary or secondary prevention indication in cardiac resynchronization therapy patients. J Cardiovasc Electrophysiol 2004;15(9):1002–9.

51. Almendral J, Arribas F, Wolpert C, et al. Dual-chamber defibrillators reduce clinically significant adverse events compared with single-chamber devices: results from the DATAS (Dual chamber and Atrial Tachyarrhythmias Adverse events Study) trial. Europace 2008;10(5):528–35.

52. Sarkozy A, Boussy T, Kourgiannides G, et al. Long-term follow-up of primary prophylactic implantable cardioverter-defibrillator therapy in Brugada syndrome. Eur Heart J 2007;28(3):334–44.

53. Sacher F, Probst V, Iesaka Y, et al. Outcome after implantation of a cardioverter-defibrillator in patients with Brugada syndrome: a multicenter study. Circulation 2006;114(22):2317–24.

54. Maron BJ, Spirito P, Shen WK, et al. Implantable cardioverter-defibrillators and prevention of sudden cardiac death in hypertrophic cardiomyopathy. JAMA 2007;298(4):405–12.

55. Marchlinski FE, Callans DJ, Gottlieb CD, et al. Benefits and lessons learned from stored electrogram information in implantable defibrillators. J Cardiovasc Electrophysiol 1995;6:832–51.

56. Woo A, Monakier D, Harris L, et al. Determinants of implantable defibrillator discharges in high-risk patients with hypertrophic cardiomyopathy. Heart 2007;93(9):1044–5.

57. Maron BJ, Shen WK, Link MS, et al. Efficacy of implantable cardioverter-defibrillators for the prevention of sudden death in patients with hypertrophic cardiomyopathy. N Engl J Med 2000;342(6):365–73.

58. Begley DA, Mohiddin SA, Tripodi D, et al. Efficacy of implantable cardioverter defibrillator therapy for primary and secondary prevention of sudden cardiac death in hypertrophic cardiomyopathy. Pacing Clin Electrophysiol 2003;26(9):1887–96.

59. Brady GH, Troutman C, Poole JE, et al. Clinical experience with a tiered therapy, multiprogrammable antiarrhythmia device. Circulation 1992; 85(5):1689–98.

60. Best PJ, Hayes DL, Stanton MS. The potential usage of dual-chamber pacing in patients with implantable cardioverter defibrillators. Pacing Clin Electrophysiol 1999;22:79–85.

61. Stein KM, Euler DE, Mehra R, et al. Do atrial tachyarrhythmias beget ventricular tachyarrhythmias in defibrillator recipients? J Am Coll Cardiol 2002; 40(2):335–40.

62. Gronefeld GC, Mauss O, Li YG, et al. Association between atrial fibrillation and appropriate implantable cardioverter defibrillator therapy: results from a prospective study. J Cardiovasc Electrophysiol 2000;11(11):1208–14.

63. Stevenson WG, Stevenson LW. Atrial fibrillation in heart failure. N Engl J Med 1999;341(12):910–1.

64. Boriani G, Biffi M, Frabetti L, et al. Cardioverter-defibrillator oversensing due to double counting of ventricular tachycardia electrograms. Int J Cardiol 1998;66(1):91–5.

65. Wolpert C, Jung W, Spehl S, et al. Case report: inappropriate discharge of an implantable cardioverter-defibrillator caused by the combined count criterion. J Interv Card Electrophysiol 1998;2(1): 53–6.

66. Weretka S, Michaelsen J, Becker R, et al. Ventricular oversensing: a study of 101 patients implanted with dual chamber defibrillators and two different lead systems. Pacing Clin Electrophysiol 2003;26: 65–70.

67. Rauwolf T, Guenther M, Hass N, et al. Ventricular oversensing in 518 patients with implanted cardiac defibrillators: incidence, complications, and solutions. Europace 2007;9(11):1041–7.

68. Occhetta E, Bortnik M, Magnani A, et al. Inappropriate implantable cardioverter-defibrillator discharges unrelated to supraventricular tachyarrhythmias. Europace 2006;8(10):863–9.

69. Schimpf R, Wolpert C, Gaita F, et al. Short QT syndrome. Cardiovasc Res 2005;67(3):357–66.

70. Hsu SS, Mohib S, Schroeder A, et al. T-wave oversensing in implantable cardioverter-defibrillators. J Interv Card Electrophysiol 2004;11(1):67–72.

71. Kowalski M, Ellenbogen KA, Wood MA, et al. Implantable cardiac defibrillator lead failure or myopotential oversensing? An approach to the diagnosis of noise on lead electrograms. Europace 2008;10(8):914–7.

72. Daoud EG, Kirsh MM, Bolling SF, et al. Incidence, presentation, diagnosis, and management of malfunctioning implantable cardioverter-defibrillator rate-sensing leads. Am Heart J 1994;128(5): 892–5.

73. Hauser RG, Kallinen LM, Almquist AK, et al. Early failure of a small-diameter high-voltage implantable cardioverter-defibrillator lead. Heart Rhythm 2007; 4(7):892–6.

74. Kolb C, Zrenner B, Schmitt C. Incidence of electromagnetic interference in implantable cardioverter-defibrillators. Pacing Clin Electrophysiol 2001;24: 465–8.

75. Pinski SL, Trohman RG. Interference in implanted cardiac devices. Part I. Pacing Clin Electrophysiol 2002;25(9):1367–81.

76. Kanagaratnam L, Pavia S, Schweikert R, et al. Matching approved nondedicated hardware to obtain biventricular pacing and defibrillation: feasibility and troubleshooting. Pacing Clin Electrophysiol 2002;25(7):1066–71.

77. Barold SS, Herweg B, Gallardo I. Double counting of the ventricular electrogram in biventricular pacemakers and ICDs. Pacing Clin Electrophysiol 2003; 26(8):1645–8.

78. Kuhlkamp V, Mewis C, Mermi J, et al. Suppression of sustained ventricular tachyarrhythmias: a comparison of D,L-sotalol with no antiarrhythmic drug treatment. J Am Coll Cardiol 1999;33(1):46–52.

79. Singer I, Al-Khalildi H, Niazi I, et al. Azimilide decreases recurrent ventricular tachyarrhythmias in patients with implantable cardioverter defibrillators. J Am Coll Cardiol 2004;43(1):39–43.

80. Dorian P, Borggrefe M, Al-Khalidi HR, et al. Placebo-controlled, randomized clinical trial of azimilide for prevention of ventricular tachyarrhythmias in patients with an implantable cardioverter-defibrillator. Circulation 2004;110(24):3646–54.

81. Connolly SJ, Dorian P, Roberts RS, et al. Comparison of beta-blockers, amiodarone plus beta-blockers, or sotalol for prevention of shocks from implantable cardioverter defibrillators: the OPTIC Study: a randomized trial. JAMA 2006;295(2):165–71.

82. Vyas AK, Guo H, Moss AJ, et al. Reduction in ventricular tachyarrhythmias with stains in the multicenter automatic defibrillator implantation trial (MADIT)-II. J Am Coll Cardiol 2006;47(4):769–73.

83. Jung W, Manz M, Pizzulli L, et al. Effects of chronic amiodarone therapy on defibrillation threshold. Am J Cardiol 1992;70(11):1023–7.

84. Manz M, Jung W, Luderitz B. Interactions between drugs and devices: experimental and clinical studies. Am Heart J 1994;127:978–84.

85. Wolbrette DL. Risk of proarrhythmia with class III antiarrhythmic agents: sex-based differences and other issues. Am J Cardiol 2003;91(6A):39D–44D.

86. Pacifico A, Hohnloser SH, Williams JH, et al. Prevention of implantable-defibrillator shocks by treatment with sotalol. D,L-sotalol implantable cardioverter-defibrillator study group. N Engl J Med 1999;340(24):1855–62.

87. Prystowsky EN. Proarrhythmia during drug treatment of supraventricular tachycardia: paradoxical risk of sinus rhythm for sudden death. Am J Cardiol 1996;78(8A):35–41.

88. Dougherty AH. Interactions between antiarrhythmic drugs and implantable cardioverter-defibrillators. Curr Opin Cardiol 1996;11(1):2–8.

89. Russo AM, Nayak H, Verdino R, et al. Implantable cardioverter defibrillator events in patients with asymptomatic nonsustained ventricular tachycardia: is device implantation justified? Pacing Clin Electrophysiol 2003;26(12):2289–95.

90. Bansch D, Castrucci M, Bocker D, et al. Ventricular tachycardias above the initially programmed tachycardia detection interval in patients with implantable cardioverter-defibrillators: incidence, prediction and significance. J Am Coll Cardiol 2000;36(2):557–65.

91. Arenal A, Almendral J, Villacastin J, et al. First postpacing interval variability during right ventricular stimulation: a single algorithm for the differential

diagnosis of regular tachycardias. Circulation 1998;98(7):671–7.

92. Brugada J, Mont L, Figueiredo M, et al. Enhanced detection criteria in implantable defibrillators. J Cardiovasc Electrophysiol 1998;9(3):261–8.

93. Higgins SL, Lee RS, Kramer RL. Stability: an ICD detection criterion for discriminating atrial fibrillation from ventricular tachycardia. J Cardiovasc Electrophysiol 1995;6(12):1081–8.

94. Swerdlow CD, Chen PS, Kass RM, et al. Discrimination of ventricular tachycardia from sinus tachycardia and atrial fibrillation in a tiered-therapy cardioverter-defibrillator. J Am Coll Cardiol 1994; 23(6):1342–55.

95. Kettering K, Dornberger V, Lang R, et al. Enhanced detection criteria in implantable cardioverter defibrillators: sensitivity and specificity of the stability algorithm at different heart rates. Pacing Clin Electrophysiol 2001;24:1325–33.

96. Garcia-Alberola A, Yli-Mayry S, Block M, et al. RR interval variability in irregular monomorphic ventricular tachycardia and atrial fibrillation. Circulation 1996;93(2):295–300.

97. Neuzner J, Pitschner HF, Schlepper M. Programmable VT detection enhancements in implantable cardioverter defibrillator therapy. Pacing Clin Electrophysiol 1995;18:539–47.

98. Rosenqvist M. Pacing techniques to terminate ventricular tachycardia. Pacing Clin Electrophysiol 1995;18:592–8.

99. Schaumann A, von zur Muhlen F, Gonska BD, et al. Enhanced detection criteria in implantable cardioverter-defibrillators to avoid inappropriate therapy. Am J Cardiol 1996;78(5A):42–50.

100. Brugada J. Is inappropriate therapy a resolved issue with current implantable cardioverter defibrillators? Am J Cardiol 1999;83(5B):40D–4D.

101. Toivonen L, Viitasalo M, Jarvinen J. The performance of the probability density function in differentiating supraventricular from ventricular rhythms. Pacing Clin Electrophysiol 1992;15(5):726–30.

102. Klingenheben T, Sticherling C, Skupin M, et al. Intracardiac QRS electrogram width—an arrhythmia detection feature for implantable cardioverter defibrillators: exercise induced variation as a base for device programming. Pacing Clin Electrophysiol 1998;21(8):1609–17.

103. Unterberg C, Stevens J, Vollmann D, et al. Long-term clinical experience with the EGM width detection criterion for differentiation of supraventricular and ventricular tachycardia in patients with implantable cardioverter defibrillators. Pacing Clin Electrophysiol 2000;23:1611–7.

104. Theuns DA, Rivero-Ayerza M, Goedhart DM, et al. Evaluation of morphology discrimination for ventricular tachycardia diagnosis in implantable cardioverter-defibrillators. Heart Rhythm 2006;3(11):1332–8.

105. Lee MA, Corbisiero R, Nabert DR, et al. Clinical results of an advanced SVT detection enhancement algorithm. Pacing Clin Electrophysiol 2005; 28(10):1032–40.

106. Gold MR, Shorofsky SR, Thompson JA, et al. Advanced rhythm discrimination for implantable cardioverter defibrillators using electrogram vector timing and correlation. J Cardiovasc Electrophysiol 2002;13(11):1092–7.

107. Swerdlow CD, Brown ML, Lurie K, et al. Discrimination of ventricular tachycardia from supraventricular tachycardia by a downloaded wavelet-transform morphology algorithm: a paradigm for development of implantable cardioverter defibrillator detection algorithms. J Cardiovasc Electrophysiol 2002;13(5):432–41.

108. Nair M, Saoudi N, Kroiss D, et al. Automatic arrhythmia identification using analysis of the atrioventricular association. Application to a new generation of implantable defibrillators. Participating centers of the Automatic Recognition of Arrhythmia Study Group. Circulation 1997;95(4):967–73.

109. Wilkoff BL, Kuhlkamp V, Volosin K, et al. Critical analysis of dual-chamber implantable cardioverter-defibrillator arrhythmia detection: results and technical considerations. Circulation 2001;103(3):381–6.

110. Korte T, Jung W, Wolpert C, et al. A new classification algorithm for discrimination of ventricular from supraventricular tachycardia in a dual chamber implantable cardioverter defibrillator. J Cardiovasc Electrophysiol 1998;9(1):70–3.

111. Theuns DA, Klootwijk AP, Goedhart DM, et al. Prevention of inappropriate therapy in implantable cardioverter-defibrillators: results of a prospective, randomized study of tachyarrhythmia detection algorithms. J Am Coll Cardiol 2004;44(12):2362–7.

112. Kolb C, Deisenhofer I, Schmieder S, et al. Long-term follow-up of patients supplied with single-chamber or dual-chamber cardioverter defibrillators. Pacing Clin Electrophysiol 2006;29(9):946–52.

113. Deisenhofer I, Kolb C, Ndrepepa G, et al. Do current dual-chamber cardioverter defibrillators have advantages over conventional single-chamber cardioverter-defibrillators in reducing inappropriate therapies? A randomized, prospective study. J Cardiovasc Electrophysiol 2001;12(2):134–42.

114. Friedman PA, McClelland RL, Balmet WR, et al. Dual-chamber versus single-chamber detection enhancements for implantable defibrillator rhythm diagnosis: the Detect Supraventricular Tachycardia Study. Circulation 2006;113(25):2871–9.

115. Theuns DA, Rivero-Ayerza M, Boersma E, et al. Prevention of inappropriate therapy in implantable defibrillators: a meta-analysis of clinical trials comparing single-chamber and dual-chamber arrhythmia discrimination algorithms. Int J Cardiol 2008;125(3):352–7.

ICD Lead Design and the Management of Patients with Lead Failure

Gautham Kalahasty, MD[a],*, Kenneth A. Ellenbogen, MD[b]

KEYWORDS

- ICD lead design • Conductors • Insulation
- Lead failure • Extraction

The implantable cardioverter defibrillator (ICD) lead is a remarkable medical device that is as critical to the function of the ICD system as the ICD itself. The mortality reduction associated with ICDs implanted for primary prevention indications has been made possible by the development of effective and reliable transvenous ICD leads. Mortality rates for implantation of transvenous ICD lead systems are currently less than 0.5%.

Since their introduction in 1993, transvenous leads have undergone rapid evolution. Despite advances in design, the high-voltage lead remains the "weakest" component of the ICD system. Long-term data from a prospective registry, published in 2007, show an overall lead survival rate of 85% at 5 years and as low as 60% at 8 years.[1] Although this study included older leads that are no longer in use (ie, Medtronic 6936, Medtronic, Minneapolis, MN, USA), it highlights the importance and limitations of ICD lead design.

Despite extensive bench, preclinical, and clinical testing, the true reliability and functional characteristics of a lead are often not known until it has been in widespread use. Lead recalls are an unfortunate reality of clinical practice and an understanding of the mechanism of lead failure is essential to proper patient management. Critical appraisal of the literature requires an understanding of lead design.

BASIC CONCEPTS

The components of a transvenous ICD lead include the conductors, insulation materials, defibrillation coils, lead electrodes, the fixation mechanism, the yoke, and lead connectors. A dual-coil, dedicated bipolar lead is shown in **Fig. 1**. The conductor is a composite metal that connects the pin (beyond the yoke) to each of the pace/sense (P/S) electrodes and to each of the coils. A bipolar ICD lead is similar to a bipolar pacing lead in that there is a tip (cathode) electrode and a ring (anode) electrode. Conductors also connect the DF-1 pin to the defibrillation coil or coils. All conductors are arranged in parallel within the lead body until they reach the yoke, where the P/S conductors and high-voltage conductors separate and terminate in the IS-1 pin or DF-1 pin, respectively. The yoke is trifurcated in the case of a dual-coil lead and is bifurcated in the case of a single-coil lead. The length of the distal (right ventricular, RV) coil is limited by the size of the right ventricle. The proximal coil (superior vena cava, SVC), if present, is generally longer. Before the development of dual-coil leads, a second coil electrode was placed in the SVC in patients with high defibrillation thresholds (DFTs). Defibrillation efficiency is in part related to the total surface area of the coils. Equal-length coils on a smaller-diameter lead have less active electrical

a Division of Cardiology, Department of Internal Medicine, Virginia Commonwealth University, Richmond, PO Box 980053, VA 23298-0053, USA
b Division of Cardiology, Cardiac Electrophysiology, Department of Internal Medicine, Virginia Commonwealth University, Richmond, VA 23298-0053, USA
* Corresponding author. Division of Cardiology, Department of Internal Medicine, Virginia Commonwealth University, Richmond, PO Box 980053, VA 23298-0053.
E-mail address: gkalahasty@mcvh-vcu.edu (G. Kalahasty).

Card Electrophysiol Clin 1 (2009) 173–191
doi:10.1016/j.ccep.2009.08.016
1877-9182/09/$ – see front matter © 2009 Published by Elsevier Inc.

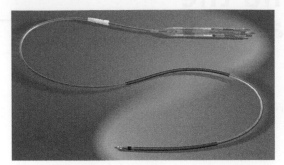

Fig. 1. Medtronic Sprint Quattro Secure ICD lead. (*Courtesy of* Medtronic, Inc; with permission.)

surface area than ones on a larger-diameter lead. Similar to pacing leads, ICD leads are made in passive fixation and active fixation versions.

Although there are many similarities, each manufacturer offers various leads with unique specifications and features. Data about older leads that are not currently being marketed, but that may still be in active service, can be found in lead "encyclopedias" published by each manufacturer or other textbooks. **Tables 1, 2** and **3** summarize key features and specifications for the most current lead models from each major US manufacturer. Some recent, but not the most current, leads may still be offered by a manufacturer to address specific patient needs or physician preference. For example, the Durata family of leads are the newest ICD leads offered by St. Jude Medical, Inc (St Paul, MN, USA); the preceding generation (Riata family) of leads is still available for implantation.

MATERIALS

The materials used in the construction of ICD leads and lead components are manufactured to high standards. Although the materials used by each of the major lead manufacturers are similar, there are some differences in how these materials are applied. Some materials, such as copolymers used for insulation, are unique to an individual manufacturer.

Conductors

The primary conductor used in most pacing and ICD leads is MP35N and silver. MP35N (Fort Wayne Metals, Fort WayneIN, USA) is a superalloy composed primarily of cobalt, nickel, chromium, and molybdenum. It has high tensile strength and is corrosion resistant. Because of its high electrical resistivity (1033 μohm-mm) MP35N is combined with efficient conductors such as silver. Single conducting filaments (wires) are made in 2 designs: a drawn brazed strand (DBS) and a drawn

filled tube. **Figs. 2** and **3** show examples of each type. The DBS design consists of the MP35N alloy stranded around the core of softer, highly conductive silver. It is brazed and drawn in the normal wire-drawing process (dies). The drawn filled tube design has a central core of silver, surrounded by MP35N and then coated with platinum or platinum-iridium. The tensile strength and electrical resistivity of this wire depends on the amount of silver in the core, which can be manufactured to the needs of the lead engineers. Both drawn filled tube wires and DSB wires can be formed into coils or twisted into cables.

MP35N is not the universal conductor for ICD leads amongst all manufacturers. The Guidant Endotak Reliance series of leads (Boston Scientific, Natick, MA, USA) use a DBS composed of silver and a version of 316LMV (Fort Wayne Metals) as the conductor for the high-voltage coil. It is composed primarily of chromium, nickel, iron, and molybdenum. 316LMV has good corrosion resistance and many metallurgical studies use it as a reference when evaluating new alloys.

Despite the sophisticated manufacturing process, MP35N can contain foreign inclusions of nitride, oxide, or carbide bodies that can negatively influence the metal fatigue life. Titanium (Ti), which is found in minute quantities in MP35N, can form Ti-carbide or Ti-nitride inclusions that are thought to promote fatigue cracking. A lead containing a modified, low-Ti MP35N alloy (US Patent #7,138,582 assigned to Medtronic, Inc) may have improved flex life. Low-Ti MP35N is not used by all manufacturers and is not yet used clinically in ICD leads.

Insulation

The materials used in ICD leads for insulation have a critical role in longevity and reliability of the lead and handling and implant characteristics. Fluoropolymers, polyurethanes, and silicone rubber are all used in various combinations within a given lead for various purposes. Fluoropolymers are fluorocarbon-based polymers with multiple strong carbon-fluorine bonds. They are characterized by a high resistance to solvents, acids, and bases. Therefore, they have maximum biocompatibility and tensile strength but their stiffness limits their use to thin coating (<0.076 mm) applications. Conductors are jacketed with a fluoropolymer layer to prevent adverse interactions with silicone tubing. Fluoropolymers will decrease the incidence of metal ion oxidation (MIO) in polyurethanes, but because ICD leads use silicone tubing, this is not the intended purpose. Examples of fluoropolymers are polytetrafluoroethylene

Table 1
Current Boston Scientific (Guidant) ICD leads

	Endotak Reliance G		Endotak Reliance SG	
Model/length (cm)	0184/59	0174/59	0180/59	0170/59
	0185/64	0175/64	0181/64	0171/64
	0186/70	0176/70	0182/70	0172/70
	0187/90	0177/90		
Fixation	Active	Passive	Active	Passive
Coils	Dual	Dual	Single	Single
Terminals	IS-1	IS-1	IS-1	IS-1
	DF-1 (2)	DF-1 (2)	DF-1	DF-1
Tip to proximal coil (cm)	18	18	NA	NA
Proximal coil active electrode surface area (mm^2)	660	660	NA	NA
Tip electrode surface area (mm^2)	5.7	2.0	5.7	2.0
Isodiametric lead diameter (mm/F)	2.7/8.1			
Coil electrode diameter (mm/F)	2.7/8.1			
Distal coil active electrode surface area (mm^2)	450			
Tip-RV coil (mm)	12			
Insulation/external overlay	Silicone rubber/proprietary lubricious coating			
DF-1 pin	Ti			
IS-1 pin	Stainless steel			
P/S conductor	MP35N, PTFE coated			
Coil material	Platinum-clad tantalum with Ti core			
Coil conductor	DBS, 316L bifilar cable, PTFE coated			
Tip electrode cover	Platinum-Iridium			
Coil electrode cover	Gore ePTFE			
Multilumen design	Asymmetric			
Sensing	Integrated bipolar			

(PTFE) (ie, Teflon, DuPont) and polyethylenetetrafluoroethylene (ETFE). Silicone rubber is a polymer that has a "backbone" of silicon-oxygen linkages. It is biocompatible and biostable. It also has high resistance to extreme temperatures and is therefore less susceptible to damage from electrocautery; it will char but not melt. Its main disadvantage is its low tensile strength, making it prone to tearing and abrasion wear. Abrasion wear comes from lead-to-lead, can-to-lead, and yoke-to-lead mechanical contact. Silicone rubber is also susceptible to cold flow (also known as creep), defined as increasing deformation under constant or cyclic compression (**Fig. 4**). It also has a high coefficient of friction, making it difficult to pass alongside other leads. Therefore, when silicone rubber is used as the primary insulation-thick layers are used and covered with a lubricious coating or polyurethane. Of the insulation materials in use, polyurethanes have the least biostability (if applied in thin layers). They are also characterized by high tear strength, high elasticity, and a low coefficient of friction. The use of polyurethanes results in limited scar formation and allows for smaller lead diameters. The observed interactions of polyurethane chemistry and body chemistry can lead to significant degradation of lead function resulting from calcification (rare), environmental stress cracking (ESC) and chain scission. ESC occurs, in part, as a result of polyurethane oxidation caused by macrophages that induce hydrogen peroxide formation to the polymer structure. Hydrogen peroxide is also produced by inflammatory cells as they make contact with the conductor, which results in oxidation-induced molecular chain breaks in the polyurethane and

Table 2
Current Medtronic ICD leads

	Sprint Quattro	Sprint Quattro Secure	Sprint Quattro Secure S
Model/length (cm)	6944/58 6944/65 6944/75 6944/100	6947/58 6947/65 6947/75 6947/100	6935/52 6935/58 6935/65 6935/75 6935/100
Fixation	Passive	Active	Active
Coils	Dual	Dual	Single
Terminals	IS-1 DF-1 (2)	IS-1 DF-1 (2)	IS-1 DF-1
Tip to proximal coil (cm)	18	18	NA
Proximal coil active electrode surface area (mm^2)	819	860	NA
Tip electrode surface area (mm^2)	1.6	5.7	5.7
Isodiametric lead diameter (mm/F)	2.7/8.1	2.9/8.7	2.8/8.4
Coil electrode diameter (mm/F)	2.7/8.1	2.9/8.7	2.8/8.4
Distal coil active electrode surface area (mm^2)	584	614	614
Tip-RV coil (mm)	8	8	8
Insulation/external overlay		Silicone rubber/polyurethane	
DF-1 pin		Stainless steel	
IS-1 pin		Stainless steel	
P/S conductor		MP35N, PTFE coated	
Coil material		Platinum clad tantalum	
Coil conductor		MP35N	
Tip electrode cover		Platinized platinum alloy	
Coil electrode cover		Silicone backfill	
Design		Asymmetric	
Sensing		Dedicated bipolar	

Table 3
St Jude Medical ICD leads

	Durata						
Model/length (cm)	7120/60 7120/65	7121/60 7121/65 7121/75	7122/60 7122/65	7130/60 7130/65	7131/60 7131/65	7170/60 7170/65	7171/60 7171/65
Fixation	Active	Active	Active	Active	Active	Passive	Passive
Coils	Dual	Dual	Single	Dual	Dual	Dual	Dual
Terminals	IS-1 DF-1 (2)	IS-1 DF-1 (2)	IS-1 DF-1	IS-1 DF-1 (2)	IS-1 DF-1 (2)	IS-1 DF-1 (2)	IS-1 DF-1 (2)
Tip to proximal coil (cm)	17	21	NA	17	21	17	21
Proximal coil active electrode surface area (mm^2)	588	588	NA	588	588	588	588
Tip electrode surface area (mm^2)	8	8	8	8	8	3.5	3.5
Isodiametric lead diameter (mm/F)			2.3/6.8				
Coil electrode diameter (mm/F)			2.3/6.8				
Distal coil active electrode surface area (mm^2)			367				
Tip-RV coil or anode (mm)			11				
Insulation/external overlay			Silicone/Optim overlay with Fast-Pass coating[a]				
DF-1 pin			MP35N and stainless steel				
IS-1 pin			MP35N and stainless steel				
P/S conductor			MP35N and MP35N drawn filled tube				
Coil material			Platinum-iridium alloy				
Coil conductor			MP35N				
Helix/cover			Platinum-iridium alloy/Ti-nitride			NA	NA
Coil electrode cover			Silicone backfill				
Multilumen design	Symmetric	Symmetric	Symmetric	Symmetric	Symmetric	Symmetric	Symmetric
Sensing	Dedicated bipolar	Dedicated bipolar	Integrated bipolar	Integrated bipolar	Integrated bipolar	Dedicated bipolar	Dedicated bipolar

[a] Optim and Fast-Pass are registered trademarks of St Jude Medical.

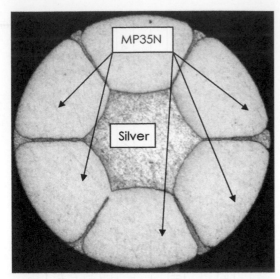

Fig. 2. Single conducting filaments (wires) are made into a DBS. (*Courtesy of* Fort Wayne Metals, Fort Wayne, MN; with permission.)

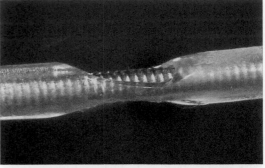

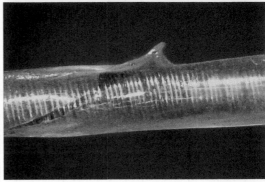

Fig. 4. Lead abrasion (*top*) and cold flow and abrasion (*bottom*). (*Courtesy of* St Jude Medical, Inc, St Paul, MN; with permission.)

MIO. Thermal instability and mechanical stresses also play a role in ESC. Polyurethane is not stable at high temperatures and is prone to melting when electrocautery is applied. Pretreating the polyurethane in an inert gas protects it against ESC. The two most common polyurethanes in clinical use today are Pellethane 80A and Pellethane 55D (Upjohn, CPR Division, Torrance, CA, USA). Pellethane 80A has been associated with increased long-term failure rates. Pellethane 55D may be more biostable but it is stiffer than Pellethane 80A.

Elast-Eon (Aortech Biomaterials, Clayton, Victoria, Australia) is a copolymer composed of silicone rubber, polyhexamethylene oxide, and polyurethane. The polyurethane is composed of methylene diisocyanate and butane diol. Elast-Eon has been designed to be used in biomedical applications because it retains the strengths of each of its primary components (tear and abrasion resistance, lubricity, flexibility, and biostability). Elast-Eon is currently exclusively used by St Jude Medical in their Durata series of ICD leads and is referred to as Optim Insulation. It is applied as a layer on top of standard silicone rubber. Although there are in vitro and in vivo animal studies as yet no large, long-term human studies have been completed.[2] At least 1 study has demonstrated that the copolymer used in these leads is not protective against thermal injury from electrocautery.[3] Other copolymers are being developed.

Although technically not an insulation material, expanded polytetraflouroethylene (ePTFE) or Gore-Tex (WL Gore and Associates, Flagstaff, AR, USA) is applied to ICD coils to prevent tissue in-growth. It has a porous structure that allows fluid ingress and therefore is not an electrical insulator, allowing for efficient defibrillation. ePTFE can prevent lead chatter from metal-metal interactions when multiple leads are present.[4] The pores are too small to allow cell penetration and help minimize fibrous tissue formation. ePTFE improves extractability without compromising electrical performance.[5,6] Most of the data are from animal

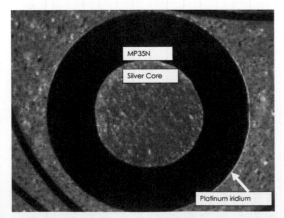

Fig. 3. Single conducting filaments (wires) are made into a drawn filled tube. (*Courtesy of* Fort Wayne Metals, Fort Wayne, MN; with permission.)

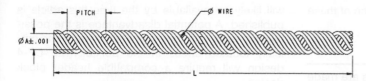

Fig. 5. The coil conductor for the cathode. Each filar has a diameter. Coil filarity is the number of separate wires with the coil. Pitch is a function of the filar diameter × the number of filars in the set + the space between filar sets. (*Courtesy of* St Jude Medical, Inc, St Paul, MN; with permission.)

studies with limited data from long-term human studies. This material is currently used only in the Guidant Reliance G series of leads. The safety and biostability of this material has been well established through its extensive use in other applications, including vascular and plastic surgery.

Defibrillation Coils, Pacing Electrodes, and Connector Pins

The metals used in defibrillation coils include platinum, iridium, tantalum, and Ti. Platinum, in particular, is known for its oxidation-corrosion resistance and biocompatibility. When combined by a process called cladding, these metal alloys offer high strength, superior conductive properties, stable thermal properties, and enhanced corrosion resistance and biocompatibility. Cladding is the metallurgical process by which dissimilar layers of metals are bonded together with no adhesives or filler materials. Combinations include platinum-clad tantalum and platinum-clad tantalum with a Ti core. Neither material has been proven to be superior to the other in clinical applications. Ti is not used by itself because it produces metallic oxides during high-voltage shocks.

The cathode and anode (of a true bipolar lead) of ICD leads are made of a platinum-iridium alloy. Although a carbon-tipped cathode has good mechanical strength and lower chronic stimulation thresholds, most manufacturers are not yet using it in their lead designs. The electrodes themselves may be coated with a substance to create

a microporous, fractal surface that increases the "electrical" surface area. These coatings include Ti-nitride, platinum black, and iridium oxide. Electrode efficiency is related to the degree of polarization that takes place at the surface.[7] Ti-nitride has the lowest polarization effect. The connector pins are made with stainless steel or Ti.

DESIGN AND CONSTRUCTION

The individual material elements used in each component have specific assembly based on the design goal. The conductors, P/S electrodes, shock coil, and yoke can be thought of as subassemblies that are then combined into an ICD lead. As will be evident later, there is significant variability in the engineering approaches taken for each component of an ICD lead. A clinical comparison of design philosophies for each component is not possible. The clinical comparison of leads is a comparison of the specific combination of design compromises that are represented in a given lead.

Conductors

Single-filament drawn filled tubes can be combined into strands and cables. Filaments are wound into cables to serve as conductors in ICD leads and pacing leads. Cabled conductors offer greater strength, fracture resistance, and redundancy than coiled conductors. Cable conductors are also not compressible. Cabled conductors are coated with a fluoropolymer to prevent insulation damage. Multipolar leads that employ cables can be made with smaller diameters than those that use coaxial coiled conductors. The number of filaments and their arrangement within a given cable vary from manufacturer to manufacturer. The structure of the P/S coil conductor of the cathode is highly variable between manufacturers. **Fig. 5** shows the structure of the coil and the characteristics that are considered by engineers. These characteristics are important because they affect the flexibility of the coil and its resistance to fracture. Wire diameter, number of filars (wires), and pitch all vary between manufacturers and between lead families of a single manufacturer. Multifilar coils offer lower electrical resistance (optimal) but may have lower fatigue life when compared with bifilar designs. There is no

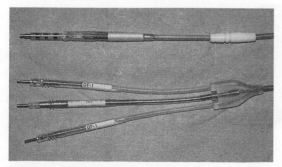

Fig. 6. Comparison of the current DF-1 connector (*bottom*) and the proposed DF-4 connector (*top*).

consensus as to the optimal combination of these factors.

Defibrillation Coil

Defibrillation coils on current ICD leads are made with round wires (Medtronic and Boston Scientific) or flat wire (St Jude Medical Durata and Biotronik). Both designs can be backfilled with silicon or covered with ePTFE. No current designs have bare coils. The shape of the wire affects the surface area and the amount of electrically active surface area, which is important for efficient defibrillation. The surface areas of various leads for the 3 domestic manufacturers are given in **Tables 1–3**. One potential advantage of flat wire coils is the more even and complete distribution of the silicone backfill, which may result in less tissue ingrowth. However, no clinical studies have shown that flat coils are superior to round coils with respect to tissue in-growth.

ICD Lead Connectors and Yoke Design

All manufacturers now follow the International Organization for Standardization (ISO) guidelines for terminal pin design. Current ICD leads have a bifurcated or trifurcated yoke with terminal pins that connect into the ICD header block. The P/S portion of the lead is terminated with an IS-1 pin and the shock coils are terminated with their respective DF-1 (ISO-11,318) pins. This design increases pocket bulk. More importantly, the yoke greatly increases the potential for lead-to-lead and lead-to-can interactions, resulting in insulation defects. The presence of 2 DF-1 pins in dual-coil leads allows for connection errors in the header block.

The next generation of ICD leads will incorporate an in-line design to form a single connector pin, the proposed DF-4 (or IS-4) connector (**Fig. 6**). Pocket bulk, and the potential for lead-to-lead interactions, will decrease. ICD leads with this design

will likely be available by the time this article is published. A potential disadvantage is the possibility of multiple component fracture from one critically located stress in the pocket. The DF-4 design will require a compatible header block design.

The ICD Lead

Early transvenous ICD leads were based on the coaxial design of pacemaker leads. In a coaxial lead design, each of the conductors is coiled around the central (cathode) coil conductor and separated by insulation (**Fig. 7**). Examples of these leads include the Medtronic Transvene 6936 and St Jude/Ventritex TVL RV 01. The central coil allows stylet insertion and helix deployment. Because of the coaxial design and the need for multiple conductors, these leads have large diameters, ranging in size from 9.7 F to 12 F. This design is more prone to conductor fracture and insulation breach and has been replaced by the multilumen design. Although no longer manufactured, many leads with this design are still in active use. For example, the Medtronic 6936 was released to the US market in 1993 and 23,700 leads were implanted. It is estimated that 3,200 leads are still in active use.

For ICD leads, the coaxial design has been replaced by the multilumen design. Similar to the coaxial design, a central coil conductor is used for the cathode and allows for stylet insertion and provides the extendable/retractable function of the helix in active fixation leads. Conductors for the anode and high-voltage coils are arranged as parallel cables and distributed around the central coil. The distribution of cables can be symmetric, as is the case for current St Jude Medical leads, or asymmetric, as is the case for current Medtronic and Boston Scientific leads (**Fig. 8**). Neither approach has been proven to be superior, but each has theoretical advantages

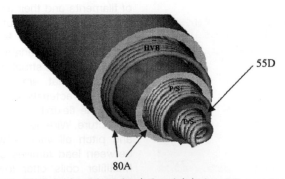

Fig. 7. The Medtronic Transvene 6936 single-coil ICD lead. Coaxial design. P/S, pace/sense; HVB, high-voltage distal coil; 80A, polyurethane 80A; 55D, polyurethane 55D.

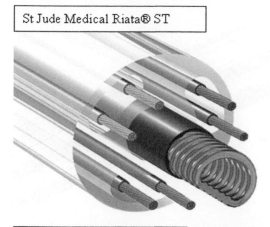

St Jude Medical Riata® ST

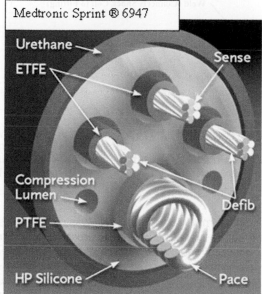

Medtronic Sprint ® 6947

Urethane

ETFE

Sense

Compression
Lumen

Defib

PTFE

HP Silicone

Pace

Fig. 8. Two examples of multilumen lead design. The St Jude Medical Riata ST has a symmetric structure whereas the Medtronic Sprint 6947 has an asymmetric structure. The cabled conductors of the Riata ST are paired and arranged in a common oversized lumen. (*Courtesy of* St Jude Medical, Inc, St Paul, MN, and Medtronic, Inc, Minneapolis, MN; with permission.)

and disadvantages. The symmetric lead design may be more prone to "stacking" of conductors when pressure is applied in any given vector across the lead diameter. Because cables are noncompressible, a symmetric design may be less flexible in any given direction than an asymmetric design. An asymmetric lead is likely to flex away from the cables preferentially, in the direction of the relatively compressible coil. Therefore, the coil and conductor may experience a variable degree of bending and binding stress, depending on the direction that the lead is flexed. Most leads are designed with one conductor for each element. The St Jude Medical Riata ST series and Durata series of leads are designed with redundant conductors that are paired into a common oversized lumen. These redundant conductors terminate at a common junction at the coil, electrode, and yoke. There is no proven advantage to this redundancy. **Fig. 9** shows dedicated bipolar and integrated bipolar leads. A true (eg, dedicated) bipolar lead has one additional conductor that is carried the entire length of the lead, extending from the anode ring to the yoke. Conductor cables are connected to the coils and ring by various methods. Connections are made at the proximal end of the SVC coil and the distal or proximal ends of the RV coil (proximal connections are shown in **Fig. 10**). Connections at the distal and proximal ends of the RV coil result in the most uniform distribution of current.[8] Current density is highest at the connection points. Uniform current delivery is thought to improve defibrillation efficiency and delivery of current to the apex is better than delivery to the annular region or the septum. All manufacturers connect the SVC coil at the proximal end. Medtronic leads are connected at the distal and proximal ends of the RV coil. St Jude Medical (Durata) leads are connected at the distal end of the RV coil. The Boston Scientific Endotak series of leads uses a proximal connection for the SVC coil and a distal connection for the RV coil.

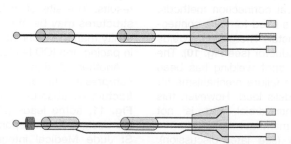

Fig. 9. A dual-coil integrated bipolar lead (*top*) and true bipolar lead (*bottom*). Note that in the integrated bipolar lead, the conductor from the distal coil bifurcates in the yoke to connect to the IS-1 and DF-1 pins.

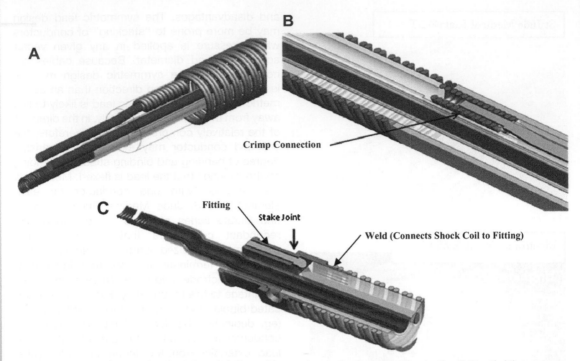

Fig. 10. Crimp coupling and stake joints. (*A*) The cable conductor (*red*) connecting to the SVC coil. (*B*) A cutaway showing the crimping of the cable conductor to small-diameter coil that expands to become the defibrillation coil. (*C*) A stake joint as the means of connection of the cable conductor to the fitting of the distal shock coil assembly. The shock coil is welded to the fitting. (*Courtesy of* Boston Scientific, Inc, Natick, MA; with permission.)

The methods used for connection include spot welding, crimp coupling, and stake joints (or a combination of these methods). Crimp coupling involves crimping the conductor coil to a platinum coupler (jacket). In some cases, this jacket is then welded to the platinum defibrillation coil. Crimp coupling can increase the rigidity of the lead at the site of coupling. This jacket is then welded to the platinum defibrillation coil. The Boston Scientific Endotak Reliance series of leads uses a crimp connection to join the cable conductor to the SVC coil and a stake connection to the join the cable conductor to the fitting of the distal shock coil assembly. The shock coil is welded to the fitting. In the Boston Scientific Endotak Reliance series of leads, only mechanical connection methods, crimping and staking, are used to make connections to the cable conductor. There are no welds directly to the cable conductor (see **Fig. 10**). The technique of resistance spot welding has been implicated as one of the failure mechanisms for the Medtronic Sprint Fidelis lead. However, this assertion remains controversial and is not substantiated by the manufacturer's returned product analysis (RPA) (see later discussion). Welding of dissimilar metals (platinum and MP35N) is a complicated materials topic and it is

an oversimplification that two dissimilar metals cannot be welded. The metals must have similar melting points and be metallurgically compatible. Metallurgical incompatibility may lead to uncontrollable weld metal cracking or a weld metal microstructure that cannot provide adequate mechanical or corrosion performance. Adjacent to the fusion boundary is a band, typically very narrow, over which there may be a steep composition and melting-point gradient caused by heat propagation. This fusion boundary region may contain microstructures that are unacceptable for service. It is also known that the technique of welding (ie, resistance spot welding or laser welding) and the use of filler metals can affect the results. The site of welding and the associated structures may be more relevant to the lead reliability than the technique. Welding is widely used in pacing and ICD leads.

Another design innovation is the use of compression lumens, which may protect against fracture by absorbing crush stress. As shown in **Fig. 11**, some leads (Medtronic Sprint Quattro) are designed with separate compression lumens. St Jude Medical integrates a common lumen around each pair of conductors in its current ICD leads. This approach was also used in the

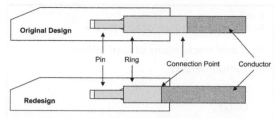

Fig. 11. The IS-1 terminal inserting into the header of original (*top*) Endotak DSP 0125 lead (Guidant/Cardiac Pacemakers Inc, St Paul, MN) and the redesigned version (*bottom*).

Medtronic Sprint Fidelis lead, which was withdrawn from the market. The Guidant (Boston Scientific) Endotak Reliance series of leads do not have separate or integrated crush lumens. There are no clinical data to suggest that the presence of compression lumens or their configuration prevents conductor fracture or affects lead reliability.

From a sensing perspective, there are 2 types of endocardial ICD leads: true (dedicated) bipolar and integrated bipolar. The true bipolar leads have separate tip and ring electrodes, similar to a standard bipolar pacing lead. Because of the presence of the ring electrode (anode), the defibrillation coil is displaced more proximally and therefore may be further from the RV apex. The gap between the tip and RV defibrillation coil is referred to as the pullback distance. An integrated bipolar lead uses the RV defibrillation coil as the anode. The primary design difference, therefore, is the need for another conductor in the lead body of the true bipolar lead. Without the intervening ring electrode, the defibrillation coil can be positioned closer to the apex.

These design differences have important clinical implications. Sensing characteristics are the most obvious consequences of these differences. An integrated bipolar lead may not be suitable for a patient with a small RV or if the high-voltage lead cannot be completely positioned across the tricuspid valve. Far-field oversensing of atrial signals may occur. Because of their similarities to standard pacing leads, true bipolar leads are expected to the have the best pacing performance with the fewest sensing errors. Some studies have cast doubt on this generalization. Data gathered at the time of implantation by Frain and colleagues showed that there was no difference in R-wave amplitude and slew rate between the two lead types. Sensing latency was longer with the true bipolar lead compared with the integrated bipolar lead. The clinical correlate is that a longer programmed atrioventricular delay may be needed

in patients with true bipolar leads.[9] When used with an automatic gain control ICD, integrated bipolar leads have been shown to yield more oversensing of high-frequency, low-amplitude, respirophasic noise transients (myopotentials).[10] This oversensing can be investigated at the time of implant by studying electrograms from the pacing system analyzer (PSA) set to the most sensitive values. This type of oversensing is important to recognize because it could lead to inappropriate tachyarrhythmia detection and therapies or pacing inhibition. Inadvertent reversal of the DF-1 terminal pins of an integrated bipolar lead in the header block can lead to inappropriate ICD shocks because of oversensing of myopotentials.[11] T-wave oversensing has been associated with true bipolar and integrated bipolar lead designs. The mechanism of gain control (fixed or automatic) within the ICD itself[12] and patient factors (ie, hypertrophic cardiomyopathy, hyperkalemia, and Brugada syndrome) can lead to T-wave oversensing.[13,14] Occasionally, the ICD lead itself needs to be replaced to manage T-wave oversensing.[15,16] In patients with cardiac resynchronization therapy (CRT) devices, it has been shown that true bipolar leads are more likely to manifest anodal stimulation and therefore can affect clinical response to CRT. Contrary to conventional thinking, Freedman and colleagues[17] showed that the rates of oversensing or undersensing did not differ between the two lead designs. However, one study demonstrated that P-wave oversensing was more common with integrated bipolar leads than with true bipolar leads.[18] The sample size in this study was small. The shorter pullback distance may give the integrated bipolar lead better defibrillation performance in selected patients. This suggestion has not been proven by clinical trials and may not be an important difference with current high-energy devices. Some newer ICDs offer electronic reconfiguration of a true bipolar lead into a functional integrated bipolar lead.

All major manufacturers produce a single- and dual-coil version of their ICD leads. Dual-coil systems are associated with reduced impedance and may lower defibrillation thresholds in some patients. Except in right-sided or abdominal implants, it is rare to use the ICD as an inactive ("cold" can) component. Although controversial, a recent study showed that placement of the proximal coil at the innominate vein-SVC junction yields lower DFTs than when the coil is at the junction of the SVC and the right atrium. This same study showed the coil separation (17 cm versus 21 cm) had no significant effect on defibrillation energy requirements.[19] Frequently, the final position of the proximal coil is dictated by the chamber sizes such that the proximal coil may reside in the right atrium entirely. Some ICD leads have widely spaced coils to maintain an SVC position for the proximal coil even in patients with severe chamber enlargement. Coil separation on the lead may not translate into true spatial separation within the heart because of the need to place the appropriate amount of redundancy. Although factors affecting defibrillation thresholds are complex and controversial, a recent meta-analysis suggested that the optimal defibrillation polarity is with the distal coil functioning as the anode.[20]

The need to place multiple leads into a single patient has highlighted the importance of lead diameter. Pacing leads range in size from 4 F to 9 F. Current ICD leads range from 6.3 F to 8.6 F. In an effort to decrease the size of the lead diameter, engineers have weighed various design compromises against their potential impact on lead function and reliability. Smaller-diameter leads have less insulation material. However, an asymmetric small-diameter lead has more insulation than a symmetric small-diameter lead. There are conflicting clinical data with respect to the incidence of lead-related complications and performance problems of small-diameter leads compared with larger-diameter leads.[21–23]

LEAD FAILURE MECHANISMS AND LEAD RECALLS

Lead failure can have more serious and immediate consequences than failure of the pulse generator. The manifestations of lead failure include high pacing or shock impedance, oversensing, undersensing, nonphysiologic interventricular (V-V) intervals, failure to capture and, less commonly, failure to defibrillate. Inappropriate shocks are the most serious expression of lead failure and can lead to morbidity and mortality.[24] Malfunction of the pulse generator can be managed by replacement but, in the case of lead failure, the management issues are more complex (see later discussion).

When considering lead materials and construction, multiple mechanisms of failure are conceivable. Lead failure can be caused by design features, implantation technique, and patient factors, in isolation or in combination. Patient-induced, repetitive, or episodic mechanical trauma to the lead can result in insulation damage and conductor fracture. Twiddler syndrome has been reported to cause both.[25] **Box 1** categorizes the locations of failure.

Failure of the fixation mechanism has been described for pacing and high-voltage leads. Individual cases of fixation problems have occurred especially with repeated extensions (and

---

> **Box 1**
> **Sites and mechanisms of lead failure**
>
> *Sites and mechanisms of lead failure*
>
> Insulation defects
>   Internal
>   Outer
> Conductor fractures
> Conductor-to-coil connection defect
> Conductor-to-electrode connection defect
> Conductor-to-terminal ring connection defect
> Fixation-mechanism defect

---

retractions). There have been no widespread problems involving this failure mechanism among ICD leads resulting in a recall.

Fracture of the high-voltage conductor is suggested by increased impedance during high-voltage therapy. The shock impedance of any failed therapy should be compared with the impedance during prior successful therapies. The impedance trends should also be analyzed. A normal measured shock impedance alone does not exclude the possibility of a fracture of the high-voltage conductor. Intraoperative troubleshooting with PSA may sometimes be needed.[26,27]

The initial design of the conductor-to-terminal ring interface of the Endotak DSP Model 0125 lead (Guidant/CPI) had a flexion point that resulted in damage to the conductor and insulation. In one series, this design characteristic resulted in a 3.5% incidence of lead fracture over a 31-month follow-up period and manifested as nonphysiologic V-V intervals.[28] The high fracture rate necessitated a redesign that allowed the connection point to be contained inside the header, thus protecting a vulnerable flexion point (see **Fig. 11**).

The Medtronic Transvene (Model 6936) is an example of an ICD lead with multiple failure mechanisms. This lead had a coaxial design that is no longer in use. According to the manufacturer, approximately 23,700 leads were implanted and an estimated 3200 are in active clinical use. Dorwarth and colleagues[29] reported a 62% lead survival at 8 years with no relationship between lead survival and patient factors or implant technique. One report suggested that conductor fracture caused by subclavian crush syndrome is a rare mechanism of failure for this lead. This finding is contrary to the RPA of the manufacturer. Lead failure rates are not linear, with a near 90%

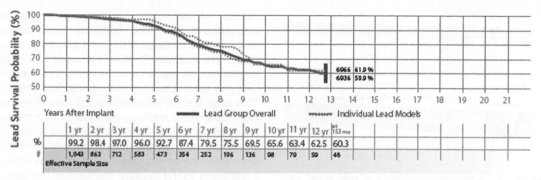

Fig. 12. Data from the product performance report showing the probability of lead survival for the Transvene 6936 ICD lead. (*Courtesy of* Medtronic, Inc, Minneapolis, MN: with permission.)

survival at 4 to 5 years and a 60% to 80% survival at 8 to 9 years (**Fig. 12**). There is a higher rate of lead failure following replacement of the pulse generator, suggesting that lead manipulation at the time of the procedure increases the risk of subsequent lead failure. In contrast to studies that showed insulation defects to be the most common mode of failure, one study from the US Food and Drug Administration (FDA) database reported that fracture of the high-voltage coil accounted for most failures (38%). This study also reported that the failure of the middle layer of polyurethane 80A (28%) was more likely than failure of the outer layer (13%).[30] MIO is thought to be responsible for the damage to the middle layer. A unique expression of failure of this lead is oversensing after an appropriate or inappropriate shock, resulting in additional inappropriate shocks. This finding may be specific to the failure of the middle insulation layer in a coaxial lead.[31] To test lead integrity at the time of generator replacement, a 1-V pacing pulse can be given between the ring and coil. A value of greater than 4.4 mA suggests that the middle insulation is intact. If this is the case, the manufacturer does not recommend replacement. However, given that the rate of lead failure seems to be higher after

generator replacement, lead replacement should also be considered at that time.

Despite the complex mechanisms of failure, the clinic impact of the Transvene 6936 is limited because of the small numbers of leads implanted and still in use today. The Medtronic Sprint Fidelis ICD lead, however, represents a larger clinical problem. An estimated 205,600 leads (Models 6930, 6931, 6948, and 6949) were implanted in the United States and an estimated 150,100 leads are in active clinical use. Most implanted leads were the dual-coil, active-fixation model 6949 lead, with 186,700 implants in the United States and 135,900 remaining in active use. **Fig. 13** shows the estimated lead survival rate at 48 months. This estimate is based primarily on the Medtronic System Longevity Study (SLS). Some attempts at sighting design and construction features to explain the mechanism of failure are speculative and based on analysis of only a few leads. These theories include an inadequate welding technique, an asymmetric arrangement of conductors leading to stacking and fracture,[32] and a coil-filar arrangement with suboptimal sheer stress tolerances. An analysis of a large number of leads is needed to make reliable conclusions and to associate (if appropriate) design characteristics with failure

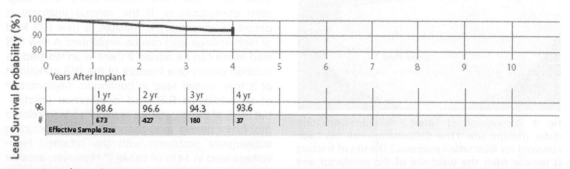

Fig. 13. Data from the product performance report showing the probability of lead survival for the Sprint Fidelis 6949 ICD lead. (*Courtesy of* Medtronic, Inc, Minneapolis, MN: with permission.)

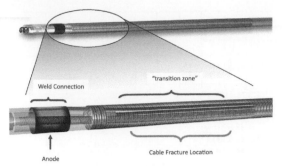

Fig. 14. The "stiffness transition and seal zone" (see text) and distal fracture site of the Sprint Fidelis ICD lead. (*Courtesy of* Medtronic, Inc, Minneapolis, MN: with permission.)

mechanisms. The manufacturer's RPA is the most useful means to understand the mechanism of lead failure. This analysis, to date, reveals that conductor fracture is the primary (90% of cases) mechanism of failure. About 10% of chronic fractures have occurred at the DF-1 connector segment or the proximal portion of the RV coil. Therefore, the inability to deliver high-voltage therapy is an uncommon expression of failure of this lead. Oversensing, loss of pacing, and inappropriate shocks are more likely presentations. The two sites of conductor fracture have been localized to the distal portion of the lead (conductor cable), near the anode (**Figs. 14** and **15**) and at the proximal

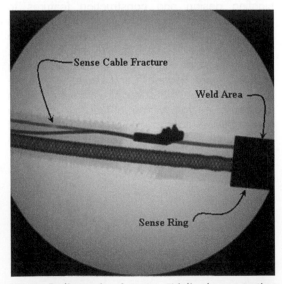

Fig. 15. Radiograph of Sprint Fidelis demonstrating distal fracture site. (The defibrillation coil has been removed for illustration purposes.) The site of fracture is remote from the weld site of the conductor and anode ring. (*Courtesy of* Medtronic, Inc, Minneapolis, MN: with permission.)

portion of the lead (conductor coil) near the anchoring sleeve. The "stiffness transition and seal zone" is the area of the lead where the transition of the relatively flexible lead body to the rigid sleeve head is made (to improve implant handling) and the lead is sealed from body fluid leakage. This is an area of transitioning stiffness of the lead body as a whole and may contribute to the fracture mechanism. It is proximal to the weld site of the conductor and anode. Propagation of heat from the weld site to the fracture sites is an unlikely contributor to the fracture mechanism because of distance. Of the proximal coil fractures, 60% have occurred immediately past the anchoring sleeve (potentially within the muscle) and 30% have occurred between the sleeve and yoke. Although the locations of these fractures have been well defined, the relationship to design and construction is yet to be defined. Furthermore, the incidence of lead fracture seems to be increasing[33] and the impact of upcoming generator replacements on the failure rate is unknown.

MANAGEMENT OF THE PATIENT WITH A FAILED ICD LEAD

The management of a patient with a failed ICD lead differs from the management of a patient with a failed pacemaker lead. Whereas programming to a unipolar pacing mode can be successful in failed pacemaker leads, such noninvasive measures have limited or no value in the management of failed ICD leads. Unipolar pacing or sensing is not an option for an ICD. Except possibly in pacemaker dependent patients, a lead fracture or insulation defect will not necessarily have immediate consequences in patients with pacemakers, but can result in inappropriate therapies in patients with ICDs.

In most cases of ICD lead failure a new lead needs to be implanted, and in some cases extraction of the existing lead is indicated. Neither strategy has been proven to be superior to the other; both can have serious short- and long-term complications. If the venous anatomy is patent or venoplasty is feasible, a new P/S lead or high-voltage lead can be implanted. A new P/S lead alone can be added if there is an isolated insulation defect or a fracture of the P/S conductor of a true bipolar lead is confirmed. Implantation of an additional P/S lead is common practice, but 28% of these patients experience lead-related problems during long-term follow-up, including subsequent problems with the retained high-voltage lead in 14% of cases.[34] However, another retrospective analysis of patients with abandoned leads by Glikson and colleagues[35] found no significant difference in the rates of sensing mal-functions, thromboembolic complications, or shocks (appropriate or inappropriate) compared with before abandonment. The addition of a second high-voltage lead can cause lead-to-lead (distal coil-to-coil) interactions and can be particularly problematic if an integrated bipolar lead is used. The effectiveness of defibrillation with the addition of another high-voltage lead caused by shunting of current to the abandoned lead is unlikely, but is theoretically possible if an insulation defect exists.[27] At least one animal model suggests this is not a concern.[36] However, defibrillation threshold testing is indicated in these patients. The presence of multiple leads crossing the tricuspid valve has not been shown to increase the risk of tricuspid regurgitation; however, lead extraction can result in an increased rate of tricuspid valve problems. Lead-to-lead interactions have also been implicated in lead fractures in areas that are otherwise mechanically stress-free.[37]

Lead extraction has become an increasingly important clinical issue and several aspects of lead design are directly relevant. The techniques of lead extraction have been described in several recent reviews.[38,39] Percutaneous lead extraction is a technically demanding practice requiring significant operator training and experience. Complications of extraction can be catastrophic, with fatal outcomes despite immediate surgical intervention.[40] Major complications include cardiac or vascular avulsion, pulmonary embolism, stroke, and death. The importance of operator experience is reflected in the changes in the published recommendations for lead extraction. The North American Society of Pacing and Electrophysiology policy statement, published in 2000,[41] recommended that a physician needs a minimum of 20 lead extractions as the primary operator under supervision of an operator who has performed in excess of 100 extractions. The recent Heart Rhythm Society (HRS) guidelines, published in 2009, recommended a minimum of 40 supervised lead extractions and at least 20 extractions per year to maintain skill.[42] Forty lead extractions may be difficult to obtain even in high-volume two-year fellowship training programs. Surgical (open-heart) extraction may be indicated in some cases, but has a survival rate comparable with percutaneous methods.[43] The reported morbidity and mortality from percutaneous lead extraction primarily reflect risks related to pacemaker-lead extraction. A European report of the experience of a single center contained only 54 ICD leads of 1032 extracted leads. There was no relationship between the type of lead extracted and the morbidity and mortality.[44]

However, another series showed a trend toward higher morbidity with ICD lead extractions.[45] The morbidity and mortality of ICD lead extraction have not been fully defined. The HRS consensus recommendations for the class I and IIa indications for a nonfunctional lead (pacing or high voltage) are summarized in **Box 2**. There are small case series of ICD leads causing intractable ventricular arrhythmias that were cured with extraction.[46] There are no examples of ICD leads (on advisory) with a failure mechanism that represents an immediate threat to patient safety if left in place. Lead extraction is indicated if there are no other options for vascular access. However, the belief that increasing lead burden increases the risk of symptomatic or asymptomatic venous occlusion has not been substantiated. For example, patients who receive cardiac resynchronization devices have not been shown to have a higher risk of venous obstruction compared with patients who receive a single-chamber ICD. Asymptomatic unilateral venous occlusion has not been shown to effect morbidity or mortality. The endovascular damage that occurs with extraction may itself predispose to venous occlusion.

Passive-fixation leads may be more difficult to extract because of excessive tissue growth around the tines. Excessive lead length in the heart increases the difficulty of extraction. Dual-coil leads are associated with more fibrosis and tissue in-growth, increasing the difficulty of extraction. Most modern ICD leads have addressed this with

---

Box 2
Indications for transvenous lead extraction (class I and IIa)

Tranvenous lead extraction may be indicated or reasonable in the following situations:

A retained lead or lead fragment that causes life-threatening arrhythmias (I)

A design characteristic or failure mechanism that poses an immediate (I) or potential (IIa) threat to the patient if the lead is left in place

A lead that interferes with the operation of the implanted device (I)

A lead that interferes with the treatment of a malignancy (I)

The implantation of another lead would result in more than 4 leads on 1 side or more than 5 leads through the SVC (IIa)

The existing lead prohibits an essential diagnostic imaging modality (eg, magnetic resonance imaging) (IIa)

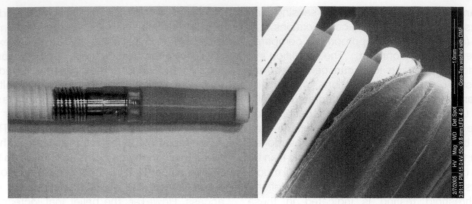

Fig. 16. Exposed bare coil as the Gore coating "slides off" on a Boston Scientific Endotak lead. (*Courtesy of* St Jude Medical, Inc, St Paul, MN; with permission.)

backfilling of the coils with medical adhesive (silicon) or covering the coils with ePTFE. The backfill and ePTFE coating methods result in easier extraction compared with bare coils. There are no clinical data comparing ePTFE with silicon backfill. There are also no clinical data suggesting that silicon backfill of flat coil leads is superior to silicon backfill of round leads with respect to extraction. Manufacturer reports regarding expected performance of any of these techniques are based on small animal studies. ePTFE coating of the coils of the current generation of leads is passive; the ePTFE is held in place by friction with the coil. If not implanted according to manufacturer recommendations, the coating may "bunch up" or "slide off," exposing bare coil (**Fig. 16**). Displacement of the ePTFE coating does not affect the electrical function of the lead. ePTFE has also been known to "bunch up" during extraction, potentially making it more difficult to remove these leads (**Fig. 17**). However, there are no clinical data suggesting that bunching of the ePTFE

material results in prolonged procedure times or adverse patient events.

Leads have been known to uncoil during extraction, resulting in failed extraction or retained components. A locking stylet is used to pull the lead from the tip during extraction. Some manufacturers have connected the cabled conductors to the body of the lead at the tip and yoke, effectively creating a built-in locking stylet (Tensi-Lock technology, Medtronic, Inc). This connection is meant as a redundancy and does not obviate the need for a true locking stylet. Ineffective sealing of the tip of the lead can allow blood into the lumen of the coil, preventing complete distal passage of any stylet.

MONITORING, DETECTING AND REPORTING OF LEAD MALFUNCTION AND FAILURE

A remarkable amount of research (bench and animal studies) and engineering skill go into the development of every pacing and defibrillation

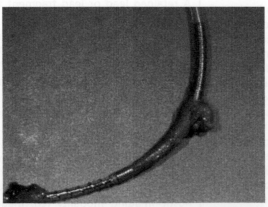
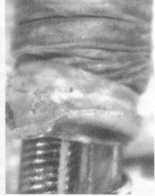

Fig. 17. Examples of the ePTFE coating "bunching-up" during extraction of a Boston Scientific Endotak lead. (*Courtesy of* Raymond H.M, Schaerf, MD, Burbank, CA.)

lead, even before premarket testing. As shown by the history of lead recalls, these practices alone are inadequate predictors of lead performance and reliability. In vivo variables and implant technique are difficult to account for. Manufacturers use a set of standard tests when assessing lead performance on the bench. Each manufacturer also uses unique tests to meet its own internal standards. Furthermore, lead design is an evolutionary process but there are no accepted definitions of a "new" lead such as to warrant a new series of clinical data or a set of industry standards.

The true incidence of lead failure is difficult to ascertain because of underreporting. Most failed leads are usually not explanted and returned to the manufacturer for analysis. Leads may be damaged during removal, complicating the analysis of the failure mechanism. Current monitoring of lead performance relies primarily on industry-based postmarket surveillance and voluntary reporting to the FDA. The MedWatch program (http://www.fda.gov/medwatch) allows physicians to report any variety of concern related to medical devices. This information is then entered into the Manufacturer and User Device Experience (MAUDE) database. In addition to underreporting and reporting bias, the utility of the MAUDE database is limited by nonvalidated entries. HeartNet is a subnetwork of the FDA's Medical Product Surveillance Network (MedSun) that focuses specifically on medical devices used in the electrophysiology laboratory. Entries are made into a publically searchable database by specialists from a large number of preselected medical facilities. Postmarket surveillance is also conducted by industry. This includes prospective registries RPA, and adverse event reports. RPA has the potential to provide insight into the mechanism of lead failure but is limited because many failed leads are abandoned and not extracted. In addition, several independent registries now exist that specifically follow ICD leads. These registries include the Danish Pacemaker and ICD registry, the United Kingdom Pacemaker and ICD Registry, the Minneapolis Heart Institute Multicenter Registry, and the National Cardiovascular Data Registry (NCDR). The data in the NCDR are derived from the Centers for Medicare and Medicaid Services (CMS) primary prevention implant data and represent more than 88% of all ICDs implanted in the United States. This will be the largest database of its kind and has the potential to yield useful information and identify uncommon lead-performance issues. Remote monitoring using proprietary Internet-based software and equipment specific to each manufacturer can provide enhanced surveillance and assist the management of individual patients.[47] For example, to identify impending lead fractures and reduce the risk of inappropriate shocks for patients with the Fidelis lead, Medtronic has made several recommendations, including enabling lead-impedance alerts and extending tachycardia detection intervals. The lead-integrity algorithm (LIA) is a downloadable RAMware (Medtronic Inc, Minneapolis, MN, USA) that should be added to all ICDs with a Fidelis lead. The LIA algorithm is effective in identifying impending fractures, but cannot capture all fractures before they present, especially if the change in impedance is less than the recommended alert level.[48,49] The HRS has recently published a set of guidelines addressing the monitoring, detecting, and reporting of lead malfunction and failure.[50] For these various systems to be effective in identifying potential lead problems, the individual clinician needs to be proactive in reporting suspected malfunctions to the regulatory agencies and to the manufacturer.

SUMMARY

The continued expansion of indications for ICD implantation and improved mortality rates for patients receiving ICDs will place increasing demand on ICD leads. They will routinely need to withstand two or perhaps three generator replacements during their service lifetime. The evolution of lead design has been influenced as much by lead failures as by successes. The last 15 years of lead design have yielded the following conclusions:

1. A multilumen ICD lead is superior to a coaxial design.
2. Conductor fracture and insulation breach are the primary mechanisms of failure.
3. Lead size, reliability, and safety are not mutually exclusive.
4. A combination of silicon and polyurethane or a copolymer is superior to silicon or polyurethane alone for insulation.
5. Engineering and design cannot completely protect against improper implant technique or patient factors.
6. The management of a patient with a failed, noninfected ICD lead should be highly individualized. Despite the evolution of lead extraction techniques, the strategy of abandoning a failed lead is not inferior to extraction.
7. A comprehensive approach from all participants and regulatory agencies is needed to identify and remove problematic leads from the market. An objective and transparent analysis of returned products is needed to identify the mechanism of failure.

ACKNOWLEDGMENTS

I would like to acknowledge Boston Scientific Inc, Medtronic Inc, and St Jude Medical Inc for technical assistance in the preparation of this article.

REFERENCES

1. Kleeman T, Becker T, Doenges K, et al. Annual rate of transvenous defibrillatin lead defects in implantable cardioverter-defibrillators over a period of >10 years. Circulation 2007;115(19):2474–80.
2. Collier TO, Kao JW. In-vivo biocompatibility and biostability of modified polyurethanes. J Biomed Mater Res 1997;36:246–57.
3. Lim KK, Reddy S, Desai S, et al. Effects of electrocautery on transvenous lead insulation materials. J Cardiovasc Electrophysiol 2009;20(4):429–35.
4. Cooper JM, Sauer WH, Garcia FC, et al. Covering sleeves can shield the high-voltage coils from lead chatter in an integrated bipolar ICD lead. Europace 2007;9(2):137–42.
5. Koplan BA, Weiner S, Gilligan D, et al. Clinical and electrical performance of expanded polytetraflouroethylene-covered defibrillator leads in comparison to traditional leads. Pacing Clin Electrophysiol 2008;31(1):47–55.
6. Wilkoff BL, Belot PH, Love CJ, et al. Improved extraction of ePFTE and medical adhesive modified defibrillation leads from the coronary sinus and great cardiac vein. Pacing Clin Electrophysiol 2005;28:205–11.
7. Neibauer MJ, Wilkoff B, Yamanouchi Y, et al. Iridium oxide-coated defibrillation electrode: reduced shock polarization and improved defibrillation efficacy. Circulation 1997;96:3732–6.
8. Lang DJ, Heil JE, Hahn SJ, et al. Implantable cardioverter-defibrillator lead technology: improved performance and lower defibrillation thresholds. Pacing Clin Electrophysiol 1995;18(3 Pt 2):548–59.
9. Frain BH, Ellison KE, Michaud GF, et al. True bipolar leads have increased sensing latency and thresholds compared with integrated bipolar configurations. J Cardiovasc Electrophysiol 2007;18(2):192–5.
10. Sweeney MO, Ellison KE, Shea JB, et al. Provoked and spontaneous high-frequency, low-amplitude, respirophasic noise transients in patient with implantable cardioverter defibrillators. J Cardiovasc Electrophysiol 2001;12(4):402–10.
11. Issa ZF. Inadvertent transposition of defibrillator coil terminal pins causing inappropriate ICD therapies. J Interv Card Electrophysiol 2008;22(1):63–8.
12. Sperry RE, Ellenbogen KA, Wood MA, et al. Failure of a second and third generation implantable cardiovertor defibrillator to sense ventricular tachycardia: implications for fixed-gain sensing devices. Pacing Clin Electrophysiol 1992;15:749–55.
13. Kapa S, Curwin JH, Coyne RF, et al. Inappropriate defibrillator shocks from depolarization-repolarization mismatch in a patient with hypertrophic cardiomyopathy. Pacing Clin Electrophysiol 2007;30(11):1408–11.
14. Otmani A, Rey JL, Leborgne L. T-wave oversensing during exercise one year after cardioverter defibrillator implantation for Brugada syndrome. Arch Cardiovasc Dis 2008;101(4):292–4.
15. Tuzcu V. Resolution of T-wave oversensing with implantable cardioverter defibrillator generator replacement in an adolescent. Pacing Clin Electrophysiol 2007;30(7):929–32.
16. Srivasthan K, Scott LR, Altemose G. T-wave oversensing and inappropriate shocks: a case report. Europace 2008;10(5):552–5.
17. Freedman RA, Petrakian A, Boyce K, et al. Performance of dedicated versus integrated bipolar defibrillator leads with CRT-defibrillators: results from a Prospective Multicenter Study. Pacing Clin Electrophysiol 2009;32(2):157–65.
18. Weretka S, Michaelsen J, Becker R, et al. Ventricular oversensing: a study of 101 patients implanted with dual chamber defibrillators and two different lead systems. Pacing Clin Electrophysiol 2003;26(1 Pt 1):65–70.
19. Gold M, Val-Mejias J, Leman RB, et al. Optimization of superior vena cava coil position and usage for transvenous defibrillation. Heart Rhythm 2008;5(3):394–9.
20. Kroll MW, Efimov IR, Tchou PJ. Present understanding of shock polarity for internal defibrillation: the obvious and non-obvious clinical implications. Pacing Clin Electrophysiol 2006;29(8):885–91.
21. Borleffs CW, van Erven L, van Bommel RJ, et al. Abstract 4695: risk of failure of implantable cardioverter defibrillator leads. Circulation 2008;118:S926.
22. Ellis CR, Rottman JN. Increased rate of subacute lead complications with small-caliber implantable cardioverter-defrillator leads. Heart Rhythm 2009;6(5):619–24.
23. Epstein AE, Baker JH 2nd, Beau SL, et al. Performance of the St. Jude Medical Riata leads. Heart Rhythm 2009;6(2):204–9.
24. Messali A, Thomas O, Chauvin M, et al. Death due to an implantable cardiovertor defibrillator. J Cardiovasc Electrophysiol 2004;15(8):953–6.
25. Budzikowski AS, Uyguanco E, Gunsburg MY, et al. Twisting until it breaks: a rare cause of ICD lead failure. Cardiol J 2008;15(6):558–60.

26. Epstein AE, Shepard RB. Failure of one conductor in a nonthoracotomy implantable defibrillator causing inappropriate sensing and potentially ineffective shock delivery. Pacing Clin Electrophysiol 1993; 16(4 Pt 1):796–800.

27. Bracke FA, Meijer A, van Gelder LM. Malfunction of endocardial defibrillator leads and lead extraction: where do they meet? Europace 2002;4: 19–24.

28. Mera F, DeLurgio DB, Langberg JJ, et al. Transvenous cardioverter defibrillator lead malfunction due to terminal connector damage in pectoral implants. Pacing Clin Electrophysiol 1999;22(12): 1797–801.

29. Dorwarth U, Frey B, Dugas M, et al. Transvenous defibrillation leads: high incidence of failure during long-term follow-up. J Cardiovasc Electrophysiol 2003;14:38–43.

30. Hauser RG, Cannom D, Hayes DL, et al. Long-term structural failure of co-axial polyurethane implantable cardiovascular defibrillator leads. Pacing Clin Electrophysiol 2002;25(6):879–82.

31. Ellenbogen KA, Wood MA, Shepard RK, et al. Detection and management of an implantable cardioverter lead failure: incidence and clinical implications. J Am Coll Cardiol 2003;41:73–80.

32. Nilsson KRJ, Hranitzky P. Early failure of a small diameter high-voltage implantable cardioverter lead. Heart Rhythm 2008;5:168–9 [author reply 169].

33. Farwell D, Green MS, Lemery R, et al. Accelerating risk of Fidelis lead fracture. Heart Rhythm 2008;5: 1375–9.

34. Wollman CG, Bocker D, Loher A, et al. Incidence of complications in patients with implantable cardioverter/defibrillator who received additional transvenous pace/sense leads. Pacing Clin Electrophysiol 2005;28(8):795–800.

35. Glikson M, Suleiman M, Luria DM, et al. Do abandoned leads pose risk to implantable cardioverter-defibrillator patients? Heart Rhythm 2009;6:65–8.

36. Fotuhi PC, KenKnight BH, Melnick SB, et al. Effect of a passive endocardial electrode on defibrillation efficacy of a non-thoracotomy lead system. J Am Coll Cardiol 1997;29:825–30.

37. Noma M, Kuga K, Matsushita S, et al. Intracardiac lead fracture in an implantable cardioverter-defibrillator. Int Heart J 2005;46(5):903–7.

38. Love CJ. Lead extraction. Heart Rhythm 2007;4: 1238–43.

39. Verma A, Wilkoff BL. Intravascular pacemaker and defibrillator lead extraction: a state-of-the-art review. Heart Rhythm 2004;1(6):739–45.

40. Krishnan SC, Epstein LM. Initial experience with a laser sheath to extract chronic transvenous implantable cardioverter-defibrillator leads. Am J Cardiol 1998;82:1293–5.

41. Love CJ, Wilkoff BL, Byrd CL, et al. Recommendations for extraction of chronically implanted transvenous pacing and defibrillator leads: indications, facilities, training. Pacing Clin Electrophysiol 2000; 24(4 Pt 1):544–51.

42. Wilkoff BL, Love CJ, Byrd CL, et al. Transvenous lead extraction: heart rhythm society expert consensus on facilities, training, indications, and patient management. Heart Rhythm 2009;6: 1085–104.

43. Camboni D, Wollmann CG, Loher A, et al. Explantation of implantable defibrillator leads using open heart surgery or percutaneous techniques. Ann Thorac Surg 2008;85:50–5.

44. Kennergren C, Bjurman C, Wiklund R, et al. A single center experience of over one thousand lead extractions. Europace 2009;11(5):612–7.

45. Agrawal SK, Kamireddy S, Nemec J, et al. Predictors of complications of endovascular chronic lead extractions from pacemakers and defibrillators: a single operator experience. J Cardiovasc Electrophysiol 2009;20:171–5.

46. Lee JC, Epstein LM, Huffer LL, et al. ICD lead proarrhythmia cured by lead extraction. Heart Rhythm 2009;6(5):613–8.

47. Spencker S, Coban N, Koch L, et al. Potential role of home monitoring to reduce inappropriate shocks in implantable cardioverter-defibrillator patients due to lead failure. Europace 2009;11(4):483–8 [Epub 2008 Dec 22].

48. Swerdlow CD, Gunderson BD, Ousdigian KT, et al. Downloadable algorithm to reduce inappropriate shocks caused by fractures of implantable cardioverter-defibrillator leads. Circulation 2008;118: 2122–9.

49. Vlay SC. Limitation of programmed alerts to predict ICD lead failures. Pacing Clin Electrophysiol 2009; 32(4):554–5.

50. Maisel WH, Hauser RG, Hammill SC, et al. Recommendations from the Heart Rhythm Society Task Force on lead performance policies and guidelines. Heart Rhythm 2009;6(6):869–85.

Remote Monitoring— The Future of Implantable Cardioverter- Defibrillator Follow-up

Michael L. Bernard, MD, PhD, Ernest Matthew Quin, MD, Michael R. Gold, MD, PhD*

KEYWORDS

- Remote monitoring • ICD • CRT • Home monitoring
- Ventricular arrhythmias

Implantable cardioverter-defibrillators (ICD) and cardiac resynchronization therapy (CRT) devices have had a significant impact on the primary and secondary prevention of sudden cardiac death.[1–4] Although these devices provide substantial clinical benefit, they impose periprocedural and long-term risks, and the need for routine surveillance. These implantable devices commit both patient and provider to long-term follow-up for monitoring of arrhythmias and normal function. Current consensus recommendations are for device checks every 3 to 6 months for the first 12 months after implantation or upgrade, followed by semiannual visits.[5,6] Over the past 5 years, the expanded indications for ICD or CRT with defibrillation capabilities (CRT-D) dramatically increased the population of patients requiring ongoing follow-up. One approach to meet the clinical demand of the post-implantation population is remote monitoring of devices. Along with reducing clinic follow-up in stable patients, remote monitoring technology has the potential to improve clinical outcomes by providing early detection of adverse events.[7–17] With reduced clinic visits and timely recognition of significant clinical entities, this new generation of ICD–CRT-D offers the potential of lower cost and more efficient care. However, new technology often begets new, and sometimes unforeseen, clinical ramifications. Adjustments to current models of patient care and the feasibility of using

advanced technology and communications in a broad patient population must be addressed. Moreover, many physicians may not be comfortable with supplanting direct patient contact with remote data transmission. The logistic, financial, and technologic aspects of remote ICD–CRT-D monitoring as well as the current clinical use of this resource will be the focus of this article.

REMOTE MONITORING HISTORY

Remote monitoring of implanted cardiac devices has been used for over 30 years.[18,19] Initially used to track pacing, sensing, and battery status of pacemakers, transtelephonic monitoring (TTM) progressed with the advance of device technology and function to provide a useful means to monitor arrhythmias and more complex pacemaker function in the outpatient setting.[20,21] The major impact of remote monitoring in pacemaker patients was the reduction of clinic visits. TTM of ICDs began in the early 1990s and was initially used as an adjunct to scheduled device-interrogation visits.[22,23] Relative to pacemaker transmissions, remote ICD interrogation included a broader array of data including ventricular tachycardia or ventricular fibrillation (VT-VF) detection parameters, VT-VF therapies, and episode counters. As ICDs and pacemakers became more sophisticated, a need for improved information

Medical University of South Carolina, 25 Courtenay Drive, ART 7031, MSC 592, Charleston, SC 29425-5920, USA
* Corresponding author.
E-mail address: goldmr@musc.edu (M.R. Gold).

Card Electrophysiol Clin 1 (2009) 193–200
doi:10.1016/j.ccep.2009.08.013
1877-9182/09/$ – see front matter © 2009 Published by Elsevier Inc.

transmission capability became apparent. With advances in both device and communications technology, modernized remote monitoring systems were developed to meet the needs of home-based device surveillance.

In 2001, Biotronik developed the first widespread remote monitoring application for ICDs, the Home Monitoring (HM)-CardioMessenger system. Medtronic added ICDs and CRTs to their CareLink Network in 2005. Boston Scientific introduced Latitude Communicator for all device products in 2006. St Jude Medical initiated HouseCall Plus for use in ICD–CRT-Ds in 2007, and has developed the Merlin.net for use with their current devices. Initial reports of remote ICD monitoring demonstrated ease of use by both clinicians and patients.[8,24] Transmissions of data via remote monitoring systems correlate well with office-based interrogations.[9,25,26] Whereas there are no trials demonstrating cardiovascular mortality or morbidity benefits, early observational studies suggest that remote monitoring can detect occult medical and device-related events leading to hastened therapeutic interventions.[10,25] In addition, remote monitoring is associated with a reduction in numbers of inappropriate shocks delivered by ICDs.[27] Many devices can also detect atrial arrhythmias and provide surveillance of heart-failure parameters.[17] Currently over 200,000 implanted ICD-CRT device recipients use remote monitoring systems.[28]

REMOTE MONITORING SYSTEMS

Although there are significant differences among the available remote monitoring systems, many features are similar across platforms. All have the ability to monitor battery status, lead function, percentage of time paced, and device settings. Additionally, each system has programmable alerts for clinical events (arrhythmias, out-of-range lead values, etc), for which the clinic or physician is notified. Each has a secure Web site that can be accessed to evaluate device data, including electrograms. An example of a stored electrogram of an episode of asymptomatic ventricular tachycardia that was pace terminated is shown in **Fig. 1.** Data transfer times vary between systems with wireless and nonwireless capabilities, and the amount of information gathered (first interrogations usually requiring longer time), but download times are usually seconds to several minutes for a routine evaluation. In the United States, four companies have systems in place: Biotronik's HM, Boston Scientific's Latitude, Medtronic's CareLink, and St Jude Medical's Merlin.net patient-care network.

Biotronik HM

Biotronik has the longest track record with home monitoring, having developed the first system in 2001. Many of the trials validating the safety and efficacy of remote monitoring systems were initiated by Biotronik. Their system transfers data from a wireless, implanted device to the Cardio-Messenger system, which relays this information to a secure Web site. This is the only available data transfer system that uses cellular technology. CardioMessenger can be placed bedside for once-daily monitoring, or it can be carried with the patient so that almost continuous monitoring for alerts is available. While monitoring via the cellular telephone, CardioMessenger is available internationally (as long as a mobile telephone signal is available); monitoring via a standard telephone jack is available in the United States. Clinical alerts are relayed by fax, email, or text message, and can be viewed on a Web site. Biotronik has extended the use of this system to some of their pacemakers.

Boston Scientific LATITUDE Patient Management System

The LATITUDE system uses the LATITUDE Communicator and a standard telephone jack; the Communicator receives telemetry from the implanted device, and transmits this data to a secure Web site. For patients with a wireless-capable implanted device, the Communicator automatically collects data from the device on a programmed schedule (up to daily); information from nonwireless systems can be downloaded weekly using a wand. Since the Communicator can transmit data via any standard telephone jack within the United States, data can be downloaded regardless of location. Boston Scientific also has the Heart Failure Management system, which includes a blood pressure monitor and weight scale that transmit information wirelessly to the Communicator. These data, and a simple patient questionnaire that asks questions regarding difficulty of breathing and development of edema, are made available for review on the secure Web site.

Medtronic CareLink Network

CareLink uses the CareLink Monitor to transfer data from the device to a secure server over a standard telephone jack for review on the Web site. The system is capable of automatic downloads from wireless devices; appointments are scheduled by clinic staff and the device automatically transfers data on scheduled dates. Programmed

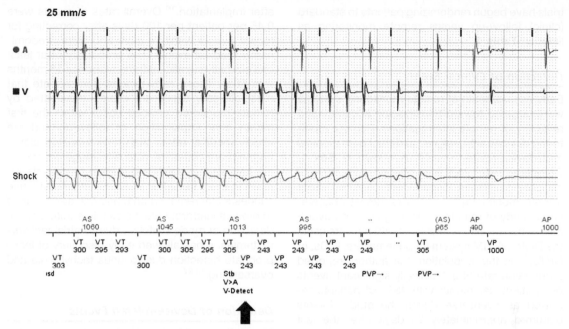

25 mm/s

A

V

Shock

AS 1060   AS 1045   AS 1013   AS 995   ..   (AS) 965   AP 490   AP 1000

VT 300 VT 295 VT 293   VT 300 VT 305 VT 295 VT 305   VP 243   VP 243   VP 243   VP 243   ..   VT 305   VP 1000

VT 303   VT 300   VP 243   VP 243   VP 243   VP 243

isd   Stb V>A V-Detect   PVP→   PVP→

Fig. 1. Latitude Patient Management electrogram report. The stored electrogram report demonstrates an episode of ventricular tachycardia and appropriate antitachycardia pacing, denoted by the arrow, which successfully terminated the arrhythmia. Note the atrio-ventricular dissociation in ventricular tachycardia.

alerts are automatically sent to the Web site, and can be transmitted to the clinic. For implants that are not capable of wireless telemetry, a wand is available; however, automatic downloads are not possible for these systems. In addition to basic device data, transthoracic impedance (OptiVol) trends, and heart rate and arrhythmia trends are available for review on the Web site.

St Jude Medical Merlin.net Patient Care Network

Merlin.net is the successor to the Housecall Plus Remote Patient Monitoring System (which is still available for the Atlas and Epic family of devices). The Merlin.net system, which services the wireless Current ICD and Promote CRT-D devices, uses the Merlin@home transmitter to download data from the implanted device, and transfers this data over a standard telephone outlet to a secure Web site. Like the other systems, it provides daily monitoring with automatic uploads, and has programmable alerts for clinical events. The format is the same as that of the Merlin programmer, which makes it easy to use for staff accustomed to using this system in a clinic setting. Alerts for significant events can be sent via email, fax, or text message. This system also has an automated patient contact system, DirectCall, which can remind patients of upcoming scheduled remote follow-ups, inform them of missed follow-ups,

notify the patient that a transmission was received and is normal, or ask the patient to call the physician's office. There is a built-in system for integration with certain electronic health record systems and device monitoring systems. Monitoring of patient data is also available through Mednet Health Care Technologies, Inc (Ewing, NJ, USA), although there is a subscription fee for this service.

CLINICAL IMPACT OF REMOTE-MONITORING SYSTEMS

Development of ICD-CRT remote monitoring stemmed from the desire to streamline postimplantation patient care and to provide a new modality to facilitate rapid detection and treatment of silent, yet significant, clinical events. To date, studies designed to assess improved outcomes are largely limited to observational investigations. Primary and secondary clinical measures included accuracy of home interrogation versus clinic interrogation, time to clinical decision, recognition of inappropriate shocks, and detection of device malfunction. The majority of available reports analyzed patients using the Biotronik HM system; however, the more recently developed brands are increasingly represented in the literature. There are currently no published reports comparing different monitoring systems. As of 2009, several trials have begun randomizing patients to standard (clinic) follow-up versus remote monitoring as listed in **Table 1**.

Detection of Clinical Events

Early assessments of remote monitoring systems were targeted toward transmission accuracy and reliability of remote interrogations. Remote monitoring devices are designed to detect both medical and device-related events as shown in **Box 1**. Compared with office interrogation, over 90% of clinically significant events were captured using remote monitoring.[9,27,29,30] The largest observational study of remote monitoring included over 3 million transmissions in over 11,000 patients using the Biotronik HM system for pacemakers, ICDs, or CRTs.[25] In this population, the authors reported a detection rate of 0.6 clinically significant events per patient per month with 48% of patients reported as event-free during the study. Events occurred approximately 26 days after the last follow up, and were mostly due to medical rather than device configuration events (86% vs 13%). A smaller observational study of over 57,148 transmissions among patients using HM for their ICD-CRTs demonstrated event detection rates of 0.14 events per patient per month with 62% and 45% of patients event free at 1 and 4 years, respectively.[31] Medical events compromised 94% of transmissions, of which 69% represented detections in the VF and VT zones. In a study of 260 ICD recipients with mean follow-up of 10 months, over 60% of HM events occurred in the first month

after implantation.[16] Overall rates of events were 0.45 per patient per 100 days after correcting for repeat events within 2 days and were predominantly medical events. The probability of at least one clinically significant transmission at 18 months was 50%. These early reports demonstrate that most clinically significant events transmitted by remote monitored devices occur within the first month after implantation or follow-up and are largely medical rather than device-related alerts. Furthermore, rates of clinically triggered events are low, with a significant portion of patients remaining event free after 1 year. Emerging evidence suggests that remote monitoring can also be used to prevent inappropriate shocks. In addition to the detection of mode switches due to atrial tachyarrhythmias, it has allowed early discovery of inappropriate detection due to sinus tachycardia and oversensing.[10,27]

Detection of Device-related Events

There is a significant body of literature describing anecdotal experience of home monitoring providing early recognition of device malfunctions and component failures, and a growing amount of data on the use of remote monitoring to assess device function. In pacemakers, for example, early lead microdislodgement has been detected leading to timely revision.[7,13] Lead fracture and lead insulation defects have been noted in ICDs.[15,32] In the largest observational report of remote monitoring in patients with pacemakers, ICDs, and CRT-Ds, consisting of 11,624 patients

Table 1
Ongoing clinical trials investigating clinical and quality measures and cost-effectiveness of remote monitoring in ICD-CRT populations

Name	Sponsor	Outcomes	Identifier
Medusa SAK	Duke University Medtronic	Patient outcomes Health care costs	NCT00606567
Monitor-ICD	Charite University, Berlin Biotronik	Clinical and cost efficacy	NCT00787683
EuroEco	Biotronik	Cost-effectiveness	NCT00776087
MORE-CARE	Medtronic	Clinical efficacy Resource use	NCT00885677
ANVITE	Biotronik	Clinical safety, efficacy	NCT00858559
EVOLVO	Medtronic	Rate of clinic visits	NCT00873899
EVATEL	Rennes University Hospital	Clinical efficacy	NCT00598026
TIM-HF	Charite University, Berlin	Mortality	NCT00543881
ConnectOptiVol	Medtronic	Heart failure outcomes	NCT00730548
QUANTUM	Biotronik	Quality of life	NCT00325221
IN-TIME	Biotronik	Prevention of hospitalization	NCT00538356

| Box 1 |
| Medical and device alerts |

Medical alerts

Supraventricular tachycardia detection

Atrial tachycardia or atrial fibrillation burden

Non-sustained ventricular tachycardia

VT detection

VF detection

Inadequate CRT pacing

Device alerts

Elective replacement interval

End of service

VT/VF detection off

Emergency pacing

High lead impedance

Low atrial or ventricular sensing

Ineffective high output shock

and including over 3 million transmissions, clinical or device events were noted an estimated 64 days earlier for patients followed at 3-month intervals, and 154 days earlier for those followed at 6-month intervals.[25] The majority of these events (86%) represented disease-related occurrences, but 66 alerts in patients with ICDs were indicators of device dysfunction. Of similar importance was the detection of greater than or equal to one ineffective 30 J shock in 271 devices. A prospective evaluation of the efficacy and reliability of remote monitoring that involved 69 patients with ICDs followed for 18 ± 9 months revealed right ventricular lead dysfunction in 8 (including lead fracture, connection or sensing defects, and lead dislodgement). Six of these 8 were detected by remote monitoring with a theoretical improvement of 1.9 ± 0.5 months in detection time for 3-month follow-up and 4.9 ± 0.5 months for 6-month follow-up schedules.[30] A significant concern remaining is the inability of current systems to measure pacing thresholds. Although this has not been extensively investigated, one prospective evaluation found 25 episodes of elevated thresholds indicative of lead dislodgement in 24 patients; none of these events was detected with the remote monitoring system.[33] Hopefully, with the increased prevalence and improvement of auto-capture algorithms in devices that automatically adjust outputs to maintain capture, pacing threshold data will become more common in remote monitoring.

Outcomes, Morbidity, and Mortality

Whereas there are little data that remote monitoring improves outcomes, several trials are currently evaluating the technology. At this time there is strong evidence that remote monitoring leads to the early detection of arrhythmias.[17,30] In one report, early detection of atrial fibrillation resulted in earlier follow-up in-clinic in 78% of patients, with initiation of anticoagulation in 36%. This resulted in a median gain in time for first intervention for atrial fibrillation of 50 days.[17] The only prospective comparison of remote monitoring against conventional follow-up revealed no significant differences in hospitalization or mortality, but did show significant cost savings.[34] In the Home CARE pilot study, a retrospective analysis of remote data from CRTs showed an increase in resting heart rate and mean heart rate over 24 hours within 7 days before hospitalization.[35] Whether this information will lead to better outcomes is under study.

Cost-effectiveness and Resource Utilization

Cost- and resource-use estimates suggest that remote monitoring could play a significant role in reduction of health care costs, and decrease the amount of time spent in follow-up. It is estimated that conversion of conventional follow-up to remote monitoring for 100 patients would result in a time-savings for a physician of 81 hours over the course of a year.[34] The estimated decrease in the cost of follow-up has been calculated at greater than $2000 over the course of 5 years in one analysis.[36] A prospective evaluation of cost-effectiveness in 41 patients showed a reduction in monitoring time for physicians from 26 minutes to 8 minutes, and a reduction in overall costs of follow-up of 41% over a 9-month evaluation period.[29] These findings have led to suggested methods for integration of remote monitoring into routine clinical practice.[33,37]

Reimbursement

Under guidelines currently in place by the Centers for Medicare and Medicaid Services, codes have been established for billing remote-device interrogation, and are the same as that for an in-person interrogation. An additional code has been established for the technical component services aspect of remote interrogation. Unlike the in-person (clinic) interrogation codes, billing for remote interrogation can occur only once per 90-day period, regardless of the number of remote interrogations that are performed; furthermore, billing for in-person interrogation is not reimbursable within this 90-day period (although codes for programming evaluation can be used during this period).

As more data become available remotely, the complexity of the organization of remote follow-up also increases. For instance, heart failure physicians may be interested in following body weight or other physiologic parameters remotely, such as transthoracic impedance or heart rate variability. However, they often do not want to follow or be responsible for arrhythmia determination of monitoring of device function. This can lead to multiple people wanting access to remote data on an individual patient. One solution for this was developed by Medtronic, where only limited data are available for those other than the primary physician caring for the device. The Cardiosight system allows health care providers who are not following device function, typically heart failure clinicians, to access physiologic parameters stored in ICD and CRT devices without risking inadvertent changes to device function. A read-only in-office device, the Cardiosight Reader, gathers up to 90 days of stored data, including OptiVol fluid trends, atrial fibrillation burden, heart rate variability, diurnal heart rates, patient activity, and percent pacing that are sent via fax to the provider. Devices that can track cardiovascular physiologic parameters, such as those using OptiVol technology, are considered Implantable Cardiovascular Monitors, ICMs. As of 2009, interrogation of ICMs once per 30 days is reimbursable and is deemed separate from interrogation of ICD-CRT functions.

Medical Legal Issues

A number of medical legal issues likely slowed the adoption of remote monitoring. For instance, physicians worry that they need to be available all day and night to address problems that may be detected. The concern is that delays in responding to an event that occurs on weekends or at night may lead to a liability risk. Some examples include the potential need for immediate attention to the onset of atrial fibrillation, lead malfunction, or shocks; this level of physician accessibility is impractical. In general, practicing within the standard of care in the community has taken precedent over unrealistic expectations of constant and immediate responsiveness by physicians. Thus, reasonable response rates are acceptable. Ownership of remote monitoring data is another interesting legal issue. When interrogated in an office, the data is part of the patient's chart. However, when remote monitoring is used, the device company is now the repository for patient data. Such data, when deidentified, are starting be used for research and clinical analyses. Health Insurance Portability and Accountability Act (HIPAA) and consent issues are typically addressed when patients are enrolled in a remote monitoring system. Finally, the security of remote data has raised some concerns from a legal perspective. Despite encryption and other technologies to protect data transmission, the "hacking" into a database or interception of transmissions could lead to significant patient safety and legal issues.

SUMMARY

Remote monitoring of ICD and CRT devices has grown dramatically over the past 5 years. It has evolved from a niche-marketing feature and curiosity to the standard of care for device follow-up. Today, nearly all modern ICD and CRT devices can be followed remotely with a significant savings of time for the patient and physician. Arrhythmias or device malfunctions can be detected more rapidly with remote monitoring, although the clinical impact of these findings is less clear. Also, other physiologic data such as intracardiac pressures, transthoracic impedance, and vital signs can be collected automatically to aid in the medical management of the patient. With the development of remote programming, clinic visits for device patients may become obsolete.

REFERENCES

1. Moss AJ, Zareba W, Hall J, et al. Multicenter Automatic Defibrillator Implantation Trial II Investigators. Prophylactic implantation of a defibrillator in patients with myocardial infarction and reduced ejection fraction. N Engl J Med 2002;346(12):877–83.
2. Bardy GH, Lee KL, Mark DB, et al. Sudden Cardiac Death in Heart Failure Trial (SCD-HeFT) Investigators. Amiodarone or an implantable cardioverter-defibrillator for congestive heart failure. N Engl J Med 2005;352(3):225–37.
3. The Antiarrhythmics Versus Implantable Defibrillators (AVID) Investigators. A comparison of antiarrhythmic-drug therapy with implantable defibrillators in patients resuscitated from near-fatal ventricular arrhythmias. N Engl J Med 1997; 337(22):1576–83.
4. Cleland JG, Daubert JC, Erdmann E, et al. Cardiac Resynchronization-Heart Failure (CARE-HF) Study Investigators. The effect of cardiac resynchronization on morbidity and mortality in heart failure. N Engl J Med 2005;352(15):1539–49.
5. Senges-Becker JC, Klostermann M, Becker R, et al. What is the "optimal" follow-up schedule for ICD patients? Europace 2005;7:319–26.

6. Epstein AE, DiMarco JP, Ellenbogen KA, et al. ACC/AHA/HRS 2008 guidelines for device-based therapy of cardiac rhythm abnormalities: a report of the American College of Cardiology/American Heart Association Task Force on Practice Guidelines (Writing Committee to Revise the ACC/AHA/NASPE 2002 guideline update for implantation of cardiac pacemakers and antiarrhythmia devices) developed in collaboration with the American Association for Thoracic Surgery and Society of Thoracic Surgeons. J Am Coll Cardiol 2008;51:e1–62.

7. Scholten MF, Thornton AS, Theuns DA, et al. Twiddler's syndrome detected by home monitoring device. Pacing Clin Electrophysiol 2004;27:1151–2.

8. Schoenfeld MH, Compton SJ, Mead RH, et al. Remote monitoring of implantable cardioverter defibrillators: a prospective analysis. Pacing Clin Electrophysiol 2004;27:757–63.

9. Varma N, Stambler B, Chun S. Detection of atrial fibrillation by implanted devices with wireless data transmission capability. Pacing Clin Electrophysiol 2005;28:S133–6.

10. Ritter O, Bauer WR. Use of "IEGM Online" in ICD patients—early detection of inappropriate classified ventricular tachycardia via Home Monitoring. Clin Res Cardiol 2006;95:368–72.

11. Santini M, Russo M, Ricci RP. Management of atrial fibrillation—what are the possibilities of early detection with home monitoring? Clin Res Cardiol 2006; 95(Suppl 3):III/10–6.

12. Res JC, Theuns DA, Jordaens L. The role of remote monitoring in the reduction of inappropriate implantable cardioverter defibrillator therapies. Clin Res Cardiol 2006;95(Suppl 3):III/17–21.

13. Loricchio ML, Castro A, Ciolli A, et al. Pacing failure de to microdislodgement of ventricular pacing lead detected by home monitoring technology. J Cardiovasc Med 2008;9:946–8.

14. Zartner P, Handke R, Photiadis J, et al. Performance of an autonomous telemonitoring system in children and young adults with congenital heart diseases. Pacing Clin Electrophysiol 2008;31: 1291–9.

15. Neuzil P, Taborsky M, Holy F, et al. Early automatic remote detection of combined lead insulation defect and ICD damage. Europace 2008;10: 556–7.

16. Nielsen JC, Kottkamp H, Zabel M, et al. Automatic home monitoring of implantable cardioverter defibrillators. Europace 2008;10:729–35.

17. Ricci RP, Morichelli L, Santini M. Remote control of implanted devices through Home Monitoring technology improves detection and clinical management of atrial fibrillation. Europace 2009;11:54–61.

18. Furman S, Escher DJ. Transtelephone pacemaker monitoring: five years later. Ann Thorac Surg 1975; 20:326–38.

19. Dreifus LS, Pennock RS, Feldman M, et al. Experience with 3835 pacemakers utilizing transtelephonic surveillance. Am J Cardiol 1975;35:133.

20. Dreifus LS, Zinberg A, Hurzeler P, et al. Transtelephonic monitoring of 25,919 implanted pacemakers. Pacing Clin Electrophysiol 1986;9:371–8.

21. Gessman LJ, Vielbig RE, Waspe LE, et al. Accuracy and clinical utility of transtelephonic pacemaker follow-up. Pacing Clin Electrophysiol 1995;18: 1032–6.

22. Anderson MH, Paul VE, Jones S, et al. Transtelephonic interrogation of the implantable cardioverter defibrillator. Pacing Clin Electrophysiol 1992;15: 1144–50.

23. Fetter JG, Stanton MS, Benditt DG, et al. Transtelephonic monitoring and transmission of stored arrhythmia detection and therapy data from an implantable cardioverter defibrillator. Pacing Clin Electrophysiol 1995;18:1531–9.

24. Joseph GK, Wilkoff BL, Thomas D, et al. Remote interrogation and monitoring of implantable cardioverter defibrillators. J Interv Card Electrophysiol 2004;11:161–6.

25. Lazarus A. Remote, wireless, ambulatory monitoring of implantable pacemakers, cardioverter defibrillators, and cardiac resynchronizatin therapy systems: analysis of a worldwide database. Pacing Clin Electrophysiol 2007;30(Suppl 1):S2–12.

26. Heidbuchel H, Pieter L, Stefaan F, et al. Potential role of remote monitoring for scheduled and unscheduled evaluations of patients with an implantable defibrillator. Europace 2008;10:351–7.

27. Spencker S, Coban N, Koch L, et al. Potential role of home monitoring to reduce inappropriate shocks in implantable cardioverter-defibrillator patients due to lead failure. Europace 2009;11:483–8.

28. Jung W, Rillig A, Birkemeyer R, et al. Advances in remote monitoring of implantable pacemakers, cardioverter defibrillators and cardiac resynchronization therapy systems. J Interv Card Electrophysiol 2008;23:73–85.

29. Raatikainen MJ, Uusimaa P, van Ginneken MM, et al. Remote monitoring of implantable cardioverter defibrillator patients: a safe, time-saving, and cost-effective means for follow-up. Europace 2008;10: 1145–51.

30. Hauck M, Alexander B, Frederik V, et al. "Home monitoring" for early detection of implantable cardioverter-defibrillator failure: a single-center prospective observational study. Clin Res Cardiol 2009;98: 19–24.

31. Theuns DA, Rivero-Ayerza M, Knops P, et al. Analysis of 57,148 transmissions by remote monitoring of implantable cardioverter defibrillators. Pacing Clin Electrophysiol 2009;32(Suppl 1):S63–5.

32. Zartner PA, Handke RP, Brecher AM, et al. Integrated home monitoring predicts lead failure in

a pacemaker dependent 4-year-old-girl. Europace 2007;9:192–3.

33. Brugada P. What evidence do we have to replace in-hospital implantable cardioverter defibrillator follow-up? Clin Res Cardiol 2006;95(Suppl 3):3–9.

34. Elsner CH, Sommer P, Piorkowski C, et al. A prospective multicenter comparison trial of home monitoring against regular follow-up in MADIT II patients: additional visits and cost impact. Comput Cardiol 2006;33:241–4.

35. Ellery S, Pakrashi T, Paul V, et al. Predicting mortality and rehospitalization in heart failure patients with home monitoring—the Home CARE pilot study. Clin Res Cardiol 2006;95(Suppl 3):29–35.

36. Fauchier L, Sadoul N, Kouakam C, et al. Potential cost savings by telemedicine-assisted long-term care of implantable cardioverter defibrillator recipients. Pacing Clin Electrophysiol 2005;28:S255–9.

37. Ricci RP, Morichelli L, Santini M. Home monitoring remote control of pacemaker and implantable cardioverter defibrillator patients in clinical practice: impact on medical management and health-care resource utilization. Europace 2008;10:164–70.

Ventricular Tachycardia Ablation—For Whom, When, and How?

Conor D. Barrett, MD[a], Luigi Di Biase, MD[b,c,d],
Miguel Vacca, MD, MSc[e], Luis Carlos Saenz, MD[e],
J. David Burkhardt, MD[b], Jeremy N. Ruskin, MD[a],
Andrea Natale, MD, FACC, FHRS[b,f,g,h,i],*

KEYWORDS

- Ventricular tachycardia • Sudden death • Ablation
- Heart disease • Entrainment

In those with structurally abnormal hearts, the occurrence of either monomorphic ventricular tachycardia (MMVT) or polymorphic ventricular tachycardia (PMVT) often carries a poor prognosis. The mechanism for MMVT in such patients most often is caused by re-entry. Significant strides have been made in the primary and secondary prevention of sudden death in such individuals with the advent of the implantable cardioverter defibrillator (ICD).[1–4] Although many trials have demonstrated the efficacy of ICDs for preventing sudden death in both the secondary and primary prevention populations, ICDs do not prevent the occurrence of the arrhythmia. That ICD discharges are associated with significant morbidity (not least psychological) and an increased mortality has been recognized.[5] Therefore, although prevention of sudden death with an ICD is of prime importance, it makes sense that preventing the recurrence of the arrhythmia, or decreasing the arrhythmic burden, would be a reasonable strategy. Traditional approaches to the treatment of recurrent ventricular tachycardia (VT), necessitating ICD shocks, have included the prescription of antiarrhythmic drugs (AADs). Of course, such medications may prove to be ineffective, untolerated or indeed proarrhythmic and associated with increased mortality.[3,6] Thus, the routine use of antiarrhythmic medications in patients with structurally abnormal hearts has not been shown to be uniformly beneficial, and for some agents, use has been shown to be dangerous. Therefore, ablation of ventricular arrhythmias in those with structurally abnormal hearts has received increasing attention over the past several years.[7,8]

Patients without evidence of cardiac structural abnormalities also may experience VT. The mechanism of VT in such patients most often is because of triggered activity or enhanced automaticity, although re-entry (including micro-re-entry) also may be mechanistically important. These so-called normal-heart VTs tend to affect younger patients, who do not have demonstrable coronary artery disease, myocardial fibrosis, or cardiomyopathy. Such VTs often are associated with symptoms, with patients complaining of palpitations to near or frank syncope. Although such VTs most often are not related to sudden death, it nonetheless has been recognized that at times premature

[a] Cardiac Arrhythmia Service, Massachusetts General Hospital and Harvard Medical School Boston, USA
[b] Texas Cardiac Arrhythmia Institute at St David's Medical Center, 1015 East 32nd Street, Suite 506, Austin, TX 78705, USA
[c] Department of Cardiology, University of Foggia, Foggia, Italy
[d] Department of Biomedical Engineering, University of Texas, Austin, TX, USA
[e] Fundation Cardio Infantil, Bogota, Colombia
[f] Division of Cardiology, Stanford University, Palo Alto, CA, USA
[g] Case Western Reserve University, Cleveland, OH, USA
[h] EP Services, California Pacific Medical Center, San Francisco, CA, USA
[i] Department of Biomedical Engineering, University of Texas, Austin, TX, USA
* Corresponding author.
E-mail address: dr.natale@gmail.com (A. Natale).

Card Electrophysiol Clin 1 (2009) 201–211
doi:10.1016/j.ccep.2009.08.003
1877-9182/09/$ – see front matter © 2009 Published by Elsevier Inc.

ventricular contractions (PVCs) can be associated with triggering of VT and/or VF, and sudden death in rare patients without discernible cardiac structural abnormalities.[9,10] Also, high-density repetitive monomorphic PVCs have been implicated in the etiology of left ventricular dysfunction, akin to tachycardia-mediated cardiomyopathy. Ablation of PVCs in such patients has been demonstrated to result in normalization of left ventricular systolic function.[11]

VT ABLATION—FOR WHOM AND WHEN?

There has been much interest in the increasing population of patients with cardiomyopathy (both ischemic and nonischemic) who develop VT. In patients with structural heart disease and defibrillators, VT can be a recurrent and incessant problem (sometimes occurring as a storm) leading to significant patient morbidity and an increased mortality and heart failure rate.[5] Many now advocate that ablation of VT should be considered early in such patients. Recent guidelines also have reinforced the concept of an earlier interventional approach for such patients.[12] According to these recently published consensus guidelines, ablation is indicated for patients with recurrent symptomatic sustained (greater than 30 seconds in duration) MMVT despite AAD therapy (or in those in whom AAD therapy is not desired or tolerated). Ablation also is indicated for those who have incessant VT (or VT storm) that is not due to a reversible cause; for VT that is felt to have caused ventricular dysfunction; for bundle-branch reentry VT; and also for that subset of patients who have been refractory to AAD therapy, who have PVCs that trigger polymorphic VT or VF. It additionally is suggested that ablation be considered an acceptable alternative to amiodarone in patients who have had a prior myocardial infarction (MI) (left ventricular ejection fraction [LVEF] greater than 30%) and a life expectancy greater than 1 year. The fact that these guidelines recommend considering ablation for patients who have had a prior MI with sustained MMVT and an LVEF greater than 35% even if they have not failed AAD therapy is a marker of the electrophysiology (EP) community's increased understanding of the mechanisms of such scar-related VT and a sign of an appreciation of the success rates of ablation when performed by experienced operators.[13–15]

In patients with structurally normal hearts, the presence of disabling symptoms traditionally has been the indication for ablation of VT (most commonly outflow tract VT). This remains the case, particularly for those patients who are intolerant of or refractory to medications or in whom such therapy is not desired. Again, a small subset of patients without structural heart disease, who have PVC-triggered PMVT or VF, in whom the trigger is felt to be amenable to ablation, should be considered for an interventional approach.[9] Thus, although the presence of symptoms in such patients is the most common indication for ablation, it is important to recognize that a small subset of patients (without demonstrable structural heart disease) may have a more sinister manifestation of such PVCs. Also patients with high PVC burden or repetitive episodes of VT (frequently nonsustained) may develop ventricular dysfunction over time. Such patients also should be considered for ablation.

VT ABLATION—PREPROCEDURAL PLANNING

The approach to ablation of VT will depend on many factors, not least being patient characteristics and the characteristics of the VT. For example, the initial approach to a presumptive epicardial scar-related VT will be different than the approach of a presumptive fascicular VT.[16] Although one may have a good sense as to the likely mechanism and substrate for a particular VT preprocedurally, the operator should be able to adapt his or her approach during the case as necessary. With all catheter ablation procedures, preprocedural planning is of utmost importance. This not only includes the basic assessment of whether structural heart disease is present, but also an assessment of the nature and severity of the structural abnormality, if present. Preprocedure imaging, of some form, is mandatory and should be performed by echocardiography at least. Many find preprocedural imaging by magnetic resonance (MR) to be helpful in the precise localization of anatomic abnormalities, including the presence of myocardial fibrosis. The utility of MR, however, is limited in this patient population, as many will have ICDs already implanted. Others have found positron emission tomography (PET) to be valuable in such patients.[17,18] Interrogation of the patient's ICD should be performed, and all available arrhythmic events should be evaluated for electrogram morphologies and VT cycle lengths. ICD therapies should be programmed off at the start of the procedure. Preprocedure analysis of all available electrocardiograms (ECGs) of clinical VTs (and during baseline rhythm) should be undertaken to aid in the localization of the likely site or region of origin of the clinical VT. Also, the ablation strategy may be altered on the basis of the interpretation of the ECG; for example, a decision may be made to map the epicardium at the start of the procedure depending upon the ECG morphology of the clinical VT.[19]

Other details of preprocedural planning are outside the scope of this article, but, in brief, include the following

- Assessment for the presence of ventricular thrombus—the presence of a mobile or acute thrombus is a contraindication to endocardial mapping
- The decision of whether to use conscious sedation or general anesthesia
- The planning for anticoagulation before, during, and after the procedure (in particular in those patients who have coexisting atrial fibrillation) and in those in whom extensive ablation is performed in the left ventricle (LV)
- The proposed access sites and the assessment for peripheral vascular and aortic valve disease if a retrograde aortic approach is to be used
- The assessment of ongoing coronary ischemia (as the treatment of this in itself may decrease or abolish the arrhythmic burden)

VT ABLATION—TECHNICAL CONSIDERATIONS

The tools available to operators are increasing in number and sophistication, and have aided in the ablation procedures. The availability of three-dimensional electroanatomical mapping systems have aided greatly in the treatment of such patients, not only in the generation of activation and voltage maps, but also in the integration with other imaging modalities (preacquired CT or magnetic resonance imaging (MRI) images or real-time intracardiac echocardiographic images). The selection of imaging modalities and mapping systems to be employed is determined largely by operator preference. Most procedures are performed with a contact mapping system; however a noncontact mapping system may be beneficial for defining the VT exit site in cases where VT is poorly tolerated. Intracardiac echocardiography (ICE) also has been proven to add advantages to these procedures, in patients with and without structural heart disease.[20] The authors have found ICE to be particularly useful in monitoring for complications (such as pericardial effusion), defining real-time cardiac anatomy in patients with structural heart disease, and also in mapping of outflow tract VTs. An example of an image obtained during catheter mapping of the coronary cusps is shown in **Fig. 1**. The choice of energy source for the ablation is limited to radiofrequency

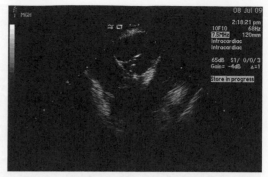

Fig. 1. An intracardiac echo image of the coronary cusps. The tip of the ablation catheter is seen in the left coronary cusp.

current (RF) or cryothermal energy. By far, most VTs are ablated with RF. For focal VTs (in structurally normal hearts), for example in the RVOT or aortic cusps, a 4mm tip catheter usually is chosen. For ablation of scar-related VTs, most operators now use an irrigated-tip catheter. If ablation is performed in the epicardial space with an open-irrigated tip catheter, periodic aspiration of the irrigating fluid must be performed. As many patients with scar-related VT have congestive heart failure, close attention must be paid to fluid volumes if such a catheter is employed during endocardial ablation. Although there are limited data with respect to cryoablation for VTs, success has been reported in some patients.[21] It is recognized that certain subsets of patients (eg, those with idiopathic dilated cardiomyopathy IDC, arrhythmogenic right ventricular cardiomyopathy [ARVC] and Chagas disease [CD]) are more likely to require an epicardial approach for elimination of VT. An example of scar in a patient with Chagas disease is shown in **Fig. 2**.

HOW—VT ABLATION STRATEGIES IN PATIENTS WITH STRUCTURAL HEART DISEASE

Patients with structural heart disease (eg, after myocardial infarction or surgical repair for congenital heart disease, dilated cardiomyopathy, ARVC, Chagas disease, sarcoid, or amyloidosis) in general have regions of definable scar.[22] VTs in such patients are more likely to be caused by re-entry than enhanced automaticity or triggered activity. Re-entry most commonly is related to those definable regions of scar (either around regions of scar or in the border zone), but bundle-branch reentry also may be seen, particularly in patients with dilated cardiomyopathy.

The approach to the ablation procedure primarily will be related to the ability to induce VT and the tolerability of induced VT. There are many mapping strategies available to the

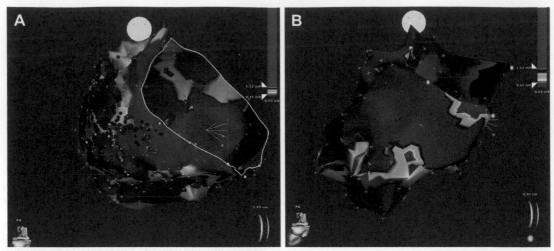

Fig. 2. Typical left ventricle posteroseptal scar in Chagas disease. Posterolateral view of a high-density epicardial (*A*) and endocardial (*B*) map obtained from a patient with Chagas disease and electrical storm showing a typical posterolateral scar with anterior and posterior extension close to the mitral annulus. The scar is mainly epicardial and basal. The endocardial surface is less affected.

operator, including substrate mapping, entrainment mapping, activation mapping, and pace mapping. For patients with scar-related VT, substrate and entrainment mapping are the preferable methods. It is advisable to exclude the diagnosis of bundle branch re-entry VT (BBR-VT) early in the case, as the treatment of this will be different (targeting the right bundle branch for ablation).

Substrate Mapping and Ablation Strategies

Mapping of the myocardial substrate is performed in a stable rhythm (eg, sinus), and it is performed to define those areas of the myocardium that could prove responsible for maintaining VT. Because induction of VT is not necessary, this is the preferred method for patients whose VTs not inducible in the EP laboratory or who have hemodynamically unstable induced VTs. Substrate mapping also typically is undertaken in patients who have multiple VTs. Many centers include substrate mapping (even in patients with hemodynamically stable VTs) as the initial component of the procedure. An electroanatomical map is generated of voltages in the ventricle. A commonly accepted approach is to define healthy myocardium as having a voltage greater than 1.5 mV and significant low voltage (scar) as less than 0.5 mV.[23] Although such regions of low voltage will correspond to regions of prior infarction in patients with an ischemic etiology, there is preponderance for low voltages to be located in the basal/peri-valvular regions in those with non-ischemic cardiomyopathy.[24] During acquisition of

the three-dimensional map, other points of interest are tagged. These regions include

Double potentials (electrograms with a long isoelectric period between them)—these potentials may define a region of electrical block

Fractionated or fragmented potentials (defined as multicomponent electrograms of a lengthy duration)—these potentials may represent important regions of slow conduction

Late potentials (which are observed later than 10 milliseconds from the terminal portion of the QRS)

Such regions later may be proven to be integral to the VT circuit. An example of an electroanatomical map with a large region of low voltage and points of fractionated and late potentials is shown in **Fig. 3**. If the substrate map was created before VT induction, then attempts at VT induction should be undertaken with programmed ventricular extrastimulation. If the resultant VT is hemodynamically stable, the operator then performs entrainment mapping of the VT. If the VT is hemodynamically unstable, it may be pace terminated or cardioverted. As in the latter scenario, if no hemodynamically stable VT is inducible, the ablation strategy will rely primarily on the substrate map. If there is foreknowledge (on the basis of a preprocedure ECG, for example) of the likely exit point of a VT, then brief periods of entrainment mapping may be possible even in those who tolerate VT relatively poorly. The correlation of observed late or

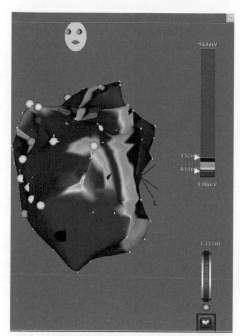

Fig. 3. An initial three-dimensional electroanatomical voltage map created of a patient with a distant history of anterior wall myocardial infarction who had received 20 implantable cardioverter–defibrillator therapies for ventricular tachycardia over the preceding week. Areas of scar (low voltage less than 0.5 mV) are shown in red. Areas of healthy myocardium (greater than 1.5 mV) are shown in purple. It is readily appreciable that a large volume of scar is present. The tagged regions near the scar border correspond to sites with fractionated, late, or split potentials.

fractionated potentials (on the substrate map) near regions of presumptive exit may permit this. Nonetheless, hemodynamically poorly tolerated VT should be terminated as quickly as possible.

After generation of the substrate map, attention is turned to modifying the substrate (usually with RF, as discussed previously). Several strategies have been described. The so-called border zone (voltages of 0.5 to 1.5 mV) can be targeted for ablation. The regions of scar can be small or quite large. Therefore entire border zone ablation in many patients would involve extensive ablation. Consequently, ablation is guided further on the basis of the electrogram properties, including regions of slow conduction and regions compatible with the location of a critical isthmus. Pace mapping at sites within the presumptive region of exit or isthmus also can be undertaken to confirm the same morphology as the observed VT. Pace mapping at sites with a long pacing stimulus to QRS interval with a resultant QRS morphology the same as the observed VT can be targeted for

ablation, as these sites may represent a critical isthmus for a re-entrant VT.[25] Furthermore, ablation can be targeted at regions of late potentials.[26,27] Because many potential exit sites may be observed, ablation usually is performed along the border zone, with additional lesions joining these sites to the region of scar (voltage less than 0.5 mV), thereby transecting the critical regions.[26,28] Thus, areas that are critical to maintaining the reentrant circuit are targeted for ablation via the substrate-guided approach to VT ablation (**Fig. 4**).

Entrainment Mapping and Ablation Strategies

In those patients who have hemodynamically stable VT, entrainment mapping is undertaken and is particularly useful. As stated previously, entrainment mapping may be performed in conjunction with substrate mapping, as the data acquired with substrate mapping will allow for more focused entrainment mapping during induced or spontaneous VT. The methodology of entrainment mapping for scar-related VT previously has been described in detail.[29] Entrainment mapping involves pacing at defined sites during VT at a cycle length slightly faster (by approximately 20 milliseconds) than the VT cycle length. The pacing current delivered ideally should be just above the pacing threshold. The responses to pacing and termination of pacing then are observed. This involves observation of the paced QRS morphology and its comparison with the VT QRS morphology, the measurement of postpacing intervals (PPIs), the observation of mid-diastolic ECGs, and the comparison of the relative timing of the stimulus to QRS with that of observed ECG to QRS. To reliably terminate VT, the critical isthmus must be ablated. This region has the characteristics of demonstrating

> Concealed fusion during entrainment (with the paced QRS having the same morphology as the VT QRS)
> A stimulation to QRS time of less than 70% of the VT cycle length, which equals the ECG to QRS time and
> A PPI that equals the tachycardia cycle length

Ablation at entrainment sites with all such characteristics most likely will result in termination of VT, with this area representing the critical isthmus for that re-entrant VT.[30,31]

Procedural End Points

Any clinical VT should be rendered noninducible at the end of the case. Attempts at induction are

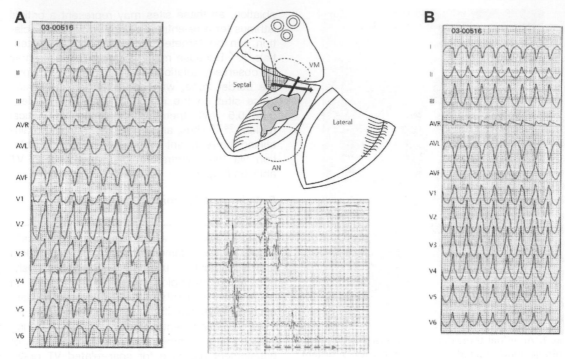

Fig. 4. Arrhythmic substrate related to the mitral annulus in Chagas cardiomyopathy. Left ventricle schema showing a peri-mitral isthmus between a posterior scar and the mitral annulus. Electrocardiogram (ECG) ventricular tachycardia morphology would depend on the exit of the circuit changing mainly from a superior axis deviation if the septum is activated first (left ECG) to an inferior axis deviation if the lateral wall is activated first (right ECG). A mitral isthmus line rendered noninducible both tachycardias. At the bottom, note the highly fragmented and late electrograms obtained at border of the scar.

made with programmed extrastimulation with up to three extra stimuli from two anatomically different sites and at two different drive trains. There remains a lack of consensus on other procedural endpoints in patients with structural heart disease undergoing VT ablation. Although some advocate the elimination of all inducible VT as a procedural end point, this remains controversial.[12]

VT ABLATION—PATIENTS WITHOUT STRUCTURAL HEART DISEASE

In contrast to patients with structural heart disease, patients with normal hearts are more likely to have enhanced automaticity or triggered activity as the mechanism for VT. This leads to the description of such VTs as focal, although localized re-entry may be mechanistically important in a small subset. Because such VTs are focal with centrifugal spread of activation, it intuitively makes sense that activation mapping will play an important role in their treatment. Consequently, activation and pace mapping are undertaken in such patients.

Activation Mapping

Activation mapping is performed easiest with the aid of an electroanatomical mapping system, which greatly aids in the localization of the site of earliest depolarization. This is represented as a color schema. The proposed successful site for ablation will be the location of earliest bipolar recording (typically approximately 30 milliseconds before QRS, with a QS on the unipolar recording). With VTs of a focal origin, it is important to ensure that all regions around the supposed early site are mapped. A wider region of early endocardial ECGs suggests a possible epicardial location of the focus. Prior to ablation at the earliest site, it is advisable to perform pace mapping also.

Pace Mapping

Pace mapping involves pacing (ideally at just suprathreshold current) at regions where the VT focus is thought to reside.[32] The resultant 12-lead ECG then is compared with the observed VT. A perfect match is one with all characteristics being identical between the paced QRS and VT QRS. Because no critical isthmus is involved, the stimulus to QRS will be shorter than that observed at successful sites for scar-related VT as discussed previously. It is advisable that comparisons are made at least at a sweep speed of 100 mm/s, so that subtle differences in QRS morphologies can be appreciated.

Specific Normal Heart VTs

Mapping and ablation strategies for different forms of normal heart VTs are considered.

Outflow tract VTs

Outflow tract VTs (OTVTs) arising from the right ventricular outflow tract (RVOT) or left ventricular outflow tract (LVOT) or coronary cusps are the most commonly encountered VTs in patients without structural heart disease. It is essential (as previously stated) that patients with structural heart disease (for example ARVD) and chanelopathies (for example Brugada syndrome) are not presumed to have OTVT, as they may demonstrate similar characteristics.[33,34]

RVOT VT is more common than LVOT-VT. Close inspection of the VT morphology is undertaken before mapping is commenced. It is recognized that RVOT-VT has an inferior axis, left bundle branch block (LBBB) morphology with an R wave transition at V4. LVOT-VT also has an inferior axis and may have a right bundle branch block (RBBB) or LBBB morphology, but with a transition by V2. R wave transition between these is indeterminate. Other important ECG characteristics include

- The observation of an M- or W-type pattern in V1 with a QS or rS in lead 1 (suggestive of an origin from the left coronary cusp) or a larger R wave in lead 1 (suggestive of a right coronary cusp origin)
- A qR pattern in V1 (suggestive of an origin at the aortomitral continuity)
- A precordial rS or RS to QRS ratio greater than 55% (suggestive of an epicardial origin) or a QS in lead 1 with the R wave in lead V2 being smaller than in lead V1 or V3 (suggestive of an epicardial location that may be ablated from within in distal great cardiac vein or anterior interventricular vein)[35–38] (**Fig. 5**).

Such a location is shown in **Fig. 6**. VT may be induced with burst pacing with or without the addition of Isoproterenol. After careful analysis of the VT morphology, an activation map is created, frequently with the aid of an electroanatomical mapping system. Pace mapping (at the cycle length of the VT) then may be performed at the sites of interest with careful attention to ensure a good or perfect (12 of 12) pace map. Best sites for ablation (usually with a 4 mm tip catheter) are those with a perfect pace map and local activation preceding surface QRS by at least 30 milliseconds.[39,40] In certain sites, however (in particular the coronary cusps), high current may be necessary to ensure capture; therefore a larger portion of myocardial capture cannot be excluded.

It is important that the operator has a sound knowledge of the anatomy and the relationship of the outflow tract tachycardia to the coronary arteries. Ablation in the cusps also carries with it the potential for subsequent valvular dysfunction and acute ostial coronary artery occlusion. Localization of the left main or right coronary arteries should be defined before ablation in the respective cusp. This may be accomplished with ICE or by a coronary angiogram. Similarly, VTs ablated from within the coronary sinus or anterior interventricular vein or after epicardial access may cause damage to the coronary arteries. An irrigated tip catheter frequently is employed in such circumstances also. Thus, knowledge of the location of these vessels is essential before lesion delivery.

Fascicular VTs in patients with normal hearts

Unlike many other VTs in patients without structural heart disease, the mechanism for fascicular VTs is re-entry in or adjacent to the fascicles of the left bundle branch (LBB). By far, most are of the left posterior fascicular type (giving a RBBB/superior axis morphology). Less common is the left anterior fascicle type (giving a RBBB/right axis morphology). Even less common is the so-called upper septal fascicular VT (giving a narrow QRS with a normal or rightward axis morphology). These tachycardias are sensitive to the administration of Verapamil. They may be targeted for ablation at sites with mid-diastolic potentials or at the VT exit site, where presystolic (Purkinje potentials) are noted. For left posterior fascicular VTs, this has been accomplished at the apical inferior septum and at the basal septum (closer to the proximal left bundle fascicle).[41–43]

Other VT locations

VTs also have been localized and ablated at the region of the mitral valve and papillary muscles and tricuspid annulus in patients with normal hearts. In nearly 10% of patients with no structural heart disease, epicardial ablation is required to successfully eliminate PVCs or VT. Triggering PVCs have been observed in different electrical disorders, including long QT syndrome, Brugada syndrome, short QT, and VF, and in patients following MI. Indeed, of particular interest are

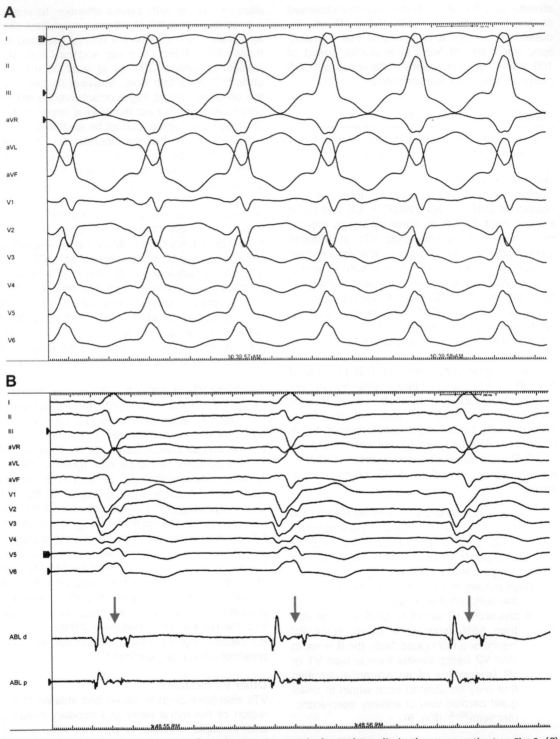

Fig. 5. (*A*) 12-Lead electrocardiogram of a spontaneous ventricular tachycardia in the same patient as **Fig. 6.** (*B*) Split potentials (*arrows*) observed in sinus rhythm (same patient as in **Fig. 6**)

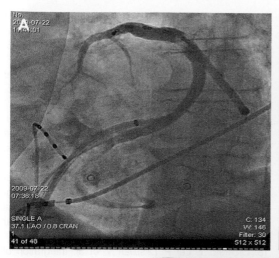
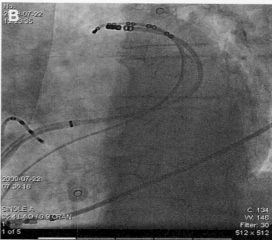
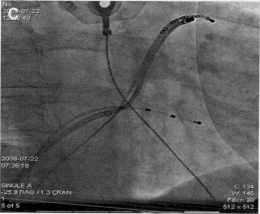

Fig. 6. (*A*) A CS venogram in the left anterior oblique view, demonstrating the great cardiac vein and anterior interventricular vein. (*B*) A similar view (left anterior oblique coronary artery) to the venogram in Fig. 6A. An externally irrigated tip ablation catheter has been advanced to the region where earliest activation of VT was observed. Ablation at this point resulted in termination of ventricular tachycardia. (*C*) The same catheter position as in 6B, but viewed in the RAO perspective.

those PVCs that have been observed to induce PMVT or VF. These may originate from the OT (as discussed previously), and they are recognized to be related to the Purkinje fibers. The latter are observed as narrow monomorphic PVCs that reliably initiate PMVT or VF (often resulting in storms in such patients). These PVCs have been targeted successfully for ablation. Because of the nature of the triggering PVC, such patients are often unstable, with frequent episodes of VF or PMVT at the time of mapping and ablation. Targeted successful sites are those with Purkinje potentials that closely precede the electrogram.[44]

SUMMARY

A diverse group of patients may manifest VT. The decision to undertake catheter ablation therapy is made for quality of life and palliation of symptoms in most patients without structural heart disease. A small subset of patients without structural heart disease may derive a mortality benefit from ablation, although this remains to be proven. In patients with structural heart disease, VT ablation can decrease the arrhythmic burden (and ICD therapies), which may have an impact not only on quality of life, but also potentially on life expectancy. Further studies will be necessary to help guide future strategies and timing of ablation therapy in this rapidly growing subset of patients.

REFERENCES

1. Connolly SJ, Gent M, Roberts RS, et al. Canadian implantable defibrillator study (CIDS): a randomized trial of the implantable cardioverter defibrillator against amiodarone. Circulation 2000;101:1297–302.

2. The Antiarrhythmics versus Implantable Defibrillators (AVID) Investigators. A comparison of antiarrhythmic drug therapy with implantable defibrillators in patients resuscitated from near-fatal ventricular arrhythmias. N Engl J Med 1997;337:1576–83.

3. Bardy GH, Lee KL, Mark DB, et al. Amiodarone or an implantable cardioverter–defibrillator for congestive heart failure. N Engl J Med 2005;352:225–37.

4. Moss AJ, Zareba W, Hall WJ, et al. Prophylactic implantation of a defibrillator in patients with myocardial infarction and reduced ejection fraction. N Engl J Med 2002;346:877–83.

5. Poole JE, Johnson GW, Hellkamp AS, et al. Prognostic importance of defibrillator shocks in patients with heart failure. N Engl J Med 2008;359:1009–17.

6. Echt DS, Liebson PR, Mitchell LB, et al. Mortality and morbidity in patients receiving encainide, flecainide, or placebo. The cardiac arrhythmia suppression trial. N Engl J Med 1991;324:781–8.

7. Reddy VY, Reynolds MR, Neuzil P, et al. Prophylactic catheter ablation for the prevention of defibrillator therapy. N Engl J Med 2007;357:2657–65.

8. Stevenson WG, Wilber DJ, Natale A, et al. Irrigated radiofrequency catheter ablation guided by electroanatomic mapping for recurrent ventricular tachycardia after myocardial infarction: the multicenter thermocool ventricular tachycardia ablation trial. Circulation 2008;16(118):2773–82.

9. Noda T, Shimizu W, Taguchi A, et al. Malignant entity of idiopathic ventricular fibrillation and polymorphic ventricular tachycardia initiated by premature extrasystoles originating from the right ventricular outflow tract. J Am Coll Cardiol 2005;46:1288–94.

10. Verma A, Kilicaslan F, Marrouche NF, et al. Prevalence, predictors, and mortality significance of the causative arrhythmia in patients with electrical storm. J Cardiovasc Electrophysiol 2004;15:1265–70.

11. Yarlagadda RK, Iwai S, Stein KM, et al. Reversal of cardiomyopathy in patients with repetitive monomorphic ventricular ectopy originating from the right ventricular outflow tract. Circulation 2005;112:1092–7.

12. Aliot EM, Stevenson WG, Almendral-Garrote JM, et al. EHRA/HRS expert consensus on catheter ablation of ventricular arrhythmias: developed in a partnership with the European Heart Rhythm Association (EHRA), a registered branch of the European Society of Cardiology (ESC), and the Heart Rhythm Society (HRS); in collaboration with the American College of Cardiology (ACC) and the American Heart Association (AHA). Heart Rhythm 2009;6:886–933.

13. Marrouche NF, Verma A, Wazni O, et al. Mode of initiation and ablation of ventricular fibrillation storms in patients with ischemic cardiomyopathy. J Am Coll Cardiol 2004;43:1715–20.

14. Verma A, Marrouche NF, Schweikert RA, et al. Relationship between successful ablation sites and the scar border zone defined by substrate mapping for ventricular tachycardia postmyocardial infarction. J Cardiovasc Electrophysiol 2005;16:465–71.

15. Saliba W, Abul Karim A, Tchou P, et al. Ventricular fibrillation: ablation of a trigger? J Cardiovasc Electrophysiol 2002;13:1296–9.

16. Schweikert RA, Saliba WI, Tomassoni G, et al. Percutaneous pericardial instrumentation for endo-epicardial mapping of previously failed ablations. Circulation 2003;108:1329–35.

17. Fahmy TS, Wazni OM, Jaber WA, et al. Integration of positron emission tomography/computed tomography with electroanatomical mapping: a novel approach for ablation of scar-related ventricular tachycardia. Heart Rhythm 2008;5:1538–45.

18. Dickfeld T, Lei P, Dilsizian V, et al. Integration of three-dimensional scar maps for ventricular tachycardia ablation with positron emission tomography-computed tomography. JACC Cardiovasc Imaging 2008;1:73–82.

19. Cesario DA, Vaseghi M, Boyle NG, et al. Value of high-density endocardial and epicardial mapping for catheter ablation of hemodynamically unstable ventricular tachycardia. Heart Rhythm 2006;3:1–10.

20. Khaykin Y, Skanes A, Whaley B, et al. Real-time integration of 2D intracardiac echocardiography and 3D electroanatomical mapping to guide ventricular tachycardia ablation. Heart Rhythm 2008;5:1396–402.

21. Di Biase L, Saliba WI, Natale A. Successful ablation of epicardial arrhythmias with cryoenergy after failed attempts with radiofrequency energy. Heart Rhythm 2009;6:109–12.

22. Mlcochova H, Saliba WI, Burkhardt DJ, et al. Catheter ablation of ventricular fibrillation storm in patients with infiltrative amyloidosis of the heart. J Cardiovasc Electrophysiol 2006;17:426–30.

23. Marchlinski FE, Callans DJ, Gottlieb CD, et al. Linear ablation lesions for control of unmappable ventricular tachycardia in patients with ischemic and nonischemic cardiomyopathy. Circulation 2000;101:1288–96.

24. Hsia HH, Callans DJ, Marchlinski FE. Characterization of endocardial electrophysiological substrate in patients with nonischemic cardiomyopathy and monomorphic ventricular tachycardia. Circulation 2003;108:704–10.

25. Brunckhorst CB, Delacretaz E, Soejima K. Identification of the ventricular tachycardia isthmus after infarction by pace mapping. Circulation 2004;110:652–9.

26. Bogun F, Good E, Reich S, et al. Isolated potentials during sinus rhythm and pace mapping within scars as guides for ablation of postinfarction ventricular tachycardia. J Am Coll Cardiol 2006;47:2013–9.

27. Arenal A, Glez-Torrecilla E, Ortiz M, et al. Ablation of electrograms with an isolated, delayed component as treatment of unmappable monomorphic ventricular tachycardias in patients with structural heart disease. J Am Coll Cardiol 2003;41:81–92.

28. Oza S, Wilber DJ. Substrate-based endocardial ablation of postinfarction ventricular tachycardia. Heart Rhythm 2006;3:607–9.

29. Stevenson WG, Khan H, Sager P, et al. Identification of re-entry circuit sites during catheter mapping and radiofrequency ablation of ventricular tachycardia late after myocardial infarction. Circulation 1993;88:1647–70.

30. El-Shalakany A, Hadjis T, Papageorgiou P, et al. Entrainment/mapping criteria for the prediction of termination of ventricular tachycardia by single radiofrequency lesion in patients with coronary artery disease. Circulation 1999;99:2283–9.

31. Bogun F, Kim HM, Han J, et al. Comparison of mapping criteria for hemodynamically tolerated, postinfarction ventricular tachycardia. Heart Rhythm 2006;3:20–6.

32. Azegami K, Wilber DJ, Arruda M, et al. Spatial resolution of pacemapping and activation mapping in patients with idiopathic right ventricular outflow tract tachycardia. J Cardiovasc Electrophysiol 2005;16: 823–9.

33. O'Donnell D, Cox D, Bourke J, et al. Clinical and electrophysiological differences between patients with arrhythmogenic right ventricular dysplasia and right ventricular outflow tract tachycardia. Eur Heart J 2003;24:801–10.

34. Haissaguerre M, Extramiana F, Hocini M, et al. Mapping and ablation of ventricular fibrillation associated with long-QT and brugada syndromes. Circulation 2003;108:925–8.

35. Bala R, Marchlinski FE. Electrocardiographic recognition and ablation of outflow tract ventricular tachycardia. Heart Rhythm 2007;4:366–70.

36. Lin D, Ilkhanoff L, Gerstenfeld E, et al. Twelve-lead electrocardiographic characteristics of the aortic cusp region guided by intracardiac echocardiography and electroanatomic mapping. Heart Rhythm 2008;5:663–9.

37. Kanagaratnam L, Tomassoni G, Schweikert R, et al. Ventricular tachycardias arising from the aortic sinus of valsalva: an under-recognized variant of left outflow tract ventricular tachycardia. J Am Coll Cardiol 2001;37:1408–14.

38. Yamada T, McElderry HT, Doppalapudi H, et al. Idiopathic ventricular arrhythmias originating from the aortic root prevalence, electrocardiographic and electrophysiologic characteristics, and results of radiofrequency catheter ablation. J Am Coll Cardiol 2008;52:139–47.

39. Coggins DL, Lee RJ, Sweeney J, et al. Radiofrequency catheter ablation as a cure for idiopathic tachycardia of both left and right ventricular origin. J Am Coll Cardiol 1994;23:1333–41.

40. Rodriguez LM, Smeets JL, Timmermans C, et al. Predictors for successful ablation of right- and left-sided idiopathic ventricular tachycardia. Am J Cardiol 1997;79:309–14.

41. Nakagawa H, Beckman KJ, McClelland JH, et al. Radiofrequency catheter ablation of idiopathic left ventricular tachycardia guided by a Purkinje potential. Circulation 2003;88:2607–17.

42. Tscuchiya T, Okumura K, Honda T, et al. Significance of late diastolic potential preceding Purkinje potential in Verapamil-sensitive idiopathic left ventricular tachycardia. Circulation 1999;99: 2408–13.

43. Nogami A, Naito S, Tada H, et al. Demonstration of diastolic and presystolic Purkinje potential as critical components on a macroreentry circuit of verapamil-sensitive idiopathic left ventricular tachycardia. J Am Coll Cardiol 2000;36:811–23.

44. Haissaguerre M, Shah DC, Jais P, et al. Role of Purkinje conducting system in triggering of idiopathic ventricular fibrillation. Lancet 2002;359: 677–8.

Index

Card Electrophysiol Clin 1 (2009) 213–218
doi:10.1016/S1877-9182(09)00026-4

Moving?

Make sure your subscription moves with you!

To notify us of your new address, find your **Clinics Account Number** (located on your mailing label above your name), and contact customer service at:

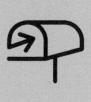

Email: journalscustomerservice-usa@elsevier.com

800-654-2452 (subscribers in the U.S. & Canada)
314-447-8871 (subscribers outside of the U.S. & Canada)

Fax number: 314-447-8029

Elsevier Health Sciences Division
Subscription Customer Service
3251 Riverport Lane
Maryland Heights, MO 63043

*To ensure uninterrupted delivery of your subscription, please notify us at least 4 weeks in advance of move.

ELSEVIER

Printed and bound by CPI Group (UK) Ltd, Croydon, CR0 4YY

03/10/2024

01040362-0004